Cardiovascular Prevention and Rehabilitation in Practice

Cardiovascular Prevention and Rehabilitation in Practice

SECOND EDITION

Edited By

Jennifer Jones

National University of Ireland, Galway, Ireland
Brunel University, Uxbridge, UK

John Buckley

University Centre Shrewsbury, Shrewsbury, UK

Gill Furze

Coventry University, Coventry, UK

Gail Sheppard

Canterbury Christ Church University, Canterbury, UK

WILEY Blackwell

Registered Office(s)
John Wiley & Sons, Inc., 111 River Street, Hoboken, NJ 07030, USA
John Wiley & Sons Ltd, The Atrium, Southern Gate, Chichester, West Sussex, PO19 8SQ, UK

Editorial Office
9600 Garsington Road, Oxford, OX4 2DQ, UK

For details of our global editorial offices, customer services, and more information about Wiley products visit us at www.wiley.com.

Wiley also publishes its books in a variety of electronic formats and by print-on-demand. Some content that appears in standard print versions of this book may not be available in other formats.

Library of Congress Cataloging-in-Publication Data
Names: Jones, Jennifer (Reader in physiotherapy), editor. | Buckley, John (Exercise physiologist), editor. | Furze, Gill, editor. | Sheppard, Gail, (Senior lecturer in health promotion/public health), editor.
Title: Cardiovascular prevention and rehabilitation in practice / edited by Jennifer Jones, John Buckley, Gill Furze, Gail Sheppard.
Other titles: BACPR cardiovascular prevention and rehabilitation
Description: 2nd edition. | Hoboken, NJ : Wiley-Blackwell, 2020. | Preceded by BACPR cardiovascular prevention and rehabilitation / [edited by] Jennifer Jones. 2014. | Includes bibliographical references and index.
Identifiers: LCCN 2019047701 (print) | LCCN 2019047702 (ebook) | ISBN 9781118458693 (paperback) | ISBN 9781118458679 (adobe pdf) | ISBN 9781118458686 (epub)
Subjects: MESH: Cardiovascular Diseases–prevention & control | Cardiac Rehabilitation–methods | Health Behavior | Healthy Lifestyle
Classification: LCC RC667 (print) | LCC RC667 (ebook) | NLM WG 120 | DDC 616.1–dc23
LC record available at https://lccn.loc.gov/2019047701
LC ebook record available at https://lccn.loc.gov/2019047702

Cover Design: Wiley
Cover Image: © crisserbug/Getty Images

Set in 10.5/13pt STIX Two Text by SPi Global, Pondicherry, India

Printed and bound by CPI Group (UK) Ltd, Croydon, CR0 4YY

10 9 8 7 6 5 4 3 2 1

Contents

Foreword   vii

List of Contributors   ix

Preface   xiii

CHAPTER 1   Cardiovascular Disease Prevention
and Rehabilitation   1
Jennifer Jones, Gill Furze, and John Buckley

CHAPTER 2   Standards and Core Components in
Cardiovascular Disease Prevention
and Rehabilitation   21
BACPR Standards Writing Group

CHAPTER 3   Delivering Quality Standards   47
Kathryn Carver

CHAPTER 4   Health Behaviour Change and Education   67
Linda Speck, Gill Furze, and Nick Brace

CHAPTER 5   Lifestyle Risk Factor Management   99
Jennifer Jones, John Buckley, and Gill Furze

CHAPTER 5A   Achieving Long-term Abstinence from
Tobacco Use in Patients in a Cardiovascular
Prevention and Rehabilitation Setting   101
Catriona Jennings and Robert West

CHAPTER 5B   Diet and Weight Management   127
Alison Atrey and Rachel Vine

CHAPTER 5C   Physical Activity and Exercise   151
John Buckley, Tim Grove, Sally Turner, and Samantha Breen

CHAPTER 6   Psychosocial Health   193
             Linda Speck, Nick Brace, and Molly Byrne

CHAPTER 7   Medical Risk Management   227
             Joe Mills, Susan Connolly, Barbara Conway,
             Marie-Kristelle Ross, Samantha Breen, and Dorothy J. Frizelle

CHAPTER 8   Long-term Management   271
             Sally Hinton, Ann Marie Johnson, and Gail Sheppard

CHAPTER 9   Audit and Evaluation   285
             Patrick Doherty, Alex Harrison, Corinna Petre, and
             Nerina Onion

CHAPTER 10   Future Prospects and International Perspectives   305
             Joe Mills, Sherry L. Grace, Marie-Kristelle Ross,
             Caroline Chessex, Robyn Gallagher, Cate Ferry, and
             Vicki Wade

             Index   313

Foreword

The International Council for Cardiovascular Prevention and Rehabilitation (ICCPR) wishes to congratulate the British Association for Cardiovascular Prevention and Rehabilitation (BACPR) on this practitioner-focused textbook. Its main aim is to take its internationally recognised Standards and Core Components and show how they can be put 'into practice'. In 1995 the UK (via the BACR) was one of only a handful of countries in the world to have produced a set of National Guidelines in the form of a textbook. Since then, the BACR (now the BACPR) have gone on to publish three editions of their Standards and Core Components (2007, 2012/2013, and 2017/2018). As BACPR was one of the three founding members of the ICCPR (along with Canada and the USA), its Standards and Core Components have always, and will continue to be, featured as an important reference in our website compilation of key cardiac rehabilitation resources (http://globalcardiacrehab.com/). These resources promulgate advocacy, value, and guidance for cardiac rehabilitation as an obligatory part of any modern or developing cardiovascular health service. One of the hallmarks of UK programmes and the BACPR's approach is delivering a large proportion of services in the community and in patients' homes, which is a model the ICCPR promotes for developing countries. We have no doubt this textbook will become a valued resource for cardiac rehabilitation and cardiovascular disease prevention specialists around the world.

Professor Sherry L. Grace CRFC
Chair, ICCPR
York University and University Health Network,
Toronto, Ontario, Canada

List of Contributors

Alison Atrey
Consultant Specialist Dietitian
CVD Management
Toronto, Ontario, Canada

Nick Brace
Principal Clinical Psychologist
Department of Health Psychology
Swansea Bay University Health Board
Neath Port Talbot Hospital
Port Talbot, UK

Samantha Breen
Allied Health Professionals Manager
Manchester Royal Infirmary and
St Mary's Hospital
Manchester University NHS
Foundation Trust
Manchester, UK

BACPR Standards Writing Group
British Association for Cardiovascular
Prevention and Rehabilitation
London, UK

John Buckley
Professor of Applied Exercise
Science
Centre for Active Living
University Centre Shrewsbury
Shrewsbury, UK

Molly Byrne
Professor in Health Psychology
Director Health Behaviour Change
Research Group
School of Psychology
National University of Ireland
Galway, Ireland

Kathryn Carver
Heart Failure Lead Nurse
Addenbrooke's Hospital
Cardiology Services
Cambridge, UK

Caroline Chessex
Associate Professor
Department of Medicine
University of Toronto
Fellowship Program Director
Division of Cardiology
University Health Network/Sinai
Health System
Toronto, Ontario, Canada

Susan Connolly
Consultant Cardiologist and
Clinical Lead
Our Hearts Our Minds Programme
for Cardiovascular Health
Western Health and Social Care Trust
Enniskillen, Northern Ireland

Barbara Conway
Associate Lecturer
Department of Health Science
University of York
York, UK

Patrick Doherty
Chair in Cardiovascular Health
Director of the National Audit of
Cardiac Rehabilitation (NACR)
Department of Health Sciences
University of York
York, UK

Cate Ferry
Manager Clinical Programs NSW
National Heart Foundation of Australia
Sydney, Australia

Dorothy J. Frizelle
Consultant Clinical Health Psychologist
& Head of Service
Executive Director for Member
Networks ACP–UK
The Mid Yorkshire Hospitals NHS Trust
Department of Clinical Health
Psychology
Dewsbury District Hospital
Dewsbury, UK

Gill Furze
Emeritus Professor in Health and
Life Sciences
Faculty of Health and Life Sciences
Coventry University
Coventry, UK

Robyn Gallagher
Professor of Nursing
Faculty of Medicine and Health
The University of Sydney
Sydney, Australia

Sherry L. Grace
Chair, International Council of
Cardiovascular Prevention and
Rehabilitation;
Professor, York University;
Sr. Scientist & Director
Cardiac Rehabilitation Research
University Health Network
University of Toronto
Toronto, Ontario, Canada

Tim Grove
Lecturer in Physiotherapy
Department of Clinical Sciences
Brunel University
Uxbridge, UK

Alex Harrison
Research Fellow
Department of Health Sciences
University of York
York, UK

Sally Hinton
BACPR Executive Director
BACPR
London, UK

Catriona Jennings
Cardiovascular Specialist Nurse
National Institute for Prevention and
Cardiovascular Health
National University of Ireland
Galway, Ireland

Ann Marie Johnson
Year of Care Facilitator
Leeds Partnerships Clinical
Commissioning
Leeds, UK

Jennifer Jones
Director of Preventive Medicine and
Cardiovascular Health
National University of Ireland
Galway, Ireland;
Reader in Physiotherapy
Department of Clinical Sciences
Brunel University
Uxbridge, UK

Joe Mills
Consultant Cardiologist
Liverpool Heart & Chest
Hospital NHS Foundation Trust
Liverpool, UK

Nerina Onion
NACR Programme Manager
Department of Health Sciences
University of York
York, UK

Corinna Petre
NACR Project Manager
Department of Health Sciences
University of York
York, UK

Marie-Kristelle Ross
Cardiologist
Hotel-Dieu de Lévis, Universite Laval
Quebec City, Quebec, Canada

Gail Sheppard
Senior Lecturer/Academic
Group Lead
Public Health and Health Promotion
Canterbury Christ Church University
Canterbury, UK

Linda Speck
Consultant Clinical Health
Psychologist and Visiting Professor
Health Psychology Service
Cwm Taf Morgannwg University
Health Board
Princess of Wales Hospital, Bridgend,
and University of South Wales, UK

Sally Turner
Physiotherapist Health
Programme Manager
Basingstoke & Alton Cardiac
Rehabilitation Charity Ltd
Alton, UK

Rachel Vine
Community Dietetic Team Manager
Leeds Community Healthcare NHS
Trust, Parkside Community
Health Centre
Leeds, UK

Vicki Wade
Senior Cultural Advisor
Rheumatic Heart Disease
Australia Menzies School of
Health Research
Casuarina, Australia

Robert West
Professor of Health Psychology
Department of Behavioural Science
and Health
Institute of Epidemiology
and Healthcare
University College London
London, UK

Preface

CARDIOVASCULAR PREVENTION AND REHABILITATION IN PRACTICE

This comprehensive book covers all the aspects of prevention and rehabilitation that are important to those who help cardiac patients to return to normal health – and also guide them to reduce to a minimum the risks of recurrence. The scope of the problem is described, followed by the nature and standards of cardiac rehabilitation (CR) and how behaviour can be changed to ensure the adoption of a healthier lifestyle. The roles of the professionals involved in treating patients leads to the need for patients to know how best to work for their own recovery.

The British Association for Cardiac Rehabilitation (BACR) was set up in 1992 and the first guidelines were published in 1995. Since then much has been achieved. In 1992 less than half of all hospitals treating heart patients had active CR programmes; today the figure is 100%. In 2000 the UK Department of Health (DoH) published the National Framework for CHD and included CR as Standard 12, ushering in the general acceptance of CR as a vital part of the management of cardiac patients. In 2010 the BACR adopted its new name, British Association for Cardiac Prevention and Rehabilitation (BACPR), to recognise its role in cardiovascular prevention together with rehabilitation. The BACPR then set out the standards and core components for cardiovascular prevention and rehabilitation in the UK. Now all centres are requested to report their performance to the National Audit of Cardiac Rehabilitation (NACR) annually using patient level data. The NACR annual report details national performance and how it is improving.

The scientific evidence base for prevention and rehabilitation is compelling – the challenge is effective implementation in everyday clinical practice. Although much has been achieved there is still much to do, both in the UK and globally, to appropriately fund service provision to levels and standards used in the underpinning research trials. In 2013 the DoH produced a Cardiovascular Disease Outcomes Strategy, which has provided guidance on the recommended percentage uptake of CR in eligible patients. Encouragingly, in the UK, uptake of CR has grown to world leading levels, but this is still only at 50%. Not only is this figure well below the recommended uptake level, there remain inequities and poor representation for women and ethnic minorities. Patients following heart surgery or an acute coronary syndrome are more likely to be included than those with exertional angina. Other presentations of atherosclerotic disease such as stroke and peripheral arterial disease are rarely included. Only a few heart failure patients receive exercise rehabilitation. Again, whilst there are improvements in the percentage of recruited patients being assessed both before and after the programme these are still not at recommended levels, and longer term outcomes are not usually measured at all.

The BACPR is working hard to improve this national picture by setting out the Standards and Core Components described in this book. These have been used to create a certification process for which all centres are invited to apply. The standards for qualifying for this certification have been set relatively low to encourage as many centres as possible to apply but so far only a minority have done so. Over time the number of centres attaining those standards, and exceeding them, should rise with the ambition of reaching 100%.

This book describes what is needed to bring the level of prevention and rehabilitation received by cardiac patients up to acceptable levels. It makes interesting and educational reading. You have got this far – now read on!

Dr Hugh Bethell
Founding President of the British Association for Cardiac Rehabilitation
(now BACPR)

Professor David Wood
President of the World Heart Federation 2017–2018 and Emeritus Professor
of Cardiovascular Medicine, Imperial College London

CHAPTER 1

Cardiovascular Disease Prevention and Rehabilitation

Jennifer Jones[1,2], Gill Furze[3], and John Buckley[4]

[1] National University of Ireland, Galway, Ireland
[2] Department of Clinical Sciences, Brunel University, Uxbridge, UK
[3] Faculty of Health and Life Sciences, Coventry University, Coventry, UK
[4] Centre for Active Living, University Centre Shrewsbury, Shrewsbury, UK

Abstract

This chapter presents the current burden of cardiovascular disease (CVD) together with the historical context of cardiac rehabilitation (CR) and its evolving evidence base. In accordance with the growing emphasis on secondary prevention and the benefits gained, including people with manifestations of atherosclerosis beyond coronary heart disease (CHD), the rationale for referring to cardiovascular prevention and rehabilitation programmes (CPRPs) in contemporary practice is discussed. Despite rehabilitation's proven benefits, participation still has much room for growth, and approaches to redress this challenge form a key feature of this chapter and textbook more widely. Finally, a brief insight into future perspectives are explored in recognition of the value of new technologies and connected health approaches that offer opportunities in the scalability of services, provide further choice, and potentially reach more people.

Keywords: *cardiovascular disease, cardiac rehabilitation, prevention, health*

Key Points

- Whilst age-adjusted mortality rates are falling in high-income countries, cardiovascular disease still remains the single largest cause of mortality in the United Kingdom (UK), Europe, and globally.
- More people are, however, surviving acute cardiovascular events, which contributes to a growing and ageing population who are living with long-term conditions.
- Cardiac rehabilitation has evolved from its traditional components of exercise, education, and psychology to now include a broadened focus on the wider physical and psycho-social lifestyle issues that lead to the underlying causes of the disease along with the related behavioural and medical management needs.
- The evidence for cardiac rehabilitation is compelling. There is now a growing emphasis, which reaches beyond outcomes of reducing morbidity and mortality, towards greater patient-centred improvements in health-related quality of life and reduced costly unplanned hospital readmissions.
- Despite the benefits, uptake to cardiac rehabilitation remains less than desirable. Programmes need to ensure to apply evidence-based approaches to increase uptake and programme adherence.
- As services develop to treat any atheromatic condition as part of a 'single family of diseases' there is a need to consider all elements of disease management and prevention within the terminology of cardiac rehabilitation.
- There is a growing interest in the use of technologies and connected health solutions in delivering successful cardiac rehabilitation, and whilst these are encouraged, novel approaches also require rigorous evaluation. As such, contemporary cardiovascular prevention and rehabilitation programmes need to participate in driving vital research to address priority health needs and inform better the prevention and management of cardiovascular disease.

1.1   RATIONALE AND AIMS

Adverse trends in non-communicable diseases (NCDs) are being seen worldwide. In low and low–middle income countries, premature mortality from cardiovascular disease (CVD) continues to rise. Whilst significant reductions are being observed across most high-income countries, CVD remains the leading cause of mortality. In addition, the number of people surviving an acute cardiac event has risen greatly resulting in a growing population living with atheromatic

CVD. Coronary heart disease (CHD) and cerebrovascular disease constitute the most important preventable NCDs and completing a cardiac rehabilitation (CR) programme is strongly recommended (Class 1 indication). A multidisciplinary CR programme aims to address the underlying causes of the disease, enable patient empowerment and self-care, and optimise health and wellbeing. Despite its demonstrated benefits and endorsement by most recognised cardiovascular societies, participation remains vastly underutilised. This chapter aims to provide a brief historical background to traditional CR and its evidence base together with a review of current perspectives and future directions. To increase uptake there is a need for services to evolve and innovate. This includes employing different modes of delivery and offering flexibility when attempting to attract either new or hitherto hard to reach 'in-scope' groups. The rationale for advocating for the provision of CPRPs as opposed to CR also features strongly. This is in recognition that preventive medicine and comprehensive intensive lifestyle and risk factor management are key if reductions in overall mortality together with a plethora of other health-related benefits are to be realised in contemporary practice.

1.2   THE BURDEN OF CVD

Atheromatic CVD remains the world's number one cause of death and disability (Global Burden of Disease 2015). Low- and middle-income countries (LMICs) are most affected and account for 80% of all CVD deaths (Bovet and Paccaud 2011). In high-income countries, although age-adjusted mortality for this disease has seen significant decline over the last 30 years, it remains the leading single disease burden. These trends concur in the United Kingdom (UK) where deaths from CVD cause more than a quarter of all deaths, or around 150 000 each year (British Heart Foundation 2018). As one of the key NCDs, the World Health Organization (WHO) has acknowledged that the prevention and/or management of CVD requires the implementation of nine different health and medical strategies, including reductions in smoking, poor nutrition/salt intake, alcohol, physical inactivity, obesity, and diabetes and hypertension, along with increasing the availability of medical and counselling therapies to prevent heart attacks and strokes and the availability of essential medicines and technologies to treat CVD and other NCDs (World Health Organization 2013). The British Association for Cardiovascular Prevention and Rehabilitation (BACPR) has identified a number of core components (British Association for Cardiovascular Prevention and Rehabilitation [BACPR] 2017; Figure 1.1) that include all of these WHO targets.

CVD is an umbrella term for all diseases of the heart and circulation, including heart disease, stroke, heart failure, cardiomyopathy, atrial fibrillation,

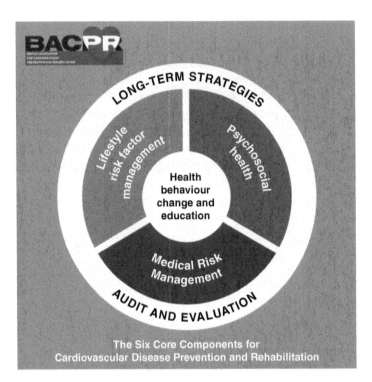

FIGURE 1.1 Core components of cardiac rehabilitation (CR) as defined by the British Association for Cardiovascular Prevention and Rehabilitation (BACPR).

peripheral arterial disease, chronic kidney disease, or any other functional disorder of the cardiovascular system. Of all CVDs, CHD is the leading cause of mortality and disease burden worldwide (WHO 2018), resulting in approximately 8.9 million deaths and 164.0 million disability-adjusted life years (DALYs) globally in 2015 (Kassebaum et al. 2016; Wang et al. 2016). In the UK specifically, CHD is responsible for around 66 000 deaths each year, an average of 180 people each day, or one every eight minutes (British Heart Foundation 2018). The total cost of premature death, lost productivity, hospital treatment, and prescriptions relating to CVD is estimated at £19 billion each year (British Heart Foundation 2018). This is highly relevant to CR, given that CHD is largely preventable with up to 90% of the risk of a first heart attack being due to nine lifestyle risk factors that can be changed (Yusuf et al. 2004). These global and national trends in mortality from CVD highlight there is a growing need for better investment in prevention-based strategies.

In high-income countries, whilst age-adjusted CVD mortality is declining morbidity is increasing, placing an escalating and untenable strain on their healthcare systems. Advances in diagnosis, revascularisation, pharmacotherapy, and overall more successful treatment of acute illness have contributed to these reductions in mortality, but simultaneously result in a growing population of people surviving acute cardiac events and living longer with chronic l,ong-term conditions, such as heart failure. Currently, there are more than 6 million new cases of CVD in the European Union (EU) and more than 11 million in Europe as a whole, every year. With almost 49 million people living with the disease in the EU, the cost to the EU economies is high at €210 billion a year (European Heart Network 2017). In the UK alone, there are an estimated 7 million people living with CVD; 2.3 million of these individuals are living with CHD – over 1.4 million men and 850 000 women (British Heart Foundation 2018). This places a growing and unsustainable burden on healthcare resources and consequently the demand for effective secondary prevention is intensifying. Availability of interventions that complement standard medical care and aim to reduce further events in those with established disease is now a pressing and urgent priority.

The burden from CVD is not solely applicable to secondary prevention. One third of apparently healthy Europeans have three or more risk factors and these risks are increasing as the population ages. The UK, like many countries in the world, is faced with a looming epidemic given the negative trends being consistently observed in diabetes and obesity. There are 3.7 million adults in the UK diagnosed with diabetes. In addition, hundreds of thousands more are living with undiagnosed Type 2 diabetes and these figures are all projected to increase (British Heart Foundation 2018). Around a quarter of adults in the UK are obese and of concern is that around 28% of children in the UK are overweight or obese. Further, growing epidemics in numbers leading a sedentary lifestyle (two out of five adults do not achieve recommended levels of physical activity), poor diet (only a quarter of adults and one in six children consume the recommended five portions of fruit and vegetables per day), persistent smoking (17% of adults), raised blood pressure (30% of all adults), and high blood cholesterol levels (50% of adults) contribute to the increasing burden and prevalence of atherosclerotic CVD (British Heart Foundation 2018). This further supports the clear need to prioritise preventive care. Distinguishing secondary from primary prevention is, to a large extent, artificial, as all patients with any form of atherosclerosis or presenting with increased multifactorial risk require lifestyle, risk factor, and therapeutic management to reduce their overall risk of developing, or having recurrent, disease.

This provides a strong rationale for opportunities for service transformation from CR to CPRP, which include the full spectrum of patients – from those with any form of established CVD, to those who are asymptomatic but at high risk of future adverse cardiovascular events.

In addition, patients with other non-infectious diseases, particularly those with chronic respiratory conditions and certain forms of cancer, may also benefit from CR (Koene et al. 2016; Lim et al. 2012). Thus, there is an opportunity to further expand the scope and influence of prevention and rehabilitation services that may, in turn, release financial resources to enable more cost-effective deployment of staff and facilities (Kaiser et al. 2013).

1.3   DEFINING CR AND CARDIOVASCULAR PREVENTION AND REHABILITATION

Since the 1960s, early prevention programmes, termed CR, have been the traditional model for delivery of secondary prevention for patients with CHD. Early programmes focused on supervised exercise to counter de-conditioning following bypass surgery and to improve exercise capacity following myocardial infarction (MI). These programmes later evolved to include an educational component (usually in a group format) aimed at educating patients about the importance of lowering multiple risk factors, including smoking, diet, and psychosocial wellbeing (Thompson and De Bono 1999).

Our knowledge about which cardiovascular risk factors to modify and methods available for modifying them have greatly expanded. Consequently, comprehensive CR in contemporary practice continues to include exercise training and education for patients with coronary artery disease *in conjunction with* a growing emphasis on prevention and strategies targeting chronic disease management. Exercise is but one sub-component of lifestyle risk factor management, and equal value should be placed on the other main components, including psychosocial health, medical risk factor management, and central to all these, health behaviour change and education. This is reflected in the BACPR's definition of CR (Box 1.1) and model of the core components for cardiovascular prevention and rehabilitation (Figure 1.1).

Over the past decade, the emphasis of CR programmes has moved towards being integrated chronic disease management and prevention programmes in order to slow disease progression, prevent future cardiac events, and maintain or enhance quality of life whilst living with the burden of underlying CVD (BACPR 2017). The BACPR (2017) grounds its goals in a comprehensive lifestyle management approach in models of behaviour change (i.e. smoking cessation, healthy nutrition, and physical activity) by using a variety of strategies (including

---

Box 1.1   What Is Cardiac Rehabilitation/Cardiovascular Prevention and Rehabilitation?

The coordinated sum of activities* required to influence favourably the underlying cause of cardiovascular disease, as well as to provide the best possible physical, mental, and social conditions, so that the patients may, by their own efforts, preserve or resume optimal functioning in their community and through improved health behaviour, slow or reverse progression of disease.

*The BACPR's six core components for CVD prevention and rehabilitation constitute the coordinated sum of activities

family-based, group-based or community-based approaches, to more structured and complex individual patient approaches). Risk factor management in terms of effective control of blood pressure, lipids, and glucose to defined targets, and the appropriate prescription and adherence to cardioprotective drugs, are now integral parts of this approach, which are inextricably linked with lifestyle behaviours and augmented by medical treatment. Finally, the psychosocial and vocational elements required to help patients to regain a life as fully as possible are also provided (Piepoli et al. 2014).

With this regard, the term 'rehabilitation' for some may have negative connotations (e.g. associated images of drug addiction or of being completely incapacitated, or people with other non-cardiac manifestations of CVD). Many programmes in the UK, Canada, and Australia have re-branded themselves to emphasise a more positive approach around patient empowerment and enhanced wellbeing by using such terms as "healthy heart programme", "action heart", "healthy hearts and minds", to name but a few. Medical fraternities in Europe and the US for over three decades have used the term 'preventive cardiology' to define such a comprehensive approach. More recently, the National Health Service for England at the National Institute for Health Care Excellence (NICE) has endorsed the concept of prevention and rehabilitation services for long-term conditions (Department of Health 2013; NICE 2013), and there are services addressing this by including people with, for example, pulmonary disease and/or cancer. Cardiovascular rehabilitation and prevention services are in a prime position to deliver these larger integrated rehabilitative services.

Internationally, the BACPR, along with its equivalent societies in Canada, the US, and Australia, have led in the founding and formation of an official alliance under the umbrella of the World Heart Federation, called the International Council for Cardiovascular Prevention and Rehabilitation (ICCPR; www.globalcardiacrehab.com). As of 2017, the ICCPR includes over 29 prevention and rehabilitation organisations from around the world with the single aim to promote a comprehensive approach to the prevention of and rehabilitation from CVD as an obligatory component to any developing cardiology service (Grace et al. 2013).

Practice Application

People following a transient ischaemic attack (TIA) and stroke or with peripheral arterial disease and many others at risk of or with manifestations of CVD can benefit from a structured CPRP but may not associate benefit if they are referred to 'CR'. Some may associate the term 'rehabilitation' with people who need help to regain function and this could impact on their attendance if they perceive themselves to be functionally well. Incorporating social marketing approaches, based on evaluating the needs and motivators of your target audience, can positively influence participation.

1.4   THE COMPELLING CASE FOR CARDIOVASCULAR PREVENTION AND REHABILITATION

CR, with a strong focus on secondary prevention, has a robust evidence base for reducing mortality and morbidity, saving healthcare costs and enhancing the quality and productivity of people's lives (Cowie et al. 2019). For overall mortality, although several recent studies, meta-analyses and recommendations of national and international guidelines suggest a beneficial effect in patients with CHD, the effect of multi-component CR in the modern era of statins and acute revascularisation remains controversial (Rauch et al. 2016).

Meta-analyses of CR trials up to 2010 showed a significant reduction in all-cause mortality but many of these trials were conducted before the modern management of acute coronary syndromes. There have been major advances in cardiology practice together with improvements in public health, which have contributed to considerably lower mortality rates following acute coronary syndromes. As a consequence, the influence that CR post MI or revascularisation may have on specifically mortality in contemporary practice is becoming more limited.

This is reflected in findings from systematic reviews and meta-analyses over time. For example, the 2011 Cochrane review involved 47 trials randomising a total of 10 794 patients and found that exercise-based CR was associated with significant reductions in overall and cardiovascular mortality and reduced hospital admissions. It was not associated with reduced risk of morbidity in terms of the risk of recurrent MI or risk of revascularisation (Heran et al. 2011). In 2016, Cochrane published an update, as there were 16 new trials, to reassess the effectiveness of exercise-based CR compared to usual care. This most recent systematic review and meta-analysis found significant reductions in cardiovascular mortality (risk ratio [RR] 0.74, 95% CI 0.64–0.86), and hospital admissions (RR 0.82, 95% CI 0.70–0.96) but no benefit in terms of total mortality (Anderson et al. 2016).

However, a further meta-analysis, including not just exercise-based CR but prevention trials as well found that CPRPs that are able to prescribe cardioprotective medications, and that intensively manage six risk factors or more, can reduce all-cause mortality and recurrent MI (Van Halewijn et al. 2017). Findings from the COURAGE trial also support the importance of managing risk factors intensively. The better the control of six protocol-specified risk factors 1 year after randomisation, the higher the probability of survival during a mean follow-up of 6.8 years. Of the four risk factor goals most strongly associated with long-term survival, three were lifestyle variables (not smoking, physical activity, and healthy diet), and the fourth variable (systolic blood pressure) was influenced by health behaviours (Maron et al. 2018).

Practice Application

Ensure your programme does not place overemphasis on the exercise component. Comprehensive programmes that actively address medical risk factor management through proactive initiation and uptitration of pharmacotherapies coupled with intensive lifestyle modification that are driven to achieve therapeutic targets and manage psychological health status have very different outcomes to exercise-focused programmes.

Certainly, mortality should not be considered the only measure of effectiveness. Reductions in unplanned hospital admissions are of great relevance, especially given the growing strains on acute services. There has been a significant reduction in acute hospital admissions (reduced from 30.7 to 26.1%, NNT 22), which is a key determinant of the intervention's overall cost-efficacy (Dalal et al. 2015; Shields et al. 2018). For individuals with a diagnosis of heart failure, CR may not reduce total mortality but does impact favourably on hospitalisation, with a 25% relative risk reduction in overall hospital admissions and a 39% reduction (NNT 18) in acute heart failure related episodes (Sagar et al. 2015). The consequences of relapse and readmission are enormous in terms of quality of life, associated morbidity, and financial impact, thus the more recent emphasis on the importance of CR for heart failure patients within national and international guidelines. In terms of direct measures of anxiety, depression, and quality of life, CR demonstrates consistently favourable outcomes for all patient groups, and for those with heart failure, a clinically relevant (and highly statistically significant) change in the Minnesota Living with Heart Failure questionnaire point score of 5.8 (Sagar et al. 2015).

Improvements in quality of life associated with CR extend to all priority patient groups (Anderson et al. 2016). Whilst optimal medical therapy and percutaneous intervention for management of CHD may add 'years to life', the potential for CR to add 'life to years' should not be under-estimated, and there is growing recognition that promotion of CR should focus upon its ability to provide cost-effective and cost-saving secondary CVD prevention (Shields et al. 2018). There are a number of strongly associated benefits, extending beyond mortality that remain very important to highlight. For example, CPRPs improve functional capacity and perceived quality of life whilst also supporting early return to work and the development of self-management skills (Anderson et al. 2016; Yohannes et al. 2010). Furthermore, those who have participated in CR after MI have shown significantly better adherence to their cardioprotective medications (Shah et al. 2009).

Practice Application

When communicating the benefits of CR, practitioners should augment their emphasis beyond just reductions in all-cause and cardiac mortality and stress the important benefits of influencing patient wellbeing in light of the growing number of surviving individuals living longer with the burden of CVD. In the context of pursuing cost savings and efficiencies in a healthcare system, the significant benefits in reduced costly hospital readmissions associated with participation in a cardiovascular prevention and rehabilitation programme should be one of the prime messages to funders, along with enhanced patient wellbeing.

1.5   SERVICE PROVISION AND UPTAKE

Although there are class IA recommendations for CR in the American Heart Association (AHA) and American College of Cardiology (ACC) management guidelines and performance measures, only around 20% of eligible patients are apparently referred in the United States (Menezes et al. 2014). Even amongst patients who are appropriately and/or automatically referred to CR, participation rates remain concerning.

Given its clinical and cost effectiveness for CVD management, it is imperative that structures are in place to maximise CR uptake, adherence, and completion. The 2017 BHF National Audit of Cardiac Rehabilitation (NACR) reported that overall mean uptake to CR in the UK has reached 51% (of all eligible patients), which brings the UK's uptake into the top 2% of countries in Europe (National Audit of Cardiac Rehabilitation 2017). Although these data represent a steady increase in uptake, a modelling study conducted by NHS Improvement in 2013 advocated that increasing uptake of CR to 65% of all eligible individuals in England would reduce emergency cardiac admissions by 30%, releasing more than £30 million per year into the NHS, which could be used within rehabilitation and re-enablement (Kaiser et al. 2013).

Predictors of sub-optimal participation include poor functional status, higher body mass index, tobacco use, depression, low health literacy, and long travel distances (Menezes et al. 2014). Furthermore, international data show unacceptable levels of modifiable risk factors at follow-up in the majority of people with CHD and other vascular disease (Kotseva et al. 2016; Steg et al. 2007). Moreover, non-attendees are less likely to believe that rehabilitation is necessary (Cooper et al. 2007) yet have higher baseline risk and poorer risk factor knowledge than those who attend (Redfern et al. 2007).

CR is effective and value for money; nevertheless, current service provision and uptake varies considerably. The application of the BACPR's six service standards aims to reduce this variation in care whilst effectively increasing participation uptake, adherence, and full programme completion (BACPR 2017). Early assessment and goal-setting together with early programme commencement are emphasised in recognition of the associated benefits in improved service uptake and potential reductions in hospital readmissions. The provision of a menu of best practice approaches run by a skilled multidisciplinary team in strong partnership (integration) between primary and secondary care is essential to improve uptake and completion rates of individualised and patient-centred programmes.

As centre-based and home-based CR do not appear to generate different outcomes, or incur substantially different healthcare costs, the CR setting can be individually tailored to patients' preferences. In some cases, home-based CR has demonstrated a higher utilisation rate (uptake, adherence, and completion), therefore services have the opportunity for innovative delivery to enhance patient recruitment (Anderson et al. 2017; Brual et al. 2012; Taylor et al. 2015).

1.6   EMPLOYING EVIDENCE-BASED APPROACHES TO INCREASE PARTICIPATION

In addition to providing choice and alternative models of service delivery such as home-based programmes, there are several important other approaches known to increase uptake and participation. If a CR clinician engages with a patient in an acute hospital setting, and begins to undertake personalised goal-setting at this point, then this may lead to higher uptake (Cossette et al. 2012).

It is also clear that the greatest benefits to programme uptake occur when participation commences early. Early programme initiation has been found to be both safe and feasible, and improves patient uptake and adherence (Aamot et al. 2010; Eder et al. 2010; Fell et al. 2016; Haykowsky et al. 2011; Maachi et al. 2007). This is a time when people are particularly receptive to changing their health behaviour and therefore avoiding delays is critically important.

In the UK, the National Audit of Cardiac Rehabilitation report highlights a mean delay of 28 days to commence an outpatient CR programme post-MI (National Audit of Cardiac Rehabilitation 2017), which may in part explain the average uptake of 51%. Commencing programme orientation within 10 days of discharge and initiating structured activity early are associated with increased uptake and improved patient outcomes (Aamot et al. 2010; Haykowsky et al. 2011; Pack et al. 2013). An early appointment to outpatient CR at hospital discharge has been shown to significantly improve attendance in a randomised, single-blind, controlled trial (Pack et al. 2013). In this comparison 148 patients with a non-surgical qualifying diagnosis for CR were randomised to receive an orientation appointment to the programme either within 10 days (early) or at 35 days (standard). The primary end point was attendance at the orientation appointment. Unlike many other studies in CR there was a good balance in sex and ethnicity; 56% of participants were male and 49% were black, with balanced baseline characteristics between groups. The median time (95% confidence interval) to orientation was 8.5 (7–13) versus 42 (35 to NA [not applicable]) days for the early and standard appointment groups, respectively ($P < 0.001$). Attendance rates at the orientation session were 77% (57/74) versus 59% (44/74) in the early and standard appointment groups, respectively, which demonstrates a significant 18% absolute and 56% relative improvement (relative risk, 1.56; 95% confidence interval, 1.03–2.37; $P = 0.022$). This simple technique could potentially increase participation in CPRPs nationwide.

A further evidence-based approach is the use of motivational invitation techniques. A review by Davies et al. (2010) included a wide variety of databases and found 10 randomised controlled trials that were suitable for inclusion (three trials of interventions to improve uptake, and seven of interventions to improve adherence). The studies evaluated a variety of techniques to improve uptake or adherence and in many studies a combination of strategies was employed. The quality of studies was generally low. All three interventions targeting uptake of CR were effective. Two of seven studies intended to increase adherence to exercise as part of CR had a significant effect (one of which was of poor quality).

The interventions evaluated included motivational letters (Wyer et al. 2001), motivational telephone contact (Hillebrand et al. 1995), and coordination of care by a trained nurse, together with patient self-monitoring of contact with health professionals (Jolly et al. 1999). The multifaceted nature of the latter trial meant that it was not possible to identify which were the active components of the intervention that brought about the increase in uptake.

Practice Application

All CPRPs should draw upon the evidence base and employ approaches that are known to increase uptake and programme completion. Early assessment and programme commencement, motivational approaches to invitation letters, and scheduled telephone contact have all been shown to be effective.

In this same review by Davies et al. (2010) seven studies of interventions to improve adherence were identified. A wide variety of techniques, and combinations of techniques, were evaluated including goal-setting, action planning, self-monitoring (of exercise, daily activities, bodyweight, heart rate, smoking, and contact with health professionals), feedback, problem-solving and coping strategies, written and oral commitment, stress management, persuasive written and telephone communication, and small group interaction and peer modelling. The majority of studies found no significant effect of the interventions on adherence. Two studies found significant effects in exercise participation following programme completion (Duncan and Pozehl 2002; Sniehotta et al. 2006). It should be noted though that the follow up period for both of these two studies was less than 12 weeks. The former trial investigated the effectiveness of an adherence facilitation intervention consisting of goal-setting, graphic feedback, and provider guidance to support adherence to home exercise in a sample of patients with heart failure. The sample consisted of 13 patients with an ejection fraction of 40% or less who were randomly assigned to either the exercise only group ($n = 6$) or the exercise with adherence facilitation group ($n = 7$). Results indicated that patients who received the intervention demonstrated higher exercise adherence and greater confidence in continuing to exercise in the future (Duncan and Pozehl 2002). However, the study sample was very small and the risk of bias was difficult to assess due to a lack of information in the study report.

Sniehotta et al. (2006) found that developing coping plans to overcome anticipated barriers together with action plans was more effective than action planning alone or usual care. Action planning alone was not more effective than usual care, suggesting that coping plans were the most important component in the combined intervention. However, randomisation was achieved by alternate allocation, which is a weak method. Adherence to exercise was self-reported and there was no information within the study report about whether those assessing outcomes were blind to the participants' treatment allocations. These factors may have introduced bias into the results of the study.

In summary, there is a wealth of data reporting on the barriers to attendance at CPRPs and possible interventions to address these. However, much of the research is of poor quality with few studies including any blinding and little consistency in the definition of adherence. Furthermore, few studies reported the effects of the interventions on clinical outcomes or health-related quality of life and none provided information about costs or resource implications. The differences between the strategies used in the studies identified mean that it is difficult to make clear recommendations. Following a review of the evidence a summary of strategies that may increase uptake and programme completion is provided in Figure 1.2. In designing an effective preventive cardiology programme these should be considered. However, further high quality research is needed.

Interventions to increase uptake	Interventions to increase adherence
• Motivational letters* • Motivational telephone contact* • Home visits* • Coordination of care by a trained nurse* • Automatic referral systems* • Inpatient visit by cardiac rehabilitation liaison* • Early programme orientation (<10 days)* • Use of lay volunteers • Offering choice • Provide transport • Care for dependents	• Planning and goal-setting* • Signed commitment or diary* • Gender-tailored programmes* • Early programme orientation*

*Supported by RCT data.

FIGURE 1.2   Summary of interventions to increase uptake and adherence to exercise-based cardiac rehabilitation (CR).

1.7   FUTURE PERSPECTIVES

In efforts to increase participation there is recognition of the need to include interventions that are targeted at reducing specific barriers to referral and participation, offering choice (e.g. home-based, evening sessions, etc.) and the use of modern technologies (internet, phone, and other communication tools). Regarding the use of innovative strategies and the value of reaching out to more people who would benefit from a CPRP, new delivery models must be adopted, especially for patients at low or low-to-intermediate risk. These include the use of telemedicine as well as internet-based, home-based (including Smartphone-based home care models), and community-based programmes to provide alternatives to conventional, medically supervised, facility-based programmes (Clark et al. 2015; Varnfield et al. 2014). Moving traditional CR out of the hospital setting and into community-based venues may increase accessibility and provides an environment removed from acute illness, thereby promoting health and wellbeing. Consequently, in a climate that is calling for innovation, it is essential for the multidisciplinary team to also be equipped to deliver and rigorously evaluate novel approaches in prevention and rehabilitation. The team must ensure to draw on the evidence base and when engaging in new approaches do so with the intention of contributing to driving vital high quality research in CVD prevention and rehabilitation. Experimental delivery models for cardiovascular prevention and rehabilitation should not be widely adopted until they have been shown to be both clinically effective and cost effective (Balady et al. 2011).

1.8   CONCLUSION

The growing burden of CVD is resulting in a greater need to address the underlying causes of atherosclerosis. CR programmes are evolving to become 'chronic disease management programmes' treating atherosclerosis as a single disease. In the United Kingdom, the Cardiovascular Outcomes Strategy (Department of Health 2013) calls for service integration and the inclusion of different clinical presentations beyond CHD, such as transient cerebral ischaemia, stroke, and peripheral arterial disease to be included. These different clinical presentations are associated with a common pathology of atherosclerosis and common underlying risk factors, particularly smoking, high blood pressure, elevated cholesterol, diabetes, obesity, and unhealthy lifestyle. Participation in a CPRP is associated with an array of improved health outcomes and, importantly, potential cost savings through reductions in unplanned hospital admissions. A 'rebranding' of CR may be required in the context of modern cardiology practice that draws on evidence-based approaches to increase uptake and programme completion together with the development, application, and evaluation of novel approaches to service delivery.

REFERENCES

Aamot, I., Moholdt, T., Amundsen, B. et al. (2010). Onset of exercise training 14 days after uncomplicated MI: a randomized controlled trial. *European Journal of Cardiovascular Prevention and Rehabilitation* 17 (14): 387–392.

Anderson, L., Sharp, G.A., Norton, R.J. et al. (2017). Home-based versus centre-based cardiac rehabilitation. *Cochrane Database of Systematic Reviews*: CD007130. https://doi.org/10.1002/14651858.CD007130.pub4.

Anderson, L., Thompson, D.R., Oldridge, N. et al. (2016). Exercise-based cardiac rehabilitation for coronary heart disease. *Cochrane Database of Systematic Reviews*: CD001800. https://doi.org/10.1002/14651858.CD001800.pub3.

Aragam, K.G., Moscucci, M., Smith, D.E. et al. (2011). Trends and disparities in referral to cardiac rehabilitation after percutaneous coronary intervention. *American Heart Journal* 161: 544–551.

Balady, G.J., Ades, P.A., Bittner, V.A. et al. (2011). Referral, enrollment, and delivery of cardiac rehabilitation/secondary prevention programs at clinical centers and beyond: a presidential advisory from the American Heart Association. *Circulation* 124: 2951–2960.

Bovet, P. and Paccaud, F. (2011). Cardiovascular disease and the changing face of global public health: a focus on low and middle income countries. *Public Health Reviews* 33: 397–415.

British Association for Cardiovascular Prevention and Rehabilitation (2017). *The BACPR Standards and Core Components for Cardiovascular Disease Prevention and Rehabilitation*, 3e. London: BACPR.

British Heart Foundation (2018). *Heart Statistics Fact Sheet*. London: BHF.

Brual, J., Gravely, S., Suskin, N. et al. (2012). The role of clinical and geographical factors in the use of hospital versus home-based cardiac rehabilitation. *International Journal of Rehabilitation* 35 (3): 220–226.

Clark, R.A., Conway, A., Poulsen, V. et al. (2015). Alternative models of cardiac rehabilitation: a systematic review. *European Journal of Preventive Cardiology* 22: 35–74.

Cooper, A.F., Weinman, J., Hankins, M. et al. (2007). Assessing patients' beliefs about cardiac rehabilitation as a basis for predicting attendance after acute myocardial infarction. *Heart* 93: 53–58.

Cossette, S., Frasure-Smith, N., Dupuis, J. et al. (2012). Randomized controlled trial of tailored nursing interventions to improve cardiac rehabilitation enrolment. *Nursing Research* 61 (2): 111–120.

Cowie, A., Buckley, J., Doherty, P. et al. (2019). Standards and core components for cardiovascular disease prevention and rehabilitation. *Heart* 105: 510–515.

Dalal, H.M., Doherty, P., and Taylor, R.S. (2015). Cardiac rehabilitation. *British Medical Journal* 351: h5000. https://doi.org/10.1136/bmj.h5000.

Davies, P., Taylor, F., Beswick, A. et al. (2010). Promoting patient uptake and adherence in cardiac rehabilitation. *Cochrane Database of Systematic Reviews* (7): CD007131. https://doi.org/10.1002/14651858.CD007131.pub2.

Department of Health (2013). *Cardiovascular Disease Outcomes Strategy: Improving Outcomes for People with or at Risk of Cardiovascular Disease*. London: Department of Health.

Duncan, K.A. and Pozehl, B. (2002). Staying on course: the effects of an adherence facilitation intervention on home exercise participation. *Progress in Cardiovascular Nursing* 17: 59–65.

Eder, B., Hofmann, P., von Duvillard, S.P. et al. (2010). Early 4-week cardiac rehabilitation exercise training in elderly patients after heart surgery. *Journal of Cardiopulmary Rehabilitation and Prevention* 30 (2): 85–92.

European Heart Network (2017). *European Cardiovascular Disease Statistics*. Brussels: EHN.

Fell, J., Dale, V., and Doherty, P. (2016). Does the timing of cardiac rehabilitation impact fitness outcomes? An observational analysis. *Open Heart* 3 (1): e000369. https://doi.org/10.1136/openhrt-2015-000369. eCollection 2016.

Global Burden of Disease (2015). Mortality and causes of death collaborators, global, regional and national age-sex specific all-cause mortality for 240 causes of death, 1990–2013: a systematic analysis of the Global Burden of Disease Study 2013. *Lancet* 385: 117–171.

Grace, S.L., Warburton, D.R., Stone, J.A. et al. (2013). International charter on cardiovascular prevention and rehabilitation: a call for action. *Journal of Cardiopulmonary Rehabilitation and Prevention* 33 (2): 128–131.

Haykowsky, M., Scott, J., Esch, B. et al. (2011). A metaanalysis of the effects of exercise training on left ventricular remodeling following myocardial infarction: start early and go longer for greatest exercise benefits on remodeling. *Trials* (92): 12. https://doi.org/10.1186/745-6215-12-92.

Heran, B.S., Chen, J.M.H., Ebrahim, S. et al. (2011). Exercise-based cardiac rehabilitation for coronary heart disease. *Cochrane Database of Systematic Reviews* (7): CD001800. https://doi.org/10.1002/14651858.CD001800.pub2.

Hillebrand, T., Frodermann, H., Lehr, D., and Wirth, V. (1995). Increased participation in coronary groups by means of an outpatient care program. *Herz Kreislauf* 27: 346–349.

Jolly, K., Bradley, F., Sharp, S. et al. (1999). Randomised controlled trial of follow up care in general practice of patients with myocardial infarction and angina: final results of the Southampton heart integrated care project (SHIP). The SHIP Collaborative Group. *British Medical Journal* 318: 706–711.

Kaiser, M., Varvel, M., and Doherty, P. (2013). *Making the Case for Cardiac Rehabilitation: Modelling Potential Impact on Readmissions*. Leicester: NHS Improvement – Heart.

Kassebaum, N.J., Arora, M., Barber, R.M. et al. (2016). Global, regional, and national disability-adjusted life-years (DALYs) for 315 diseases and injuries and healthy life expectancy (HALE), 1990–2015: a systematic analysis for the global burden of disease study 2015. *Lancet* 388 (10053): 1603–1658.

Koene, R.J., Prizment, A.E., Blaes, A., and Konety, S.H. (2016). Shared risk factors in cardiovascular disease and cancer. *Circulation* 133: 1104–1114. https://doi.org/10.1161/CIRCULATIONAHA.115.020406.

Kotseva, K., Wood, D., De Bacquer, D. et al. (2016). EUROASPIRE IV: A European Society of Cardiology survey on the lifestyle, risk factor and therapeutic management of coronary patients from 24 European countries. *European Journal of Cardiovascular Prevention and Rehabilitation* 23: 636–648.

Lim, S.S., Vos, T., Flaxman, A.D. et al. (2012). A comparative risk assessment of burden of disease and injury attributable to 67 risk factors and risk factor clusters in 21 regions, 1990–2010: a systematic analysis for the Global Burden of Disease Study 2010. *Lancet* 380: 2224–2260. https://doi.org/10.1016/S0140-6736(12)61766-8.

Maachi, C., Fattirolli, F., Molino Lova, R. et al. (2007). Early and late rehabilitation and physical training in elderly patients after cardiac surgery. *American Journal of Physical and Medical Rehabilitation* 86: 826–834.

Maron, D.J., Mancini, G.B.J., Hartigan, P.M. et al. (2018). Healthy behavior, risk factor control, and survival in the COURAGE trial. *Journal of the American College of Cardiology* 72: 2297–2305.

Menezes, A.R., Lavie, C.J., Milani, R.V. et al. (2014). Cardiac rehabilitation in the United States. *Progress in Cardiovascular Diseases* 56: 522–529.

National Audit of Cardiac Rehabilitation (2017). *Annual reports 2007 to 2017.* University of York, British Heart Foundation and NHS Digital http://www.cardiacrehabilitation.org.uk/reports.htm.

National Institute of Health and Care Excellence (2013). *CG172 Secondary Prevention Post Myocardial Infarction.* London: Royal College of Physicians.

Pack, Q.R., Mansour, M., Barboza, J.S. et al. (2013). An early appointment to outpatient cardiac rehabilitation at hospital discharge improves attendance at orientation: a randomized, single-blind, controlled trial. *Circulation* 127: 349–355.

Piepoli, M., Corra, U., Adamopoulos, S. et al. (2014). Secondary prevention in the clinical management of patients with cardiovascular diseases. Core components, standards and outcome measures for referral and delivery. *European Journal of Preventive Cardiology* 21: 664–681.

Rauch, B., Davos, C.H., Doherty, P. et al. (2016). The prognostic effect of cardiac rehabilitation in the era of acute revascularisation and statin therapy: a systematic review and meta-analysis of randomized and non-randomized studies – The Cardiac Rehabilitation Outcome Study (CROS). *European Journal of Preventive Cardiology* 23 (18): 1914–1939.

Redfern, J.R., Ellis, E.R., Briffa, T., and Freedman, S.B. (2007). High-risk factor level and prevalence and low-risk factor knowledge in patients not accessing cardiac rehabilitation after acute coronary syndrome. *Medical Journal of Australia* 86: 21–25.

Sagar, V.A., Davies, E.J., Briscoe, S. et al. (2015). Exercise-based rehabilitation for heart failure: systematic review and meta-analysis. *Open Heart* 2: e000163. https://doi.org/10.1136/openhrt-2014-000163.

Shah, N.D., Dunlay, S.M., Ting, H.H. et al. (2009). Long-term medication adherence after myocardial infarction: experience of a community. *The American Journal of Medicine* 122: 961–913.

Shields, G., Wells, A., Doherty, P. et al. (2018). Cost-effectiveness of cardiac rehabilitation: a systematic review. *Heart* Published Online First: doi: https://doi.org/10.1136/heartjnl-2017-312809.

Sniehotta, F.F., Scholz, U., and Schwarzer, R. (2006). Action plans and coping plans for physical exercise: A longitudinal intervention study in cardiac rehabilitation. *British Journal of Health Psychology* 11: 23–37.

Steg, P.G., Bhatt, D.L., Wilson, P.W.F. et al. (2007). One-year cardiovascular event rates in outpatients with atherothrombosis. *Journal of the American Medical Association* 297: 1197–1206.

Taylor, R.S., Dalal, H., Jolly, K. et al. (2015). Home-based versus centre-based cardiac rehabilitation. *Cochrane Database of Systematic Reviews*: CD007130. https://doi.org/10.1002/14651858.CD007130.pub3.

Thompson, D.R. and De Bono, D.P. (1999). How valuable is cardiac rehabiltation and who should get it? *Heart* 82: 545–546.

Van Halewijn, G., Deckers, J., Tay, H.Y. et al. (2017). Lessons from contemporary trials of cardiovascular prevention and rehabilitation. *International Journal of Cardiology* 232: 294–303.

Varnfield, M., Karunanithi, M., Lee, C.K. et al. (2014). Smartphone-based home care model improved use of cardiac rehabilitation in post myocardial infarction patients: results from a randomised controlled trial. *Heart* 100: 1770–1779.

Wang, H., Naghavi, M., Allen, C. et al. (2016). Global, regional, and national life expectancy, all-cause mortality, and cause-specific mortality for 249 causes of death, 1980–2015: a systematic analysis for the global burden of disease study 2015. *Lancet* 388 (10053): 1459–1544.

World Health Organization (2013). *Global Action Plan for the Prevention and Control of NCDs 2013–2020*. Geneva: World Health Organization.

World Health Organization (2018). *World Health Statistics 2018: Monitoring Health for the SDGs, Sustainable Development Goals*. Geneva: World Health Organization.

Wyer, S.J., Earll, L., Joseph, S. et al. (2001). Increasing attendance rates at a cardiac rehabilitation programme: an intervention study using the theory of planned behaviour. *Coronary Health Care* 5: 154–159.

Yohannes, A.M., Doherty, P., Bundy, C., and Yalfani, A. (2010). The long-term benefits of cardiac rehabilitation on depression, anxiety, physical activity and quality of life. *Journal of Clinical Nursing* 19: 2806–2813.

Yusuf, S., Hawken, S., Ounpuu, S. et al. (2004). INTERHEART study Investigators. Effect of potentially modifiable risk factors associated with myocardial infarction in 52 countries (the INTERHEART study): case-control study. *Lancet* 364: 937–952.

CHAPTER 2

Standards and Core Components in Cardiovascular Disease Prevention and Rehabilitation

BACPR Standards Writing Group

British Association for Cardiovascular Prevention and Rehabilitation, London, UK

Abstract

This chapter presents the current Standards and Core Components for Cardiovascular Disease Prevention and Rehabilitation from the British Association for Cardiovascular Prevention and Rehabilitation (BACPR). These aim to define cardiovascular prevention and rehabilitation services, operationally, through six standards and six core components for assuring a quality service of care using a multidisciplinary biopsychosocial approach. The six standards aim to ensure that service commissioners, providers, and health professionals are aware of the requirements for providing a multidisciplinary team that is competent and thus clinically effective, cost effective, and ultimately cost saving as a result of preventing hospital readmissions. The six core components, delivered as a coordinated sum of activities, aim to best influence uptake, adherence, quality of life, and long-term healthier living.

Keywords: *cardiovascular disease, cardiac rehabilitation, prevention, standards, core components, audit*

Cardiovascular Prevention and Rehabilitation in Practice, Second Edition.
Edited by Jennifer Jones, John Buckley, Gill Furze, and Gail Sheppard.
© 2020 John Wiley & Sons Ltd. Published 2020 by John Wiley & Sons Ltd.

Key Points

- Cardiovascular prevention and rehabilitation programmes (CPRPs) are effective and value for money; nevertheless, current service provision, uptake, and quality vary considerably.
- The British Association for Cardiovascular Prevention and Rehabilitation (BACPR) Standards and Core Components for Cardiovascular Disease Prevention and Rehabilitation sets out six core standards and six core components to: ensure more equitable care, improve uptake, and enhance quality of service provision.
- Early assessment and goal-setting together with early programme commencement are emphasised in recognition of the associated benefits in improved service uptake and potential reductions in hospital readmissions.
- The provision of a menu of best practice approaches run by a skilled multidisciplinary team in strong partnership (integration) between primary and secondary care is essential to improve uptake and completion rates of individualised and patient-centred programmes.
- The illustrative model of the six core components represents health behaviour change and education as central and integral to all of the other components, as well as equal emphasis on the delivery of care in lifestyle risk factor management, psychosocial health, medical risk factor management and cardioprotective therapies.
- On programme completion it is imperative for effective long-term management that each service has defined pathways for continuity of care that ultimately leads to the best possible levels of self-management and secondary prevention.
- Audit and evaluation is given major importance; being included as both a standard and core component.

2.1   RATIONALE AND AIMS

Given that cardiovascular prevention and rehabilitation (CR) is recognised as a clinically and cost-effective therapeutic intervention in cardiovascular disease management (Chapter 1), its low uptake remains of concern (National Audit for Cardiac Rehabilitation 2017). Within the United Kingdom, variation between countries and regions is evident with considerable heterogeneity seen in key indicators, such as time from referral to commencement of CR and assessment completion rates. Large differences between the regions demonstrate gross inequality of provision and considerable variation in the quality of care being delivered. The BACPR sets out six core standards and six core components that aim to reduce this variation in care whilst effectively increasing service uptake, programme completion, and quality of provision (BACPR 2017). The following chapter presents these standards and core components, setting the scene for subsequent chapters that concentrate on enabling their implementation in order to realise the benefits in accordance with the associated evidence base.

2.2 SIX STANDARDS TO ACHIEVE HIGH QUALITY CARDIOVASCULAR PREVENTION AND REHABILITATION

The six standards for cardiovascular prevention and rehabilitation are:

1. The delivery of six core components by a qualified and competent multidisciplinary team, led by a clinical coordinator.
2. Prompt identification, referral, and recruitment of eligible patient populations.
3. Early initial assessment of individual patient needs, which informs agreed personalised goals that are reviewed regularly.
4. Early provision of a structured CPRP, with a defined pathway of care, which meets the individual's goals and is aligned with patient preference and choice.
5. Upon programme completion a final assessment of individual patient needs and demonstration of sustainable health outcomes.
6. Registration and submission of data to the National Audit for Cardiac Rehabilitation (NACR) and participation in the National Certification Programme (NCP_CR).

Important notes:

- Within the standards criteria the word 'shall' is used to express a requirement that all programmers are expected to comply with (Grade A/B recommendations based on the highest quality evidence available and recognised as best practice). The word 'should' is used to express a recommendation that is recognised as desirable (Grade C/D recommendation).
- In some cases, these recommendations may exceed the current minimum standards required for the National Certification Programme, which set annual targets based on national averages.

Performance indicators associated with meeting the minimum standards required for programme certification can be found at: www.bacpr.com

Standard 1

The Delivery of Six Core Components by a Qualified and Competent Multidisciplinary Team, Led by a Clinical Coordinator

- Each programme shall deliver the six essential core components to ensure clinically effective care and achieve sustainable health outcomes as presented in Section 2.3.
- The team shall include a senior clinician who has responsibility for coordinating, managing, and evaluating the service. This also includes: resource and financial management for the service; collaboration with NHS data analysts to successfully draw on all available funding and identify any savings arising from reduced hospital admissions; and engagement with funding and commissioning bodies.
- There shall be an appropriately qualified and competent named lead for each of the core components. These practitioners who lead each of the core components should be able to demonstrate that either they or their delivery team have appropriate training, professional development, qualifications, skills and competency for the component(s) for which they are responsible. Practitioners should use the BACPR Competencies Frameworks, where available.
- The team shall include a physician who has sustained interest, commitment, and knowledge in cardiovascular disease prevention and rehabilitation
- The delivery of the core components requires expertise from a range of different professionals working within their scope of practice. The composition of each team may differ but collectively the team shall have the necessary knowledge, skills, and competencies to meet the standards and deliver all the core components. Patients' benefit from access to a wide range of specialists, which most typically may include:
  - Dietitian
  - Exercise specialist
  - Nurse specialist
  - Occupational therapist
  - Pharmacist
  - Physician with special interest in prevention and rehabilitation
  - Physiotherapist
  - Practitioner psychologist.
- There shall be dedicated administrative support.

- The cardiovascular prevention and rehabilitation team shall actively engage and collaborate with the patient's/client's wider care team (e.g. general practitioners, practice nurses, cardiovascular disease specialist nurses, sports and leisure instructors, social workers, and educationalists) to create a truly comprehensive approach to long-term management.
- When designing, evaluating, and developing programmes, service users should also be included in this process.

Standard 2

Prompt Identification, Referral, and Recruitment of Eligible Patient Populations

(a) Patient Identification

- The following priority patient groups shall be offered a CPRP irrespective of age, sex, ethnic group, and clinical condition.
  - acute coronary syndrome
  - coronary revascularisation
  - heart failure.
- Programmes should also aim to offer this service to other patient groups known to benefit:
  - stable angina, peripheral arterial disease, post-cerebrovascular event
  - post-implantation of cardiac defibrillators and resynchronisation devices
  - post-heart valve repair/replacement
  - post-heart transplantation and ventricular assist devices
  - adult congenital heart disease (ACHD).
- It is recognised that asymptomatic individuals who have been identified as high cardiovascular risk for CVD events are likely to benefit from the same professional lifestyle interventions and risk factor management as those that currently qualify for CPRPs. In addition, risk factors for cardiovascular disease are largely shared with the wider spectrum of non-communicable diseases such as cancer, chronic obstructive pulmonary disease, and atrial fibrillation (Koene et al. 2016; Lim et al. 2012). Existing cardiovascular prevention and rehabilitation services, if appropriately

resourced, are in a strong position to provide high quality, cost-effective interventions to individuals both with and without established CVD. CPRPs should demonstrate an ambition to broaden their offer and initiate discussions with commissioners locally.

- It is recognised that local policy may be required to address priority groups in the first instance to reduce variation, ensuring consistency and equity of access. These standards, however, advocate investment in cardiovascular prevention and rehabilitation services so as to ensure all patient groups ultimately benefit.

(b) Patient Referral

- An agreed and coordinated patient referral and/or recruitment process shall be in place so that all eligible patients are identified and invited to participate.
- CPRPs shall receive the referral of an eligible patient either during the inpatient stay or within 24 h of discharge. Referrals sent within a community setting or following a day case intervention shall be received by the CPRP within 72 h of the individual being identified as eligible.
- Prior to discharge, all eligible hospitalised patients should be encouraged by a healthcare professional to attend and complete a CPRP.

(c) Recruitment

- Upon receipt of referral, all patients deemed eligible shall be contacted within 3 working days to review their progress and discuss enrolment.
- A mechanism of re-offer and re-entry should be put in place where patients initially decline.

Standard 3

Early Initial Assessment of Individual Patient Needs, which Informs Agreed Personalised Goals that Are Reviewed Regularly

- The initial assessment shall commence within 10 working days of receipt of referral.

- The initial assessment is deemed complete when documentation of all the following has taken place:
  - Demographic information and social determinants of health
  - Medical history, current health status and symptoms, together with a review of any relevant investigations
  - Lifestyle risk factors (exposure to tobacco, adherence to a cardio-protective diet, body composition, physical activity status, and exercise capacity)
  - Psychosocial health (anxiety, depression, illness perception, social support, psychological stress, sexual wellbeing, and quality of life)
  - Medical risk management (control of blood pressure, lipids and glucose, use of cardioprotective therapies, and adherence to pharmacotherapies).
- Additional parameters should be assessed on an individual basis and may include psychosocial factors such as anger, hostility, substance misuse, and occupational distress.
- Even if the initial assessment cannot be completed in its entirety (e.g. exercise capacity assessment temporarily contraindicated) this shall not delay the assessment of the remaining elements or the commencement of a formal CPRP.
- The initial assessment shall identify each individual's needs, using validated measures that are culturally sensitive and also take account of associated co-morbidities.
- The assessment shall identify any physical, psychological, or behavioural issues that have the potential to impact on the patient's ability to make the desired lifestyle changes.
- The assessment shall include formal risk stratification for exercise utilising all relevant patient information (e.g. LVEF, history of arrhythmia, symptoms, functional capacity).
- The written care plan should include a defined pathway of care which meets the individual patient needs, participation preferences, and choices.
- Patients shall receive on-going assessment throughout their CPRP and a regular review of their goals, with adjustments agreed and documented where required.

Standard 4

Early Provision of a Structured CPRP, with a Defined Pathway of Care, which Meets the Individual's Goals and Is Aligned with Patient Preference and Choice

- A CPRP shall be deemed underway once patient goal(s) have been identified and appropriate interventions have begun. This should occur immediately following completion of the initial assessment (Standard 3) and shall occur within 10 working days of receipt of referral.
- In instances where there may be wait-time delays to commence group-based exercise, such as a patient presenting with a contraindication to exercise, this shall not delay initiating management strategies in other relevant core components.
- In order to maximise uptake, completion, and outcomes, CPRPs shall deliver a menu-based approach to meet a patient's individual needs. This should include choice in terms of venue (e.g. home, community, hospital) and scheduling of sessions (e.g. early mornings, evening, and weekends).
- CPRPs can be delivered using a variety of modes (e.g. centre-based, home-based, manual-based, web-based, etc.). Irrespective of mode of programme delivery:
  - Interventions provided are evidence-based and address the individual's needs across all the relevant core components.
  - Patients shall have access to the multidisciplinary team as required.
  - Patients shall be supported to participate in a personalised structured exercise programme at least 2 to 3 times a week, designed specifically to increase physical fitness. This requires documented evidence of regular review, goal-setting, and exercise progression.
  - There shall be documented interaction between the patient and the multidisciplinary team, lasting a minimum of 8 weeks.

Standard 5

Upon Programme Completion a Final Assessment of Individual Patient Needs and Demonstration of Sustainable Health Outcomes

- In order to demonstrate effective health outcomes and ascertain the extent to which a patient's goals have been achieved, a formal assessment shall be performed at programme completion, which includes all the initially assessed components:

- Lifestyle related risk factors (exposure to tobacco, adherence to a cardioprotective diet, body composition, physical activity status, and exercise capacity).
- Psychosocial health (anxiety, depression, illness perception, social support, psychological stress, sexual wellbeing, and quality of life).
- Medical risk management (control of blood pressure, lipids and glucose, use of cardioprotective therapies, and adherence to pharmacotherapies).
- Any additional parameters assessed initially should be reassessed formally upon programme completion. For example, additional psychosocial factors such as anger, hostility, substance misuse, and occupational distress.
- Data from the final assessment shall be formally recorded for evaluation of outcome measures and audit.
- Final assessment shall be used to identify any unmet goals as well as any newly developed or evolving clinical issues. This shall assist the formulation of long-term strategies.
- Within 10 working days of programme completion, the primary care provider (and the referral source where relevant) shall be provided with a pre/post comparison of the patient's risk factor profile together with current medications and a summary of the long-term strategies proposed. A copy shall also be provided to the patient.

Standard 6

Registration and Submission of Data to the NACR and Participation in the National Certification Programme

- Formal audit and evaluation of the cardiovascular prevention and rehabilitation service shall include individual data on clinical outcomes and patient experience and satisfaction as well as data on service performance.
- In order to clearly demonstrate clinical outcomes every service shall routinely submit the required audit data to NACR each year.
- Every cardiovascular prevention and rehabilitation service should strive to meet requirements for the National Certification Programme and submit their data to the certification panel. Once achieved, CPRPs should maintain their certification status.

2.3   THE CORE COMPONENTS

A key aim of a CPRP, through the core components, is not only to improve physical health and quality of life but also to equip and support people to develop the necessary skills to successfully self-manage. Delivery should adopt a biopsychosocial evidence-based approach, which is culturally appropriate and sensitive to individual needs and preferences.

Figure 2.1 illustrates the six core components, which include:

1. Health behaviour change and education
2. Lifestyle risk factor management:
   - Physical activity and exercise training
   - Healthy eating and body composition
   - Tobacco cessation and relapse prevention
3. Psychosocial health
4. Medical risk management
5. Long-term strategies
6. Audit and evaluation.

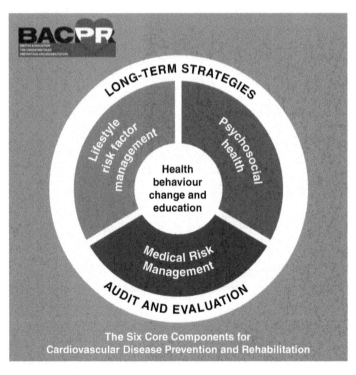

FIGURE 2.1   The British Association for Cardiovascular Prevention and Rehabilitation (BACPR) model for cardiovascular disease prevention and rehabilitation.

Practitioners who lead each of the core components must be able to demonstrate that they have appropriate training, professional development, qualifications, skills, and competency for the component(s) for which they are responsible (Standard 1). BACPR aims to be a resource for providing guidance on the knowledge, skills, and competences required for each of the components.

2.3.1 Health Behaviour Change and Education

In meeting individual needs, health behaviour change and education are integral to all the other components of cardiovascular prevention and rehabilitation. Adopting healthy behaviours is the cornerstone of prevention and control of cardiovascular disease.

2.3.1.1 Health Behaviour Change

To facilitate effective behaviour change, cardiovascular prevention and rehabilitation services should ensure:

- The use of health behaviour change interventions and key behaviour change techniques underpinned by an up-to-date psychological evidence-base_ENREF_29 (National Institute for Health and Care Excellence 2014a).
- The provision of, or access to, training in communication skills for all staff, which may include motivational interviewing techniques and relapse prevention strategies.
- The provision of information and education to support fully informed choice from a menu of evidence-based locally available programme components. Offering choice may improve uptake and adherence to cardiovascular prevention and rehabilitation (Dalal et al. 2009; Taylor et al. 2015).
- They address any cardiac or other misconceptions (including any about cardiovascular prevention and rehabilitation) and illness perceptions that lead to increased disability and distress (French et al. 2006; Furze et al. 2005; Stafford et al. 2009).
- Support for patients (and significant supporting others), including goal-setting and pacing skills, and exploring problem-solving skills, in order to improve long-term self-management.
- Regular follow up to assess feedback and advise on further goal-setting (Institute of Medicine 2003).
- Where possible, the patient identifies someone best placed to support them (e.g. a partner, relative, close friend). The accompanying person should be encouraged to actively participate in CPRP activities whenever possible, to maximise patient recovery and health behaviour change, whilst also addressing their own health behaviours (Franks et al. 2006; Moser and Dracup 2004; Wood et al. 2008).

2.3.1.2 Education

Education should be delivered not only to increase knowledge but importantly to restore confidence and foster a greater sense of perceived personal control. As far as possible, education should be delivered in a discursive rather than a didactic fashion. It is not enough to simply deliver information in designated education sessions; health behaviour change needs to be achieved simultaneously and fully integrated into the whole service.

Attention should be paid to establishing existing levels of knowledge and to assessing the learning needs (of individuals and groups), and subsequently tailoring information to suit assessed needs.

- Patients (and significant supporting others) should be encouraged to play an active role in the educative process, sharing information in order to maximise uptake of knowledge.
- Education should be culturally sensitive and achieve two key aims:
  - To increase knowledge and understanding of risk factor reduction
  - To utilise evidence-based health behaviour change theory in its delivery.

  Incorporation of both aspects of education increases the probability of successful long-term maintenance of change.
- The educational component should be delivered using high quality and varied teaching methods that take account of different learning styles and uses the best available resources to enable individuals to learn about their condition and management. Information should be presented in different formats using plain language and clear design, and tailored to the learning needs identified during assessment (Knowles et al. 2015).
- The educational component of cardiovascular prevention and rehabilitation should empower individuals to better manage their condition. Topics may include:
  - Pathophysiology and symptoms
  - Physical activity, healthy eating, and weight management
  - Tobacco cessation and relapse prevention
  - Self-management and behavioural management of other risk factors including blood pressure, lipids, and glucose
  - Medical and pharmaceutical management of blood pressure, lipids, and glucose
  - Psychological and emotional self-management
  - Social support and other contextual factors
  - Activities of daily living (ADL)
  - Occupational/vocational factors

- Resuming and maintaining sexual relations and dealing with sexual dysfunction
- Surgical interventions and devices
- Cardiopulmonary resuscitation
- Additional information, as specified in other components.

2.3.2 Lifestyle Risk Factor Management

Physical activity and exercise, together with a healthy diet and avoidance of obesity and exposure to all forms of tobacco, represents a lifestyle that is strongly associated with good cardiovascular health. All patients should have the opportunity to discuss their concerns across all of these lifestyle risk factors as relevant. Achievement of the lifestyle targets, as defined by the most up to date Joint British Societies Guidelines, should utilise evidence-based health behaviour change approaches led by specialists in collaboration with the multidisciplinary team. Supporting individuals in developing self-management skills is the cornerstone to long-term cardiovascular prevention and rehabilitation.

2.3.2.1 Physical Activity and Exercise Training

- Staff leading the exercise component of cardiovascular prevention and rehabilitation should be appropriately qualified, skilled, and competent (British Association for Cardiovascular Prevention and Rehabilitation Exercise Professionals Group (BACPR-EPG) 2011).
- Baseline assessment of physical fitness shall be carried out to inform risk assessment, tailor the exercise prescription and aid goal-setting (American Association of Cardiovascular and Pulmonary Rehabilitation (AACVPR) 2013; Association of Chartered Physiotherapists in Cardiac Rehabilitation (ACPICR) 2015; Balady et al. 2007; Piepoli et al. 2014).
- Best practice standards and guidelines for physical activity and exercise prescription shall be used (American Association of Cardiovascular and Pulmonary Rehabilitation (AACVPR) 2013; Association of Chartered Physiotherapists in Cardiac Rehabilitation (ACPICR) 2015; Balady et al. 2007).
- Risk stratification, based upon clinical features and baseline exercise capacity shall be undertaken (Association of Chartered Physiotherapists in Cardiac Rehabilitation (ACPICR) 2015). This will then determine the appropriate:
  - Exercise prescription, ADL guidance, and support
  - Staffing levels and skills (British Association for Cardiovascular Prevention and Rehabilitation Exercise Professionals Group (BACPR-EPG) 2011)

- Resuscitation support and provision will be in line with current Resuscitation Council UK/BACPR guidance (Resuscitation Council (UK) 2013)
- Choice of venue (home/community/hospital).
- Patients should receive individual guidance and advice on ADLs together with a tailored activity and exercise plan with the collective aim to increase physical fitness as well as overall daily energy expenditure and decrease sedentary behaviour. The activity and exercise plan should be identified with the patient, take account of their co-morbidities, and should be sensitive to their physical, psychosocial (cognitive and behavioural) capabilities and needs.

2.3.2.2   Healthy Eating and Body Composition

- Staff leading the dietary component of cardiovascular prevention and rehabilitation should be appropriately qualified, skilled, and competent.
- All patients shall have a baseline assessment of their dietary habits, including concordance with a cardioprotective diet and measurement of their weight, body mass index, and waist circumference.
- The focus of advice should be on making healthy dietary choices to reduce total cardiovascular risk and improve body composition.
- Misconceptions about nutrition, dieting, and weight cycling should be addressed and corrected (British Nutrition Foundation 1999; Tylka et al. 2014).
- Patients should receive personalised dietary advice that is sensitive to their culture, needs and capabilities coupled with support to help them achieve and adhere to the components of a cardioprotective diet as defined by the most up to date Joint British Societies and National Institute for Health and Care Excellence (NICE) guidelines (JBS3 Board 2014; National Institute for Health and Care Excellence 2010a, 2013b).
- Patients with additional co-morbidities leading to more complex dietary requirements should be assessed and managed individually by a registered dietitian.
- Weight management may form an important component in cardiovascular prevention and rehabilitation and could include:
  - Weight gain (e.g. in debilitated patients)
  - Weight loss, which where appropriate and in relation to excess fat, is best achieved through a combination of increased physical activity and reduced caloric intake (Shaw et al. 2006)
  - Weight maintenance (e.g. in those who have recently quit smoking [Aubin et al. 2012] or those with heart failure).

- It may be appropriate to refer to the appropriate specialists for pharmaco-therapy and/or bariatric surgery in order to co-manage weight loss (National Institute for Health and Care Excellence 2006).

2.3.2.3 Tobacco Cessation and Relapse Prevention

Staff delivering the tobacco cessation and relapse prevention component of car-diovascular prevention and rehabilitation should be appropriately qualified, skilled, and competent in keeping with the NHS Centre for Smoking Cessation and Training Standard, which is available for download from their website – www.ncsct.co.uk (NHS Centre for Smoking Cessation and Training (NCSCT) n.d.).

- Current and past tobacco use should be assessed in all patients, including whether they are a current user or recent quitter, their history of tobacco use, past quit attempts, and exposure to second hand smoke.
- In patients who are currently using tobacco, frequency and quantity of use should be quantified. In addition, motivation to quit and a measure of nicotine dependence should be assessed, together with identifying psychological co-morbidities like depression and tobacco use by others at home.
- At the first assessment, medical advice to quit should be reinforced and a quit plan discussed that proposes the use of pharmacological support and follow-up counselling within the prevention and rehabilitation service. Every effort should be made to assist individuals to achieve complete ces-sation of all forms of tobacco use, with repeat assessment of progress with cessation at every visit (National Institute for Health and Care Excellence 2006, 2008; Rice and Stead 2008).
- Patient preference is a priority regarding the choice of aids to use in tobacco cessation. The use of evidence-based therapies like varenicline and combination long- and short-acting nicotine replacement therapy (NRT) is considered the gold standard, however non-medical nicotine delivery devices like e-cigarettes should also be considered as evidence is building for their efficacy. Guidance for cessation advisers can be found in the NHS Centre for Smoking Cessation and Training (NCSCT) e-cigarette briefing (McEwen and McRobbie 2016).
- Preventing relapse is vital and may include prolonging the use of NRT and varenicline beyond the usual duration, and/or e-cigarettes in cases where cessation has been problematic. Risk of relapse is higher when an individual lives, socialises, or works closely with others who use tobacco, therefore encouraging quit attempts in partners/spouses/friends/children may be helpful.

2.3.3 Psychosocial Health

People taking part in cardiovascular prevention and rehabilitation may have many different emotional issues, and a comprehensive, holistic assessment is crucial to achieving the desired outcomes. Every patient should be screened for psychological, psychosocial, and sexual health and wellbeing as ineffective management can lead to poor health outcomes (Dickens et al. 2008; Kronish 2006; Shibeshi et al. 2007).

- Staff leading the psychosocial health component should be appropriately qualified, skilled, and competent.
- All patients should undergo a valid assessment of:
  - Psychological distress, for example, anxiety and depression (using an appropriate tool – Hospital Anxiety and Depression Scale (HADS) is available through the NACR)
  - Quality of life (using an appropriate tool – Dartmouth COOP and Minnesota Living with Heart Failure (MLWHF) are available through the NACR)
  - Psychological stressors
  - Illness perceptions and self-efficacy for health behaviour change
  - Adequacy of social support (covered in Dartmouth COOP – available through NACR)
  - Alcohol and substance misuse.
- Services should help patients to increase awareness of ways in which psychological development, including illness perceptions, stress awareness and improved stress management skills can affect subsequent physical and emotional health.
- Attention should be paid to social support, as social isolation or lack of perceived social support is associated with increased cardiac mortality (Mookadam and Arthur 2004). Whereas appropriate social support is helpful, overprotection may adversely affect quality of life (Joekes et al. 2007).
- Levels of psychological intervention (for psychological distress):
  - Cardiovascular prevention and rehabilitation teams are best placed to deal with the normal range of emotional distress associated with a patient's precipitating cardiac event.
  - Where appropriately trained psychological practitioners exist within the cardiovascular prevention and rehabilitation team, individuals with clinical levels of anxiety or depression related to their cardiac

event can be managed within the service. In the absence of dedicated psychological support in the team, or where individuals have signs of severe and enduring mental health problems, referrals should be made to appropriately trained psychological practitioners, and the GP should be informed (National Institute for Health and Care Excellence 2009, 2011a; Whalley et al. 2011).

- Services should be aware of patients with problems related to alcohol misuse or substance misuse and offer referral to an appropriate resource.
- It is also important to consider vocational advice and rehabilitation/ financial implications and to establish an agreed referral pathway to appropriate support and advice.
- Sexual health issues are also common with cardiovascular disease, and can negatively impact quality of life and psychological wellbeing (Günzler et al. 2009; Træen and Olsen 2007).
- Every patient should be provided with the opportunity to raise any concerns they may have in relation to sexual activity and/or function. Assessment of patients' sexual concerns can be beneficial (Steinke et al. 2013).
- Concerns or issues raised on assessment should be addressed through sexual counselling and medical management where indicated (Steinke et al. 2013; Steinke and Swan 2004; Tra Levine et al. 2012).
- Health issues should be offered referral to an appropriate resource (Steinke et al. 2013; Steinke and Swan 2004; Tra Levine et al. 2012).

2.3.4 Medical Risk Management

- Staff leading the medical risk management component of cardiovascular prevention and rehabilitation services should be appropriately qualified, skilled, and competent. Ideally an independent prescriber should be part of the multidisciplinary team.
- Best practice standards and guidelines for medical risk factor management (blood pressure, lipids, and glucose) (JBS3 Board 2014; National Institute for Health and Care Excellence 2011b, 2013b, 2014b, 2015), optimisation of cardioprotective therapies, and management of patients with implantable devices (Association of Chartered Physiotherapists in Cardiac Rehabilitation (ACPICR) 2015; National Institute for Health and Care Excellence 2010b, 2014c) should be used.
- Assessment should include:
  - Measurement of blood pressure, lipids, glucose, HR, and rhythm
  - Current medication use (dose and adherence)

- Patients' beliefs about medication as this affects adherence to drug regimens (Byrne et al. 2005)
- A discussion regarding sexual activity/function (pending patient's willingness to discuss)
- Implantable device settings where applicable.
- During the CPRP, blood pressure and glucose should be regularly monitored with the aim of helping the individual to reach the targets defined by national guidelines by programme completion (JBS3 Board 2014; National Institute for Health and Care Excellence 2010a, 2011b, 2014b, 2015).
- Key cardioprotective medications are prescribed according to current guidance.
- Cardioprotective medications should be up-titrated during the programme so that evidence-based dosages are achieved.
- Cardiovascular prevention and rehabilitation staff should be involved with initiation and/or titration of appropriate pharmacotherapy, either directly through independent prescribing by a member of the multidisciplinary team or agreed protocols/patient group directives or through liaison with an appropriate healthcare professional (e.g. cardiologist, primary care physician).
- Erectile dysfunction in cardiovascular patients is typically multifactorial with vascular disease, psychogenic factors, and medication all acting as potential contributors. Individuals with erectile dysfunction should be considered for medication review and appropriate referral made where indicated.
- Maintaining guideline levels of blood pressure and glucose is also important for safe exercise.
- In people with implantable devices, such as implantable cardiac defibrillators and/or cardiac resynchronisation therapy:
  - Devices can have an impact on psychological and physical function and exercise ability, which should be considered within the individualised programme and may require additional expertise (Association of Chartered Physiotherapists in Cardiac Rehabilitation (ACPICR) 2015; Fitchet et al. 2003; Lewin et al. 2001).
  - Liaison with specialist cardiac services is important (e.g. arrhythmia nurse specialist, electrophysiologist, and cardiac physiologist).
- Cardiovascular prevention and rehabilitation services also provide an opportunity to identify patients who may benefit from an implantable device (National Institute for Health and Care Excellence 2014c).

2.3.5   Long-Term Strategies

By the end of the CPRP the patient should have:

- Undergone assessment and reassessment as identified in Standards 3 and 5.
- Participated in a tailored programme that encompasses the core components.
- Identified their long-term management goals.

2.3.5.1   Patient Responsibilities

- By the end of the programme patients will have been encouraged to develop full biopsychosocial self-management skills and so be empowered and prepared to take ownership of their own responsibility to pursue a healthy lifestyle. Carers, spouses, and family should also be equipped to contribute to long-term adherence by helping and encouraging the individual to achieve their goals.
- Patients and their families should be signposted and encouraged, where appropriate, to join:
  - Local heart support groups
  - Community exercise and activity groups
  - Community dietetic and weight management services
  - Tobacco and smoking cessation services.
- Promoting ongoing self-management strategies could also include online applications or tools and self-monitoring resources.

2.3.5.2   Service Responsibilities

- Patients should be supported to plan and implement self-management strategies to help them transition from the CPRP and continue to work towards minimising their risk of cardiovascular disease progression following programme completion.
- Upon programme completion there should be a formal assessment of lifestyle risk factors (physical activity, diet, and tobacco use as relevant), psychological and psychosocial health status, medical risk factors (blood pressure, lipids, and glucose), and use of cardioprotective therapies together with long-term management goals. This should be communicated by discharge letter to the referrer and the patient as well as those directly involved in the continuation of healthcare provision.

- There should be communication and collaboration between primary and secondary care services to achieve the long-term management plan.
- Patients should be registered onto GP Practice CHD/CVD registers.

2.3.6   Audit and Evaluation

The NHS and its services are required, through NICE Guidance, to offer CR to all eligible patients and in doing so they are duty bound to audit their performance locally and supply data to ensure equity of service delivery nationally. Although uptake to CR is improving the quality of the services delivered is not unified across the UK.

The BACPR recommends that every CPRP should formally audit and evaluate their service, which can be achieved through using the NACR directly or through upload of data if collected on local provider software. The BACPR include the contribution of data to the NACR as a standard as this plays a key role in monitoring the quality of service delivery and influencing and informing national policy. Data entered directly or uploaded to NHS Digital (the organisation that hosts NACR data) should include both individual and service level data based on assessment and including outcomes.

Service level audit should therefore include the collection of data to meet the following aims:

- Monitor and manage patient progress
- Monitor cardiovascular prevention and rehabilitation service resources
- Evaluate programmes in terms of clinical and patient-reported outcomes
- Benchmarking against local, regional, and national standards
- Provide measures of performance and quality for commissioners and providers of cardiovascular prevention and rehabilitation services
- Contribute to the national audit functions
- Present and share cardiovascular prevention and rehabilitation outcomes in both clinical and patient formats.

Where service resources and service design permits, the BACPR encourages cardiovascular prevention and rehabilitation teams to provide one year follow-up data as part of the audit. NHS Digital-NACR has the capability and capacity to capture this data within their online software. The ability to report at 12 months requires a high level of integration and communication between secondary and primary care, which can be achieved without duplication of work if carried out within the NHS Digital-NACR software, which is integrated along the patient journey.

2.3.6.1   National Certification Programme for Cardiac Rehabilitation

The BACPR and the NACR launched a joint National Certification Programme for Cardiac Rehabilitation (NCP_CR) in 2016 with an aim to ensure that all programmes are working to agreed clinical standards. The new 2017 standards and core components are aligned with data requirements for the NCP_CR (Furze et al. 2016).

The BACPR encourages all programmes to submit data and register for the NCP_CR so that patients, wherever they live, can be confident that the services on offer meet agreed minimum standards. The ultimate goal is for all CR programmes to deliver services in line with the standards and core components in this document; however, at present, most programmes are working towards the minimum standards as outlined in the NCP_CR (Doherty et al. 2017). Future NACR reports will incorporate the extent by which programmes are meeting NCP_CR criteria.

REFERENCES

American Association of Cardiovascular and Pulmonary Rehabilitation (AACVPR) (2013). *Guidelines for Cardiac Rehabilitation and Secondary Prevention Programs*, 5e. Champaign, IL: Human Kinetics.

Association of Chartered Physiotherapists in Cardiac Rehabilitation (ACPICR) (2015). *ACPICR Standards for Physical Activity and Exercise in the Cardiac Population*. ACPICR. http://acpicr.com/publications.

Aubin, H.-J., Farley, A., Lycett, D. et al. (2012). Weight gain in smokers after quitting cigarettes: meta-analysis. *British Medical Journal* 345: e4439. https://doi.org/10.1136/bmj.e4439.

Balady, G.J., Williams, M.A., Ades, P.A. et al. (2007). Core components of cardiac rehabilitation/secondary prevention programs: 2007 update: a scientific statement from the American Heart Association Exercise, Cardiac Rehabilitation, and Prevention Committee, the Council on Clinical Cardiology; the Councils on Cardiovascular Nursing, Epidemiology and Prevention, and Nutrition, Physical Activity, and Metabolism; and the American Association of Cardiovascular and Pulmonary Rehabilitation. *Circulation* 115 (20): 2675–2682.

British Association for Cardiovascular Prevention and Rehabilitation Exercise Professionals Group (BACPR-EPG) (2011). *Position Statement: Essential competences and minimum qualifications required to lead the exercise component in early cardiac rehabilitation*. London: BACPR. www.bacpr.com.

British Association for Cardiovascular Prevention and Rehabilitation (2017). *The BACPR Standards and Core Components for Cardiovascular Disease Prevention and Rehabilitation*, 3e. London: BACPR. www.bacpr.com.

British Nutrition Foundation (1999). *Obesity: The Report of the British Nutrition Foundation Task Force*. London: Blackwell Science.

Byrne, M., Walsh, J., and Murphy, A.W. (2005). Secondary prevention of coronary heart disease: patient beliefs and health-related behaviour. *Journal of Psychosomatic Research* 58: 403–415.

Dalal, H.M., Wingham, J., Evans, P. et al. (2009). Home based cardiac rehabilitation could improve outcomes. *British Medical Journal* 338 (12, 1): 1921.

Dickens, C., McGowan, L., Percival, C. et al. (2008). New onset depression following myocardial infarction predicts cardiac mortality. *Psychosomatic Medicine* 70: 450–455.

Doherty, P., Salman, A., Furze, G. et al. (2017). Does cardiac rehabilitation meet minimum standards: an observational study using UK national audit? *Open Heart* 3: e0005. http://openheart.bmj.com/content/4/1/e000519.

Fitchet, A., Doherty, P.J., Bundy, C. et al. (2003). Comprehensive cardiac rehabilitation programme for implantable cardioverter-defibrillator patients: a randomised controlled trial. *Heart* 89 (2): 155–160.

Franks, M., Stephens, M.A.P., Rook, K.S. et al. (2006). Spouses' provision of health-related support and control to patients participating in cardiac rehabilitation. *Journal of Family Psychology* 20 (2): 311–318.

French, D.P., Cooper, A., and Weinman, J. (2006). Illness perceptions predict attendance at cardiac rehabilitation following acute myocardial infarction: a systematic review with meta-analysis. *Journal of Psychosomatic Research* 61: 757–767.

Furze, G., Doherty, P., and Grant-Pearce, C. (2016). Development of a UK National Certification Programme for cardiac rehabilitation (NCP_CR). *British Journal of Cardiology* 23: 102–105.

Furze, G., Lewin, R., Murberg, T.A. et al. (2005). Does it matter what patients think? The relationship between changes in patients' beliefs about angina and their psychological and functional status. *Journal of Psychosomatic Research* 59: 323–329.

Günzler, C., Kriston, L., Harms, A., and Berner, M.M. (2009). Association of sexual functioning and quality of partnership in patients in cardiovascular rehabilitation – a gender perspective. *The Journal of Sexual Medicine* 6 (1): 164–174.

Institute of Medicine (2003). *Priority Areas for National Action: Transforming Healthcare Quality*, 52. Washington, DC: National Academies Press.

JBS3 Board (2014). Joint British Societies' consensus recommendations for the prevention of cardiovascular disease (JBS3). *Heart* 100 (Suppl 2): ii1–ii67. http://heart.bmj.com/content/100/Suppl_2/ii1.short.

Joekes, K., Maes, S., and Warrens, M. (2007). Predicting quality of life and self-management from dyadic support and overprotection after myocardial infarction. *British Journal of Health Psychology* 12: 473–489.

Knowles, M.S., Holton, E.F., and Swanson, R.A. (2015). *The Adult Learner: The Definitive Classic in Adult Education and Human Resource Development*, 8e. Burlington, MA: Elsevier.

Koene, R.J., Prizment, A.E., Blaes, A., and Konety, S.H. (2016). Shared risk factors in cardiovascular disease and cancer. *Circulation* 133 (11): 1104–1114.

Kronish, I.M. (2006). Persistent depression affects adherence to secondary prevention behaviors after acute coronary syndromes. *Journal of General Internal Medicine* 21: 1178–1183.

Lewin, R.J., Frizelle, D.J., and Kaye, G.C. (2001). A rehabilitative approach to patients with internal cardioverter-defibrillators. *Heart* 85 (4): 371–372.

Lim, S.S., Vos, T., Flaxman, A.D. et al. (2012). A comparative risk assessment of burden of disease and injury attributable to 67 risk factors and risk factor clusters in 21 regions, 1990–2010: a systematic analysis for the Global Burden of Disease Study 2010. *The Lancet* 380 (9859): 2224–2260. http://www.sciencedirect.com/science/article/pii/S0140673612617668.

McEwen, A., McRobbie, H., on behalf of the National Centre for Smoking Cessation and Training (NCSCT) and Public Health England (2016). *Electronic Cigarettes: A Briefing for Stop Smoking Services*. NCSCT: Dorchester www.ncsct.co.uk/publication_electronic_cigarette_briefing.php.

Mookadam, F. and Arthur, H. (2004). Systematic overview: social support and its relationship to morbidity and mortality after acute myocardial infarction. *Archives of Internal Medicine* 164 (14): 1514–1518.

Moser, D.K. and Dracup, K. (2004). Role of spousal anxiety and depression in patients' psychosocial recovery after a cardiac event. *Psychosomatic Medicine* 66: 527–532.

National Audit of Cardiac Rehabilitation (2017). *Annual Statistical Report. Vol 6*. London: British Heart Foundation. http://www.cardiacrehabilitation.org.uk/reports.htm.

National Institute for Health and Care Excellence (2006). *Obesity Guidance on the Prevention, Identification, Assessment and Management of Overweight and Obesity in Adults and Children. CG43*, Updated 2013. London: NICE. www.nice.org.uk/CG43NICE.

National Institute for Health and Care Excellence (2008). *Smoking Cessation Services in Primary Care, Pharmacies, Local Authorities and Workplaces, Particularly for Manual Working Groups, Pregnant Women and Hard to Reach Communities. PH10*. Updated 2013. London: NICE. http://guidance.nice.org.uk/PH10.

National Institute for Health and Care Excellence (2009). *Depression in Adults with a Chronic Condition. CG 91*. London: NICE. www.nice.org.uk/guidance/CG91.

National Institute for Health and Care Excellence (2010a). *Unstable Angina and NSTEMI: The Early Management of Unstable Angina and Non-ST-Segment-Elevation Myocardial Infarction. CG94*. Updated 2013. London: NICE. www.nice.org.uk/CG94.

National Institute for Health and Care Excellence (2010b). *Chronic heart failure: management of chronic heart failure in adults in primary and secondary care.* CG108. London: NICE. Available at: http://www.nice.org.uk/CG108.

National Institute for Health and Care Excellence (2011a). *Common Mental Health Problems: Identification and Pathways to Care. CG123.* London: NICE. www. nice.org.uk/guidance/cg123.

National Institute for Health and Care Excellence (2011b). *Hypertension. CG127.* Updated 2016. London: NICE. http://guidance.nice.org.uk/CG127.

National Institute for Health and Care Excellence (2013a). *Cardiac Rehabilitation Services: Commissioning Guide.* London: NICE. www.nice.org.uk/guidance/qs9/ resources/cardiac-rehabilitation-services-commissioning-guide-304110253.

National Institute for Health and Care Excellence (2013b). *Myocardial Infarction: Cardiac Rehabilitation and Prevention of Further Cardiovascular Disease. CG172.* London: NICE. www.nice.org.uk/guidance/cg172.

National Institute for Health and Care Excellence (2014a). *Behaviour Change: Individual Approaches. PH49.* London: NICE. www.nice.org.uk/guidance/ph49.

National Institute for Health and Care Excellence (2014b). *Cardiovascular Disease: Risk Assessment and Reduction, Including Lipid Modification: CG181.* Updated 2016. London: NICE www.nice.org.uk/guidance/cg181.

National Institute for Health and Care Excellence (2014c). *Implantable Cardioverter Defibrillators and Cardiac Resynchronisation Therapy for Arrythmias and Heart Failure: TA314.* London: NICE www.nice.org.uk/guidance/ta314.

National Institute for Health and Care Excellence (2015). *Type 2 Diabetes in Adults: Management. NG28.* Updated 2016. London: NICE. www.nice.org.uk/ guidance/ng28.

National Institute for Health and Clinical Excellence (2006). *Brief Interventions and Referral for Smoking Cessation: Guidance. PH1.* London: NICE. http://guidance. nice.org.uk/PH1.

Papadikas, S. and McKewen, A. (eds.) (2018). *NCSCT Training Standard: Learning Outcomes for Training Stop Smoking Practitioners. 3rd Edition.* Dorchester, UK: National Centre for Smoking Cessation and Training (NCSCT) https://www. ncsct.co.uk/pub_training-resources.php.

Piepoli, M.F., Corrà, U., Adamopoulos, S. et al. (2014). Secondary prevention in the clinical management of patients with cardiovascular diseases. Core components, standards and outcome measures for referral and delivery: a policy statement from the cardiac rehabilitation section of the EACPR. Endorsed by the Committee for Practice Guidelines of the European Society of Cardiology. *European Journal of Preventive Cardiology* 21 (6): 664–681.

Resuscitation Council (UK) (2013). *Requirements for resuscitation training and facilities for supervised cardiac rehabilitation programmes.* Resuscitation Council (UK). http://www.resus.org.uk/cpr/requirements-for-resuscitation-training.

Rice, V.H. and Stead, L.F. (2008). Nursing interventions for smoking cessation. *Cochrane Database of Systematic Reviews* (1): CD001188. https://doi.org/10.1002/14651858.CD001188.pub3.

Shaw, K., Gennat, H., O'Rourke, P., and Del Mar, C. (2006). Exercise for overweight or obesity. *Cochrane Database of Systematic Reviews* 18 (4): CD003817.

Shibeshi, W.A., Young-Xu, Y., and Blatt, C.M. (2007). Anxiety worsens prognosis in patients with coronary artery disease. *Journal of the American College of Cardiology* 49: 2021–2027.

Stafford, L., Berk, M., and Jackson, H.J. (2009). Are illness perceptions about coronary artery disease predictive of depression and quality of life outcomes? *Journal of Psychosomatic Research* 66 (3): 211–220.

Steinke, E.E., Jaarsma, T., Barnason, S.A. et al. (2013). Sexual counselling for individuals with cardiovascular disease and their partners: a consensus document from the American Heart Association and the ESC Council on Cardiovascular Nursing and Allied Professions (CCNAP). *Circulation* 128 (18): 2075–2096. https://doi.org/10.1161/CIR.0b013e31829c2e53.

Steinke, E.E. and Swan, J.H. (2004). Effectiveness of a videotape for sexual counseling after myocardial infarction. *Research in Nursing & Health* 27: 269–280.

Taylor, R.S., Dalal, H., Jolly, K. et al. (2015). Home-based versus centre-based cardiac rehabilitation. *Cochrane Database of Systematic Reviews* 8 http://dx.doi.org/10.1002/14651858.CD007130.pub3.

Tra Levine, G.N., Steinke, E.E., Bakaeen, F.G. et al. (2012). Sexual activity and cardiovascular disease: a scientific statement from the American Heart Association. *Circulation* 125 (8): 1058–1072. https://doi.org/10.1161/CIR.0b013e3182447787.

Træen, B. and Olsen, S. (2007). Sexual dysfunction and sexual well-being in people with heart disease. *Sexual and Relationship Therapy* 22: 193–208.

Tylka, T.L., Annunziato, R.A., Burgard, D. et al. (2014). Weight-inclusive versus weight-normative approach to health: evaluation the evidence for prioritizing well-being over weight loss. *Journal of Obesity* 2014: 983495. http://dx.doi.org/10.1155/2014/983495.

Whalley, B., Rees, K., Davies, P. et al. (2011). Psychological interventions for coronary heart disease. *Cochrane Database of Systematic Reviews* 10 (8): CD002902. http://onlinelibrary.wiley.com/doi/10.1002/14651858.CD002902.pub3/full.

Wood, D.A., Kotseva, K., Connolly, S. et al. (2008). Nurse-coordinated multidisciplinary, family-based cardiovascular disease prevention programme (EUROACTION) for patients with coronary heart disease and asymptomatic individuals at high risk of cardiovascular disease: a paired, cluster-randomised controlled trial. *Lancet* 371: 1999–2012.

CHAPTER 3

Delivering Quality Standards

Kathryn Carver

Addenbrooke's Hospital Cardiology Services, Cambridge, UK

Abstract

This chapter considers how each of the standards presented in Chapter 2 can be met, and demonstrates ways in which cardiovascular prevention and rehabilitation teams have problem solved and developed their services to meet these standards. This does not offer a single solution to implementation of the standards; instead it offers a variety of approaches that individual services can consider and then apply or further adapt to ensure a comprehensive cardiovascular prevention and rehabilitation programme (CPRP) is available to all eligible patients in their locality. The examples used vary from simple to very complex and are offered for practitioners to consider when presented with some of the challenges often faced by services.

Keywords: *standards, quality, service delivery, certification*

Cardiovascular Prevention and Rehabilitation in Practice, Second Edition.
Edited by Jennifer Jones, John Buckley, Gill Furze, and Gail Sheppard.
© 2020 John Wiley & Sons Ltd. Published 2020 by John Wiley & Sons Ltd.

Key Points

- The British Association for Cardiovascular Prevention and Rehabilitation (BACPR) Standards and Core Components (2017) provide the gold standard by which good practice in cardiovascular disease prevention and rehabilitation can be recognised.
- There is no uniform way of delivering cardiovascular disease prevention and rehabilitation.
- Each of the BACPR standards is discussed and practice examples given of different ways to meet them.
- The concept of 'minimum standards' is considered and the development of certification of meeting these minimum standards is outlined.

3.1   RATIONALE AND AIMS

As outlined in Chapter 2, the third edition of the BACPR standards aims to refocus health professionals, patients, service providers, and commissioners about the level of service that should be expected of a cardiovascular prevention and rehabilitation programme (CPRP) (BACPR 2017). Greater emphasis is placed on robust markers of the structure and content of CPRPs. The rationale for this chapter is to support CPRP staff to think about and assess how their programme meets the standards and changes that they can make to improve their service. This chapter provides examples of how to maintain evidence-based practice and how to meet each of the standards in turn, and will later introduce the concept of 'minimum standards' as used in the BACPR/National Audit of Cardiac Rehabilitation (NACR) certification guidance.

3.2   MAINTAINING EVIDENCE-BASED PRACTICE

There is a responsibility on the multidisciplinary team to keep up to date with emerging evidence, have a process in place to disseminate this information, and then adapt their practice as necessary. Clinical guidance, for example from the National Institute for Health and Clinical Excellence (NICE) or BACPR, has a regular review cycle; however, new evidence is continually emerging and for complex and multifaceted services, such as cardiovascular rehabilitation (CR), there needs to be a mechanism for highlighting this. It can be helpful to join national associations (e.g. BACPR, the British Cardiovascular Society, the Association of Chartered Physiotherapists in Cardiac Rehabilitation, Canadian Association for Cardiovascular Prevention and Rehabilitation) as well as international bodies (e.g. European Association of Preventive Cardiology) as they identify evidence and highlight it to members through regular communications. It also may be worth considering setting up a regular electronic search for new evidence using popular search engines and incorporating a regular review of new journal articles into multidisciplinary team meetings, as highlighted in Practice Example 1.

Practice Example 1

Responding to the Evidence Base

One service identified a member of their multidisciplinary team as a 'champion' of bringing the latest evidence around cardiovascular disease prevention and rehabilitation to the attention of the rest of the team. They now coordinate a monthly journal club lasting 20 minutes in which different members of the team volunteer to discuss a recent article. This element of their service has been running for a year and the team admit it took at least six months for this to be an embedded and valued part of the service. Key to its success was having a champion who was prepared to undertake the bulk of the early presentations and help colleagues prepare for their presentations. This preparation could range from searching for new evidence, helping the individual critically analyse an article, or identifying the implications for practice. Changes to practice from this initiative were small to start with, such as rephrasing a patient letter to make it more motivational. The team are now considering a major redesign of the exercise component of their programme. The champion of this initiative reports that the biggest change over the time is that 'the multidisciplinary team can now critically review their service without it feeling like a personal assault on individual members because the evidence supports change or maintenance of current practice'.

This chapter will approach each of the standards in turn.

3.3   STANDARD 1: THE DELIVERY OF SIX CORE COMPONENTS BY A QUALIFIED AND COMPETENT MULTIDISCIPLINARY TEAM, LED BY A CLINICAL COORDINATOR

Each programme should deliver the six essential core components to ensure clinically effective care and achieve sustainable health outcomes (Chapter 2). Services need to identify how best to deliver the six core components within their local area. Is the service going to deliver all the components in their entirety or will they access other local providers to provide key elements? The Department of Health's 'Cardiovascular Outcomes Strategy' (Department of Health 2013) recognises the value of integrated service models and the importance of 'joined up' approaches to the provision of care in order to avoid duplication of effort, improve efficiency, and achieve better patient outcomes.

Practice Example 2

Addressing all Six Core Components

One CPRP identified that their local smoking cessation service provided a comprehensive, high quality service via local drop-in centres and general practices. The provision of the core component for smoking cessation was achieved through the regular attendance of smoking cessation specialist staff from this local service to the rehabilitation programme. To complement this specialist input, all members of the multidisciplinary team were trained to undertake brief interventions as recommended by NICE (2006). Additionally, referral to this specialist team was facilitated by developing an electronic referral system requiring just three clicks from their computers.

Around the globe, guidance recommends that CR should be delivered by an appropriately skilled and qualified multidisciplinary team (BACPR 2017; Balady et al. 2011; Piepoli et al. 2014). The Skills for Health Workforce Report (2011) cited the drive for effective use of resources, regulations about staff working hours, and different management and funding approaches influencing how the workforce is organised as the key drivers in the development of multidisciplinary teams in recent years. The effectiveness of team working is shown in a systematic review of 29 studies of multidisciplinary strategies for management of heart failure, which reported that these strategies reduce hospitalisations with heart failure. Follow-up by multidisciplinary teams reduced mortality and hospitalisations from any cause (McAlister et al. 2004).

There is no one aim of a multidisciplinary team but their functions include:

- Ensuring that all patients receive timely treatment and care for all of the core components of CR from appropriately skilled professionals
- Continuity of care
- Provision of adequate information and support for patients
- Facilitate communication between primary, secondary, and tertiary care
- Collection of reliable data for audit and research
- Monitor adherence to clinical guidelines
- Promote the effective use of resources
- Improve participants' working lives through the provision of opportunities for learning and development.

There is an on-going debate as to which professions need to be part of the cardiovascular prevention and rehabilitation multidisciplinary team. This section will not resolve this debate but it does aim to help the service lead identify who they might need as members.

In considering the make-up of the multidisciplinary team the competency of practitioners to deliver the core components must become a higher priority than the individual professional groups represented. Each core component should be led by an individual who is competent in delivering that component, who would be responsible, and accountable, for driving that element of the service forwards. The component lead is responsible for ensuring that other members of the multidisciplinary team, irrespective of their professional group, understand their contribution to that component and are competent in their role within the delivery of the component.

The nature of good multidisciplinary team working is that there is a blurring at the edges of roles with some overlapping of function between members. This is reflected in BACPR's commitment to fully describing the competences required for delivery of each of the core components, rather than relying on specific professional roles. As an example, the BACPR Core Competences for the Physical Activity and Exercise Component (BACPR 2012) enable clinical coordinators to identify the training needed for the lead(s) of this component to be fully competent in its delivery. It also recognises that other staff may be required to lead on some elements of the same core component. For example, the Physical Activity component, mentioned above, includes a section on managing the unwell patient. If the person identified to lead on this core component is a non-clinically trained exercise professional, the clinical coordinator would need to identify a clinically competent person (such as a specialist nurse) to lead on this one element within the full component.

Approaches to achieving a multidisciplinary team vary from centre to centre and will most likely be driven by the size and make-up of the population that the service is required or commissioned to serve, as this will influence the number of staff required. Large services with a greater number of whole time equivalent staff have more flexibility to recruit across the professional groups than smaller teams whose core individuals may have to develop a wider range of competences and contract-in specific smaller blocks of time from other professional groups to meet their service needs. However, it must be noted that to be a multidisciplinary team requires that there be more than two professions involved in delivery of the programme. BACPR have mandated that, in order to achieve certification of meeting minimum standards, at least three professions must be represented within the team. Adopting a competency-based approach will give all services, irrespective of their size, a better chance of delivering high quality care.

There is a need to identify the competences required to deliver the cardiovascular prevention and rehabilitation service. This may vary from service to service and over time, e.g. offering a rehabilitation programme to those with heart failure or with an ICD in situ will require the development of new skills and competences for those who have previously been delivering a service purely for patients post-MI or following revascularisation. Whether that is through new staff members or by developing the skills of the current multidisciplinary team is a matter for each service. Every time a member of the team leaves it is a useful exercise to undertake a review of competences and multidisciplinary team mix to best meet the needs of the patients accessing the service. The clinical coordinator should have the autonomy and skills to lead a review of the staffing and skill mix.

Practice Example 3

Defining Roles in the Multidisciplinary Team

A simple and practical approach is to prepare an Excel spreadsheet with the elements of the BACPR core components on the vertical axis and all the current professions represented in the CPRP team on the horizontal axis. In a more comprehensive form, you would use the full competency identifying lead and supporting roles for each element. You can then identify where there are training gaps and potential skill mix gaps. From there you can develop a strategy to make the necessary changes over time.

Every team must include a senior clinician who has responsibility for coordinating, managing, and evaluating the service. This coordination role should not be underestimated as it requires expertise in leadership, management, and budgeting skills to lead a multidisciplinary team, often consisting of part-time members, to deliver a comprehensive service to an increasingly complex population. Integrating a multidisciplinary team requires an understanding of individual professional roles and how they contribute to the overall aim of the service, and the ability to mobilise the team to effectively deliver a patient-centred approach that addresses all six core components. The coordinator requires excellent communication skills and knowledge of the service to discuss issues ranging from service provision and commissioning to complex clinical scenarios, in addition to often leading on core components within the scope of their professional practice.

The clinical coordinator leading the cardiovascular prevention and rehabilitation service should be fully involved in financial and budgetary considerations for the service, which may include monitoring progress against agreed performance indicators. This will require an understanding of the financial systems used within the health organisation. To achieve this, the clinical coordinator may need to be proactive in seeking out individuals in the organisation responsible for monitoring the finances of the CPRP service. It is important to receive regular information on the budget and have regular, at least monthly, meetings with finance and operational managers to monitor this throughout the year. If the organisation provides in-house courses on finance and budgeting it is worth accessing them in order to understand if the budget meets the full cost of delivering the commissioned service and to take action if it is not. Monitoring the service contract should be a part of audit, and submission of data to the NACR is a standard inclusion in many current service specifications.

3.4 STANDARD 2: PROMPT IDENTIFICATION, REFERRAL, AND RECRUITMENT OF ELIGIBLE PATIENT POPULATIONS

The eligible groups identified in the BACPR Standards and Core components (BACPR 2017) include all the cardiovascular conditions that could potentially benefit from a CPRP (Chapter 2). In reality, health service economics have resulted in CPRPs often being prioritised and restricted to certain groups. Those patients with an acute coronary syndrome event with or without revascularisation are most typically included with variation in the inclusion of other manifestations of cardiovascular disease, such as heart failure, transient ischaemic attack, and stable angina.

The Cardiovascular Disease Outcome Strategy (DH 2013) calls for atherosclerosis to be treated as a 'single family of diseases' and recognises the benefits of a structured comprehensive prevention and rehabilitation programme being provided more widely than coronary heart disease (CHD). All CPRPs should be highlighting the benefits of their services for all eligible patient groups (Chapter 2) at every opportunity, and seeking investment and opportunities for reconfiguration to achieve this.

For CPRPs that are restricted and unable to accommodate all eligible patient groups it is important there are processes in place to manage those individuals who are not deemed eligible. It may be that there are mechanisms by which a general practitioner or the patient themselves may appeal. Auditing the number of suitable referrals that the service has not been able to accommodate can support a case for increased access in the future. The minimum standards that were developed for certification initially included requirements for programmes to be delivered to people post-MI, revascularisation, and for heart failure. As more programmes deliver to the existing minimum standards, the conditions regarded as mandatory for inclusion as part of the minimum standards will be increased, with the aim over time of the majority of programmes meeting the full range of conditions given in the BACPR standards (2017).

Practice Example 4

Improving Access to Cardiac Rehabilitation

In one locality the CPRP was unable to accommodate all of those eligible to attend. The service lead opened discussions with the lead for pulmonary rehabilitation. Plans are now underway to run a combined pulmonary and heart failure exercise class with the education component for each group running in parallel.

There needs to be a pathway that ensures consistency and equity of access irrespective of the referral pathway or qualifying condition. The NACR has consistently reported low uptake for CPRPs year on year with large variance in uptake across the core conditions of MI, revascularisation, and heart failure (BHF NACR 2018), a finding which is echoed internationally (Clark et al. 2015). NICE guidance on secondary prevention after an MI (NICE 2013) makes very clear recommendations around recruitment to a comprehensive CPRP programme. This includes the use of automated referral systems. Identify the main referral sources to the service and establish a relationship with them, taking time to agree how referrals are sent and the information expected to be included in this referral.

Practice Example 5

Managing Referrals

One local service received 70% of their referrals from the regional tertiary centre. The CPRP team in the tertiary centre collated the referrals for distribution to local centres by their administrative assistant who only worked on a Friday. The result of this work pattern was that 30 or more referrals would arrive on Friday with nothing on other days of the week. This naturally impacted on the workload of the local centre. Discussion between the two CPRP leads resulted in the individual wards in the tertiary centre referring emergency patients such as those with primary percutaneous coronary intervention (PPCI), acute myocardial infarction (AMI), and non-ST segment elevation myocardial infarction (NSTEMI) directly with referrals for those undergoing elective procedures such as percutaneous coronary intervention (PCI) or cardiac surgery continuing to be referred on a Friday. This spread the referral rate across the week for the local service and ensured those who had undergone an emergency procedure were contacted the day after discharge. The group of patients undergoing elective procedures were advised by the tertiary centre they would be contacted by their local CPRP in the week following discharge, reducing the pressure on the local service.

Within your service you need to have a process for managing referrals to ensure there is timely contact and invitation to commence the CPRP. Patients should be contacted within three operational days of receipt of referral and ideally be attending their initial assessment within 10 working days of discharge or diagnosis in the case of those not admitted to hospital (Chapter 2). Achieving this standard should be formally monitored. If an influx of referrals or staff sickness prevents achieving this standard then ensure it is recorded and action taken.

The recruitment strategy needs to be carefully planned and considered as a marketing exercise if uptake is to be increased. Evidence suggests that if a first contact is with a clinician rather than an administrator then uptake is higher (Halcox et al. 2011), this needs to be considered when looking at the multidisciplinary team make-up and developing a business case for improvements. Patients who are not known to the service could be contacted by a personal motivational letter from the clinical lead, as this has been shown to be effective (Grace et al. 2006, 2012). However, having a template letter prepared and sent out by an administrator may well be an effective use of staff in this situation.

Multidisciplinary team staff involved in recruiting patients to a CPRP can enhance their opportunities for successful recruitment if they have skills in motivational interviewing and basic marketing techniques. If training is required consider accessing a formal course or looking within your organisation for informal training. Accessing the marketing department may be useful in developing programme materials. Similarly, if available, trained counsellors and psychologists can be highly valuable in advising on methods of communication with regards to invitation to join the programme.

3.5   STANDARD 3: EARLY INITIAL ASSESSMENT OF INDIVIDUAL PATIENT NEEDS WHICH INFORMS THE AGREED PERSONALISED GOALS THAT ARE REVIEWED REGULARLY

Early initial assessment for a CPRP is recommended. This is ideally within 10 working days wherever possible. For those who have had an MI, uptake has been shown to dramatically improve if attendance to the programme begins within 10 days of discharge (NICE 2013). This initial assessment should include formally assessing the individual's health behaviour change status, lifestyle and medical risk factors, and psychosocial health. An initial assessment is only complete once each of these components has been reviewed. It may not be possible to fully assess all elements very early in the rehabilitation journey, for example, activity levels may be assessed at an early stage but fitness/functional capacity assessment with risk stratification might be undertaken later in the pathway if the patient is not yet ready to participate in the exercise component.

All patients should undergo functional assessment in order to ensure an appropriate exercise prescription. This applies equally to patients undertaking home- or centre-based programmes.

Practice Example 6

Early Assessment

One programme, a finalist from the British Heart Foundation Celebrating CR Awards (2011), undertakes their initial assessment during the inpatient stay and uses these to set personalised goals for health behaviour change in the immediate post-discharge phase. This method of service implementation improves uptake to the core CPRP.

Patient-focused SMART goals should be set immediately following an initial assessment and these will form the basis for on-going assessment throughout the patient journey with adjustments agreed and documented where required. Documentation tools such as personal health plans and patient-held progress records are useful adjuncts to the review process.

Practice Example 7

On-Going Review

One programme undertakes regular review of progress towards individual goals during the final 15 minutes of the exercise programme when participants remain under supervision for safety reasons (Association of Chartered Physiotherapists in Cardiac Rehabilitation [ACPICR] 2015). The team identify the participants for review in advance of the class and offer the individual a one to one review with a member of the team.

3.6   STANDARD 4: EARLY PROVISION OF A STRUCTURED CPRP, WITH A DEFINED PATHWAY OF CARE, WHICH MEETS THE INDIVIDUAL'S GOALS AND IS ALIGNED WITH PATIENT PREFERENCE AND CHOICE

The most recent NICE guidance on secondary prevention after an MI (CG172) recommends offering CR during the inpatient phase for those who have had an MI, additionally it recommends that their first appointment at a CPRP be within 10 days of discharge (NICE 2013). Early initiation of a CPRP has been shown to increase adherence and completion of CR (Pack et al. 2013).

Developing a high-level pathway for the patient journey through a CPRP is beneficial. This should be based on seven stages (see below).

Stages of CR (BACPR 2017):

- Stage 0: Identify and refer patient
- Stage 1: Manage referral and recruit patient to cardiac rehabilitation programme
- Stage 2: Assess patient for cardiac rehabilitation
- Stage 3: Develop patient care plan
- Stage 4: Deliver comprehensive cardiac rehabilitation programme
- Stage 5: Conduct final assessment
- Stage 6: Discharge and transition to long-term management.

3.6.1   Identifying and Referring Patients

Stage 0: teams should take a 'refer all' approach when considering referral to a CPRP and assume that the service will offer to all who are eligible. This blanket referral provides the receiving teams with evidence of unmet needs if the service cannot provide a CPRP to all eligible patients. This information can be used when developing a business case to increase resources to enable all eligible patients to be offered a CPRP.

3.6.2   Manage the Referral and Recruitment of Patients

Service commissioners may set timeframes within which they expect patients to be offered and recruited to a comprehensive CPRP and it is likely that this will be audited. This will include ensuring that those who initially turn down or are not yet ready to participate in CR are re-offered a start date within a reasonable time frame. NICE CG172 (NICE 2013) highlights a range of motivational and supportive measures undertaken in a bid to increase uptake and adherence to CR through appropriate offer and re-offer strategies and includes studies demonstrating the effectiveness of electronic, written, and telephone contact strategies. The strategy adopted should reflect issues that local services may have with referral and recruitment.

Increasing technology and secure shared networks such as nhs.net can be used very effectively if both Stage 0 and Stages 1–6 providers can access it. Referrals can be made via fax or post if they are going to non-NHS providers. The tools and technology used to recruit patients should again be based on local need and no one approach is going to appeal to everyone. Traditional postal methods of sending letters may not be motivating to those who utilise IT throughout their day but electronic communication and web-based programmes will be challenging to fully utilise in areas with poor internet speeds.

3.6.3 Assessing for and Delivering a Comprehensive CPRP

After assessment of the patient's needs in terms of the core components, it is important to ensure a defined pathway of care that meets these needs but also aligns with patient preference and choice. A menu-based approach, delivered in easily accessible venues, provides for the greatest chance of uptake and adherence to the CPRP. Choice in terms of venue (including home) and time (e.g. early mornings and evenings) are examples of a menu-based approach on how to best meet a patient's individual needs.

Practice Example 8

Offering Choice
Many services deliver both group and home-based CPRPs with additional resources such as weight management and walking groups to those with a wide range of cardiac conditions. The additional resources were developed in response to the needs of their local populations.

The different components of the CPRP should be available as individual elements. There may be reasons why individuals cannot access the exercise component immediately after their event. However, if the education component can be accessed this offers support and information to individuals in what is often a lonely and frightening period in their recovery.

Practice Example 9

Embracing Technology
One service based in Leicester offers a web-based CPRP called 'Activate Your Heart' in addition to their core CPRP. Web-based, mobile approaches and the use of technology are likely to become increasingly popular and CPRPs are encouraged to embrace new ways of working. Exploring with patients the strategies that work for them will increase uptake and adherence to ensure a greater number of patients access and complete a CPRP.

3.6.4 Standard 5: Upon Programme Completion, a Final Assessment of Individual Patient Needs and Demonstration of Sustainable Health Outcomes

The final assessment has traditionally been one of the areas CPRP teams have struggled to undertake, with only 63% of individuals receiving a follow-up assessment in the latest NACR report (BHF NACR 2018). Final assessments are important in providing the individual participant with a formal record of their time in the CPRP and demonstrating their progress against the goals they set at the start. Final assessments, when communicated to the primary care team, give baseline data against which future progress can be assessed at CHD annual reviews.

Programme completion includes a formal reassessment of the individual's health behaviour change status, lifestyle and medical risk factors (including re-assessment of functional capacity), psychosocial health, and cardioprotective medications. Further, the end of programme assessment should additionally include a long-term management plan. It is essential that relevant signposting and, where possible, facilitated introduction is undertaken to long-term support programmes, such as community-based exercise classes delivered by trained and qualified exercise instructors, weight management programmes, and smoking cessation services. The data collected during these assessments has both clinical and audit value, as much of the data can be included in the NACR dataset and be used for review of effectiveness of interventions within the team and locality.

This information should be communicated to all involved in the on-going care of the patient, in particular the primary care team. Communication in the form of a discharge letter to the GP is usually part of the service specification and a recommended outcome by NICE (2013).

Practice Example 10

Undertaking a Final Assessment

In one programme the final assessment occurs during the week prior to their last attendance. The individual attends the assessment at the programme venue when all of the initially assessed components, including a sub-maximal exercise test, are repeated. Progress against goals is reviewed and a long-term management plan is agreed with the patient. The CPRP team then prepare the outcome report and discharge letter for that individual prior to their final session. The patient is given a copy of this document and agrees the content of the letter, which will be sent to their GP, thus increasing their ownership of the long-term management plan. This also ensures the primary care team receive the information within the 10 working days set within the BACPR standards (2017).

Final assessment results when combined in a database provide the CPRP with evidence of its own effectiveness and enable Standard 6 to be achieved. It is questionable whether clinical outcomes can be demonstrated without such a database. The data also enables the CPRP to target service improvement projects at specific areas where clinical outcomes are not optimised.

3.6.5   Standard 6: Registration and Submission of Data to the NACR and Participation in the National Certification Programme (NCP_CR)

The rationale behind this standard is to provide CPRP services with a mechanism for reviewing the clinical effectiveness of their programme at both a local and national level, and to use these data to ensure that the service meets national certification or accreditation criteria.

3.6.6   Audit

The availability of reliable data to measure clinical outcomes in order to assess both the cost and clinical effectiveness of CR services is increasingly required by those who commission services. The NACR database is now housed within the Health and Social Care Information Centre, which has helped to improve the quality of the data gathered, and is now the accepted mechanism for audit of CR outcomes across the majority of the UK. This does mean that administrative support to submit data to the NACR should be considered as an important role within the multidisciplinary team. Internationally, there are also drives to develop registry-based national audit schemes, for example in Canada (Grace et al. 2015) and Australia (Redfern et al. 2014).

Practice Example 11

Aligning your Data with NACR

Step 1: Assess the patient information currently collected within the CPRP and compare this against the dataset for the national audit.

If there are missing data fields within your information, what would it take to collect these? Small alterations can be easily made, but others may require planned changes:

- The data for many fields may match but is not recorded in a style that is aligned to the NACR. You need to plan a review of your documentation (see step 2).
- Changes to clinical practice may be required to collect the data. In this scenario you may need to consider a full review of your CPRP (see step 3).

Step 2: Reviewing your documentation to align with the NACR dataset.

All of the NACR data may be collected but it appears on your service documentation in a different order or format. If administrative staff enter and submit the data to NACR it makes sense to align documentation with the NACR dataset so that fields appear on your documentation in an order similar to the NACR dataset to reduce the time spent leafing through documents looking for a specific field. It may be helpful to consider using the NACR dataset as the core document and build a personalised set of documents from there. This can seem a time-consuming process but the rewards in terms of time saved at the data submission stages will be worthwhile.

Step 3: Reviewing your service to align it with the NACR dataset.

If there are compulsory fields in the NACR dataset that are not currently collected during the CPRP you may need to consider changes to practice and review the service as a whole. Audit and reporting on outcomes is an inescapable fact in modern healthcare and if the data requested by service commissioners is not available then unfortunately the service will be at risk. Plan a team event where you can work on this together and consider if you are going to run this yourselves or seek the support of a facilitator experienced in the change management process.

Step 4: Entering and submitting data.

In considering how to collect and submit data to the NACR, it is advisable to discuss this with both the NACR team and the audit/IT team within your own organisation. The NACR team are highly experienced in working with different IT systems and are a valuable resource when undertaking the background work prior to commencing data submission.

Changes that need to be made in order to collect audit data and meet criteria for certification may require development of a business case. This is a proposal that details the way in which a service plans to meet a service specification to provide cardiovascular prevention and rehabilitation to the local population. This business case can be either to secure and develop your existing service or to create a new service. The business case will be submitted to the designated decision-making body so it is important the evidence and particularly the budget required is clearly presented. Ensuring all the information required is included can be challenging as it is not a task frequently undertaken by clinical practitioners. The service commissioners may provide the template required; however, if this is not the case, the BHF have produced a template to support the development of a business case. It is always worthwhile to look at other examples of business cases to help identify the best way to present your case. The BHF business case toolkit can be found online at: https://www.bhf.org.uk/for-professionals/healthcare-professionals/resources-for-your-role/business-case-toolkit

Operational and finance managers are expected to support production of a business case but the lead practitioner needs to ensure that it is realistic and reflects all the costs involved in providing a comprehensive CPRP, for example: non-pay costs such as venue, IT, equipment, patient education material, transport, pathology, interpreter services, team training and professional development, and any capital development.

3.6.7 Certification

Schemes to certify that CPRP meet minimum standards are being developed in various countries across the world, following the lead of the USA, which initiated their peer-led scheme in 1998 (Sanderson et al. 2004).

3.6.8 Certification in the UK

The annual statistical reports from NACR have strongly and repeatedly highlighted that CR is often not delivered to the standards given with the previous BACPR Standards and Core Components (2012), and yet it was difficult for a programme to demonstrate to their patients, managers, and service commissioners that they were delivering rehabilitation to a good standard. This led to BACPR and NACR to collaborate on developing a programme to certify whether a CPRP met minimum standards.

3.6.9 What Are 'Minimum Standards'?

An expert group discussed what would be considered good practice in meeting the standards and how could this be demonstrated in an effective and transparent way. Convened in 2014 and using the second edition of the BACPR standards (2012) they reached consensus that six of the seven standards could be included in the assessment of minimum standards. These minimum standards would be derived using, where possible, the national median for an outcome taken from the most recent NACR report. These have now been aligned to ensure consistency with the latest BACPR standards (2017).

Examples of the minimum standards include the following:

- The multidisciplinary team – the latest BACPR standards (BACPR 2017) reflect the consensus from the expert group that the 'minimum' would be three different professions.
- The BACPR standards state that early assessment should occur ideally within 10 working days of discharge or diagnosis. However, the average waiting time from initiating event to assessment 1 varies hugely across the UK. To overcome this, it was decided to use the national median waiting time given in the most recent version of the NACR report as the standard to meet for certification.

As more programmes meet the national median outcomes given as the minimum standards, this will have the effect of improving that median figure. In this way, cardiovascular prevention and rehabilitation across the UK will continue to improve.

The full guidance on certification of CPRPs that meet minimum standards (and includes the most recent version of the minimum standards) is available from education@bacpr.com.

3.7 CONCLUSION

This chapter has considered how to maintain evidence-based practice, and has discussed, using examples from practice, how each of the six standards can best be delivered. The ideas given within this chapter will hopefully help staff in CPRPs across the UK to consider service improvements (some simple, some complex) that could ensure that their service continues to be commissioned, and provide patients with the gold standard care that they deserve.

REFERENCES

Association of Chartered Physiotherapists in Cardiac Rehabilitation (ACPICR) (2015). *ACPICR Standards for Physical Activity and Exercise in the Cardiac Population*. London: ACPICR http://acpicr.com/publications.

BACPR (2011). *Celebrating Cardiac Rehabilitation*. London: BACPR https://www.bacpr.com/resources/CCR_Awards_2011_booklet_270511.pdf (accessed 20 July 2016).

BACPR (2012). *The BACPR Standards and Core Components for Cardiovascular Disease Prevention and Rehabilitation*, 2e. London: BACPR.

BACPR (2017). *The BACPR Standards and Core Components for Cardiovascular Disease Prevention and Rehabilitation*, 3e. London: https://www.bacpr.com/resources/BACPR_Standards_and_Core_Components_2017.pdf

BACPR Exercise Professionals Group (BACPR-EPG) (2012). *Core Competences for the Physical Activity and Exercise Component for Cardiovascular Disease Prevention and Rehabilitation Services*. London: BACPR. http://www.bacpr.com/resources/BACPR_Core_Comp_PA_Exercise_web_FINAL_NOV_12_2.pdf

Balady, G.J., Ades, P.A., Bittner, V.A. et al. (2011). Referral, enrollment, and delivery of cardiac rehabilitation/secondary prevention programs at clinical centers and beyond: a presidential advisory from the American Heart Association. *Circulation* 124 (25): 2951–2960.

BHF National Audit of Cardiac Rehabilitation (2018). *Quality and Outcomes Report 2018*. London: British Heart Foundation. www.cardiacrehabilitation.org.uk/nacr/reports.htm

Clark, R.A., Conway, A., Poulsen, V. et al. (2015). Alternative models of cardiac rehabilitation: a systematic review. *European Journal of Preventive Cardiology* 22 (1): 35–74.

Department of Health (2013). *Improving Cardiovascular Disease Outcomes Strategy*. London: HMSO https://www.gov.uk/government/publications/improving-cardiovascular-disease-outcomes-strategy (accessed 28 October 2017).

Grace, S.L., Angevaare, K.L., Reid, R.D. et al. (2012). Effectiveness of inpatient and outpatient strategies in increasing referral and utilization of cardiac rehabilitation: a prospective, multi-site study. *Implementation Science* 7: 120.

Grace, S.L., Krepostman, S., Brooks, D. et al. (2006). Referral to and discharge from cardiac rehabilitation: key informant views on continuity of care. *Journal of Evaluation in Clinical Practice* 12 (2): 155–163.

Grace, S.L., Parsons, T.L., Heise, K., and Bacon, S.L. (2015). The Canadian Cardiac Rehabilitation Registry: inaugural report on the status of cardiac rehabilitation in Canada. *Rehabilitation Research and Practice* 2015 https://doi.org/10.1155/2015/278979.

Halcox, J., Lindsay, S., Begg, A. et al. (2011). Lifestyle advice and drug therapy post myocardial infarction: a survey of UK current practice. *British Journal of Cardiology* 18: 178.

McAlister, F.A., Stewart, S., Ferua, S., and McMurray, J.J. (2004). Multidisciplinary strategies for the management of heart failure patients at high risk of admission: a systematic review of randomised trials. *Journal of the American College of Cardiology* 44 (4): 810–819.

National Institute for Health and Care Excellence (2013). *NICE Clinical Guideline CG172. Secondary Prevention in Primary and Secondary Care for Patients Following a Myocardial Infarction*. London: NICE. www.nice.org.uk/CG172.

National Institute for Health and Clinical Excellence (2006). *NICE PH1. Brief Interventions and Referral for Smoking Cessation Guidance*. London: NICE. http://guidance.nice.org.uk/PH1.

Pack, Q.R., Mansour, M., Barboza, J.S. et al. (2013). An early appointment to outpatient cardiac rehabilitation at hospital discharge improves attendance at orientation: a randomized, single-blind, controlled trial. *Circulation* 127 (3): 349–355.

Piepoli, M.F., Corrà, U., Adamopoulos, S. et al. (2014). Secondary prevention in the clinical management of patients with cardiovascular diseases. Core components, standards and outcome measures for referral and delivery: a Policy Statement from the Cardiac Rehabilitation Section of the European Association for Cardiovascular Prevention & Rehabilitation. Endorsed by the Committee for Practice Guidelines of the European Society of Cardiology. *European Journal of Preventive Cardiology* 21 (6): 664–681.

Redfern, J., Hyun, K., Chew, D.P. et al. (2014). Prescription of secondary prevention medications, lifestyle advice, and referral to rehabilitation among acute coronary syndrome inpatients: results from a large prospective audit in Australia and New Zealand. *Heart* 100 (16): 1281–1288. https://doi.org/10.1136/heartjnl-2013-305296.

Sanderson, B.K., Southard, D., Oldridge, N., and Writing Group (2004). AACVPR consensus statement: outcomes evaluation in cardiac rehabilitation/secondary prevention programs. *Journal of Cardiopulmonary Rehabilitation* 24 (2): 65–79.

Skills for Health (2011). *Key Changes in the Healthcare Workforce: Rapid Review of International Evidence.* London: Department of Health.

CHAPTER 4

Health Behaviour Change and Education

Linda Speck[1], Gill Furze[2], and Nick Brace[3]

[1] Health Psychology Service, Cwm Taf Morgannwg University Health Board, Princess of Wales Hospital, Bridgend and University of South Wales, UK
[2] Faculty of Health and Life Sciences, Coventry University, Coventry, UK
[3] Department of Health Psychology, Swansea Bay University Heath Board, Neath Port Talbot Hospital, Port Talbot, UK

Abstract

This chapter will explain what we mean by health behaviour change and outline the underpinning concepts. It will introduce major principles for supporting health behaviour change in cardiovascular prevention and rehabilitation programmes (CPRPs), and describe the key skills, techniques, and processes required. Consideration will be given to incorporation of these factors in the delivery of CPRPs. The chapter will also consider the delivery of effective health education, including the key principles of adult learning and suggestions for group education sessions.

Keywords: *health behaviour change, health education, cardiovascular prevention and rehabilitation*

Cardiovascular Prevention and Rehabilitation in Practice, Second Edition.
Edited by Jennifer Jones, John Buckley, Gill Furze, and Gail Sheppard.
© 2020 John Wiley & Sons Ltd. Published 2020 by John Wiley & Sons Ltd.

Key Points

- Health behaviour change and education underpin the successful delivery of all of the other core components.
- In order to promote health behaviour change, cardiovascular prevention and rehabilitation professionals need to understand the major theoretical assumptions and concepts with which it is underpinned. Some of these are outlined in this chapter.
- Key principles, skills, techniques, and processes to support health behaviour change are highlighted, along with practice examples.
- The core principles that support adult learning are outlined with suggestions offered for successful delivery of group education, and for the development of educational materials.

4.1   RATIONALE AND AIMS

The British Association for Cardiovascular Prevention and Rehabilitation (BACPR) Standards and Core Components (2017b) recognise that all of the components for successful cardiovascular prevention and rehabilitation are underpinned by health behaviour change and education. The aim of this chapter is to help cardiovascular prevention and rehabilitation health professionals to understand how they might effectively encourage heath behaviour change within the delivery of all components of a cardiovascular prevention and rehabilitation programme (CPRP). The chapter gives an overview of the key knowledge, skills, and processes required to support health behaviour change and to deliver effective patient education, with practice examples, that can be adapted and developed to suit the needs of individual services.

4.1.1   What Do We Mean by Health Behaviour Change?

The term health behaviour relates to all behaviours and activities that people engage in that have the potential to impact upon their health status. These can be healthful (health protective or health maintaining), or they can be unhealthy (with potential for harming health status). Whilst long-term health is a priority for some, it is by no means the main focus for all. Unhealthy behaviours may be perceived to have significant short-term benefits, such as stress relief, comfort, time out, or acquiescence to peer pressure. What is important is to assess what individuals understand healthy behaviour to be, and what behaviours they are undertaking in order to try to become, or remain, healthy.

4.1.2 Why Is this Component Necessary?

Health behaviour underpins the modifiable risk factors for heart disease such as smoking, engagement in physical activity and exercise, and dietary intake. Certain behaviours identified as unhealthy are major reasons why people develop cardiovascular disease (CVD), and changing such behaviours is the key to reducing future risk of further CVD. Furthermore, evidence is clear that 'significant events or transition points in people's lives present an important opportunity for intervening ... because it is then that people often review their own behaviour' (NICE 2007, p. 7). Later National Institute for Health and Clinical Excellence (NICE) guidance suggests that health professionals need to 'recognise the times when people may be more open to change, such as when recovering from a behaviour-related condition (for example, following diagnosis of cardiovascular disease)' (NICE 2014, p. 15). This offers enormous potential for modification of behaviours identified as unhealthy at the time that people present to CPRPs.

Health behaviour impacts not only on lifestyle risk factors, but is also a mediating factor in the efficacy of medical, surgical, and pharmacological approaches. Improvements in drug therapies abound, yet adherence to drug regimes can be seen as a health behaviour issue, with as many as 60% of those with CVD not adhering to treatment recommendations (Baroletti and Dell'Ofano 2010). Cardiac related surgical techniques have improved very significantly in recent years, yet re-occlusion of arteries remains a significant problem (Ho et al. 2008). This is why the BACPR Standards (2017b) cite health behaviour change as a central focus for future development of cardiovascular prevention and rehabilitation services.

4.1.3 Who Will Lead the Component within the Cardiovascular Prevention and Rehabilitation Programme?

Supporting health behaviour change is the responsibility of every member of the cardiovascular prevention and rehabilitation team. However, whilst every member of the team would benefit from an understanding of effective techniques to support successful behaviour change, the person who leads this component should be appropriately qualified, skilled, and competent, as defined within the 'Core Competences for the Health Behaviour Change and Education Component for Cardiovascular Disease Prevention and Rehabilitation Services' (BACPR 2017a). It is important that the lead not only has an understanding of *what* they are doing but also fully understands the evidence base underpinning *why* they are doing it.

4.2 HEALTH BEHAVIOUR CHANGE – THEORETICAL FOUNDATIONS

Traditionally, information about recommended lifestyle changes has been provided, trusting that this will be sufficient for people to make appropriate health behaviour changes. Unfortunately for many, simply having the correct information ensures neither adherence to healthful behaviour, nor healthful behaviour change (NICE 2014, p. 40). In order for individuals to make changes it is important to understand why they engage in unhealthy behaviours. People make sense of situations within their particular social contexts via their cognitions or thought processes. There is a large body of research underpinned by psychosocial theories, which goes some way to predicting and explaining health behaviour choices, thereby increasing understanding of effective methods of change. Health behaviour change techniques must be based on psychological theory and be evidence-based. Although there are a number of different psychological models that seek to explain health behaviour there is consensus about the most influential variables, as accounted for in the major theorists' model (Figure 4.1).

The three major variables that account for behaviour are:

1. *Intention* to undertake the behaviour
2. *Skills* needed to perform the behaviour
3. Presence or absence of *environmental constraints.*

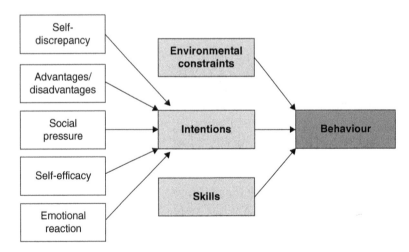

FIGURE 4.1 Major theorists' model (Conner and Norman [2007]. Reproduced with permission of Scientific Research Publishing Inc.).

1. *Intentions*: These are influenced by a number of factors, namely; (i) self-efficacy, (ii) social pressure, (iii) perceived advantages or disadvantages of the behaviour, (iv) emotional reaction, and (v) self-discrepancy (see Conner and Norman 2007).

   (i)   Self-efficacy. An essential concept within all major health behaviour change models, originally conceived by Bandura (1986). Recognition that there is a difference between merely understanding that certain actions will result in specific outcomes and one's perceived capability to perform these actions is crucial within health behaviour change. Self-efficacy comprises two particularly useful components, outcome expectancies and efficacy expectations, which may be utilised in cardiovascular prevention and rehabilitation.

   (a)   Outcome expectancies relate to beliefs that certain actions will result in specific outcomes. For example, 'I believe that giving up smoking will decrease my chances of having a second heart attack'.

   (b)   Efficacy expectations (self-efficacy) relate to beliefs in one's capability to perform certain actions, e.g. 'I believe that I can give up smoking'.

   It is important not only to improve understanding of the need for change but also to increase self-efficacy for change. People with high levels of self-efficacy for a certain health behaviour change are more likely to engage in it, which further bolsters self-efficacy to continue (Bandura 1997). A person cannot be classified as being either generally 'high' or 'low' in self-efficacy, as perceived self-efficacy will vary across behaviours and situations for each individual. Knowledge of both efficacy and outcome expectations will best predict behaviour.

   (ii) Social pressure. The social context of health behaviour should not be underestimated. Other people play an important part in considering health behaviour change. Partners, family members, and also friends can have a considerable influence. For instance, stopping smoking can be very difficult if your family and friends continue to smoke.

   (iii) Advantages/disadvantages of the behaviour. People may review some of the advantages and disadvantages of both maintaining and changing their behaviour without much conscious awareness. The benefits of a specific behaviour need to outweigh the costs for that behaviour in order for it to be amenable to change. Unfortunately, this is rarely a comprehensive and considered process. An individual's active assessment of the 'pros' and 'cons' of undertaking a specific behaviour can help to facilitate change.

(iv) Emotional reaction. If the emotional reaction to undertaking a particular behaviour is perceived to be more positive than negative, it is more likely to influence intention to change. If an individual experiences considerable anxiety simply thinking of making a change, there will be considerable reluctance to even take the first step by forming the intention to do so.

(v) Self-discrepancy. When the behaviour identified to be changed is consistent with a person's self-image they are more likely to think of undertaking that change. For instance, if someone had previously eaten a healthy diet but in recent years had stopped doing so, perhaps because of chaotic work patterns, it is more likely that healthy eating will be reinstated as it more closely corresponds with their self-image.

2. *Skills*: Without the necessary skills to adopt a new behaviour it will be unrealistic to make that change. For instance, despite forming the intention to swim regularly, unless a person is actually able to swim, this will be unachievable.

3. *Environmental constraints*: These are important to recognise whenever considering health behaviour change. Despite strong intentions to change there might be extraneous factors hindering successful implementation.

Having a strong intention to change, together with the required skills and presence of a facilitative environment, will foster the right conditions for successful change. Making successful health behaviour changes can fail for many different reasons and is dependent on individual circumstances. One of the major stumbling blocks is progressing from developing intentions to change into enacting tangible health behaviour change.

Some understanding of psychosocial theories of health behaviour change will better inform interactions with people in relation to their health behaviours, as well as gaining more insight into relevant structured approaches to facilitating health behaviour change.

4.3 HEALTH BEHAVIOUR CHANGE – ADDITIONAL CONCEPTS

4.3.1 Habit Formation

The repeated performance of health behaviours in specific situations, determined by the motivation to do so, may lead to cued habit formation (see Lally and Gardner 2013). The intention stage may then be bypassed, as health behaviours become automatic in nature with specific environmental cues activating them.

There is no 'one size fits all' approach to the facilitation of health behaviour change, as individual differences and the diverse contexts in which people live mean that effectiveness of interventions is variable. Therefore, we can only offer broad principle guidance on which cardiovascular prevention and rehabilitation practice might be best based.

4.3.2   Implementation Intentions

Whilst intentions are the best single predictor of health behaviour, there remains significant discrepancy in translating intention into actual behaviour (Gollwitzer 1993). Sheeran (2002) reported that intention to perform a particular goal accounted for only 28% of the likelihood of behaving in a manner consistent with the intention. Research has highlighted that there are a number of methods that can increase the likelihood of an individual carrying out an intended behaviour. This includes exploration of how individuals might implement healthful behaviours and consideration of the difficult situations in which healthful behaviour may be undermined.

Implementation intentions are formed as 'if–then' plans that define how individuals will behave in relation to their identified goals (e.g. 'if my friend offers me an unhealthy snack at break time, then I will choose a piece of fruit instead'). Such plans are considered to increase the chances of automatic desirable behavioural responses to critical cues, thereby reducing the need for deliberation over whether, or how, to act consistently with intentions.

Implementation intentions have been demonstrated to be helpful both in initiating and maintaining goal-related behaviour (Gollwitzer and Oettingen 2011), and have been shown to significantly increase the likelihood of attaining a wide range of life goals (Gollwitzer and Sheeran 2006). With direct relevance to cardiovascular rehabilitation, a meta-analytic study from Adriaanse et al. (2011) reported a key finding that implementation intentions that aimed to increase healthy eating behaviour were significantly more effective than those that aimed to extinguish unhealthy eating. Additionally, Luszczynska (2006) demonstrated the effectiveness of implementation intentions in increasing adherence to physical activity sessions over an eight month period following a CPRP. The effectiveness of the intervention appeared to be mediated by whether people continued to use planning strategies over the duration of the study. Those who continued to make plans about when, how often, where, and with whom they would engage in physical activity sessions were more likely to have carried out their goal intentions in the longer term. For implementation intentions to be maximally effective it would appear that a strong commitment to a goal, adequate self-efficacy, and continued self-regulatory plans would appear to be imperative.

4.3.3   Motivational Interviewing

Given the vast media coverage of cardiac risk factors and healthy lifestyles, there are few people totally unaware of what constitutes healthy behaviour. Consequently, the principal challenge for health professionals is not always convincing people of the need to change but helping them to commit to change and to initiate the first steps towards life-long maintenance. Incorporating principles of motivational interviewing into cardiovascular prevention and rehabilitation settings can help people form intentions to make health behaviour changes and also translate intention into action. Despite public awareness of the impact of lifestyle choices on future health, there is often ambivalence about change, due to uncertainty about potential benefits, with some unwilling to relinquish pleasurable behaviours.

Motivational interviewing is a 'client-centred, directive style for enhancing intrinsic motivation to change by exploring and resolving ambivalence', (Miller and Rollnick 2002). It is primarily a communication style rather than a set of techniques, although there are specific skills involved in motivational interviewing.

4.3.4   Solution-focused Approaches

Much of healthcare centres around the question of what is wrong and why, and adopts the position of fixing what is wrong. Indeed cardiac interventions follow this model. Solution-focused approaches (deShazer 1985; Miller et al. 1996) are more interested in intrinsic skills and solutions that people possess in order to improve their situation. Rather than focusing attention on problems, these approaches prefer to consider incidences where problems do not occur, and recreate these conditions in future, in order to identify solutions. This focuses on using a person's pre-existing competencies in order to identify where solutions to problems might lie. It is suggested that cardiovascular prevention and rehabilitation is most effective if it is centred in the present and future, underpinned by the belief that focusing on what is already working and how further progress can be achieved, utilising the skills and knowledge that people have already acquired. This changes the nature of conversations in cardiovascular prevention and rehabilitation from problems to solutions, which it is posited is more likely to lay the foundations for more effective health behaviour change.

4.3.5   Illness Representations

Those attending cardiovascular prevention and rehabilitation are active recipients of care, trying to attain a common-sense understanding of their condition and integrate new information from health professionals and elsewhere into beliefs and ideas that have been developed through previous experience.

Beginning with the self-regulation model of illness, developed by Leventhal and colleagues (1980, 1984), illness representations consider how people are actively trying to make sense of what has happened to them, how it will affect them in future, and what can be done to ameliorate the negative effects of a cardiac condition. It recognises that health messages can be distorted and misunderstood in circumstances where they challenge pre-existing beliefs and ideas, potentially impacting upon how individuals might perceive different aspects of their cardiovascular prevention and rehabilitation.

4.3.6   Rapport Building

Rapport building is a vital factor in early contact with patients who will be 'in the system' for a significant period of time. It is not achievable, or indeed desirable, to present all the possibilities of cardiovascular prevention and rehabilitation to a person in a single consultation. Therefore, it is essential that practitioners work to help individuals feel understood, to ensure that they understand that rehabilitation is about negotiation and collaboration, and that rehabilitation has something of benefit to offer them, without judging them for previous behaviours.

Patients may often be expecting 'the usual lecture about smoking', and it is useful to discuss their expectations of consultations first, to clarify any possible misunderstandings. Practitioners in motivational interviewing highlight the spirit of motivational interviewing as an important aspect of the approach. This is described as 'a collaborative conversation about behaviour change' (Rollnick et al. 1999, p. 32), rather than telling people what is best for them, and this can be a useful guide as to how practitioners might approach rehabilitation consultations.

4.3.7   Effective Communication

Central to cardiovascular prevention and rehabilitation success is effective communication. Ley (1997) recommended that communication needed to be in a language that patients understand, presented with minimal complexity, that care should be taken when offering information that is inconsistent with an individual's own understandings of the situation, and that quality information exchange involves a process of checking the person's understandings following the presentation of new information. This information exchange has been described by motivational interviewing theorists as the 'elicit–provide–elicit' principle.

Indeed, it is now widely accepted that people are not passive recipients of health information, but are actively trying to integrate information into their pre-existing health-related frame of reference and that their pre-existing ideas and beliefs impact on the way that new information is perceived or processed. This is shown by research into illness representations and cardiac misconceptions.

4.4 HEALTH BEHAVIOUR CHANGE – TRANSLATING THEORY INTO PRACTICE

4.4.1 Motivational Interviewing

Principles of motivational interviewing are now quite widely employed in helping people to consider making health behaviour changes. Four important principles of motivational interviewing have been identified, as follows:

1. Expressing empathy – often using active, reflective listening, primarily expressing an understanding of the person's perspective
2. Rolling with resistance – resisting the urge to be confrontational whilst acknowledging an understanding of the reasons for the resistance
3. Supporting self-efficacy – building confidence to change but also avoiding telling people what they should do
4. Developing discrepancy – highlighting how current behaviour doesn't fit in with what a person might be stating he/she really wants to do.

The motivational interviewing approach recognises that:

- The decision to change resides with the patient rather than the practitioner (you cannot make someone change unless they truly wish to)
- The role of the practitioner is to guide rather than to be the expert, with the relationship being collaborative and more of a partnership.
- The aim is to elicit and enhance intrinsic motivation rather than attempting to persuade someone to make changes
- Information is not imposed and there is instead an information exchange with the practitioner resisting the temptation to assume the expert role.

Central to the provision of information is the notion of asking permission to discuss health behaviour change, not assuming the right to do so. This may be a significant departure from traditional consultations of an 'expert' telling someone what they should do and becoming frustrated when behaviour change is not forthcoming. Fully involving individuals in consultations and encouraging ownership is essential and key to establishing effective health behaviour change.

Related concepts are *importance* and *confidence*. If we do not see a change as important, or we are not confident that we can achieve change, then we are less likely to succeed than those people who see the change as important and are confident that they will succeed.

4.4.2   Cardiac Misconceptions and Illness Representations

> **Case Example**
>
> **Jane**
>
> Jane was treated with primary percutaneous cardiac intervention for a myocardial infarction last year. She had been very careful since then to look after herself; she hadn't bothered with cardiovascular prevention and rehabilitation as 'it wasn't for people like me - I don't do gyms'. She was careful with her diet, rested as much as possible and made sure that she never got worked up about anything. Because her level of fitness had fallen due to her lack of exercise, she was finding that she was able to do less and less as she got too breathless, and she felt low in mood as she didn't have the grandchildren over very often in case they got too boisterous – which meant she didn't see her family very much at all.

Jane's story is not uncommon. She had built a set of beliefs about her heart disease and how to live with it that meant that she adopted an unhealthy and significantly restricted lifestyle, resulting in a great reduction in her fitness, and leading to low mood. In the 1960s the Australian government funded a large study to find out why so many men were not returning to work after a myocardial infarction. They found that 50% of the men experienced unwarranted distress and disability, often caused by misconceptions about their condition (Wynn 1967). Further work in Norway in the 1980s reported that people with cardiac misconceptions had reduced quality of life and felt less in control of their condition after a myocardial infarction than people with fewer misconceptions (Maeland and Havik 1989). People who hold more common misconceptions are found to be significantly less active, and also experience increased symptoms of anxiety and depression. Where cardiac misconceptions are reduced or modified, cardiovascular prevention and rehabilitation outcomes improve (Furze et al. 2005).

4.4.3   Managing Misconceptions

Research has shown that health professionals rarely ask people what they believe about their conditions, which means that individual beliefs remain private, and misconceptions or unhelpful illness representations are not dispelled (Petrie and Weinman 1997). Simple questionnaires can be used to assess illness representations, such as the Brief Illness Perception Questionnaire (Broadbent et al. 2006) and the Cardiac Beliefs Questionnaire (Furze et al. 2009). These can be included in the assessment process to highlight whether someone has misconceptions or potentially unhelpful beliefs. Alternatively, questioning people about their understanding of their condition and how it might best be managed or controlled, using questions similar to those included in the Brief Illness Questionnaire or the Cardiac Beliefs Questionnaire is simple and can be effective and enlightening.

Where unhelpful beliefs or misconceptions are highlighted, gentle challenging of these understandings may help to adjust perceptions of what might be healthful behaviours. Questioning how misconceptions were developed and offering information to adjust any misunderstandings might form the basis of a sensitive approach to managing such situations. If questions are used to encourage individuals to think through their misconceptions, in order to reach their own conclusions about appropriate lifestyle choices, this can be more effective than simply giving information which is incongruent with original beliefs.

4.5   BRINGING IT ALL TOGETHER – GOAL-SETTING AS A PRACTICAL EXAMPLE

Careful goal-setting is fundamental for promoting health behaviour change within cardiovascular prevention and rehabilitation, and is used here as an example to illustrate how cardiovascular prevention and rehabilitation practice may be informed by the principles of health behaviour change.

4.5.1   Principles of Goal-setting

Goal-setting can begin at first point of contact. Skilful practitioners will understand the importance of working with individuals to identify meaningful goals for that person. They will also recognise that initial rehabilitation takes place over a period of several months, and subsequently continues for life. Therefore, consideration of goals, goal-setting, and goal achievement is bound to change over time. For example, when lying in a hospital bed, rehabilitative goals may be small, and immediate. Once people have been discharged from hospital, goals may be centred on beginning to re-establish routines. Several weeks on, during a CPRP, goals may, or may not, have developed significantly, and may look rather different.

However, at any stage of rehabilitation, eliciting personal values and attempting to link specific goals to those values is engaging for that person, and appears to be more effective than simply repeating pre-determined goals that relate directly to the professional agenda. Patient-focused goals do not, however, have to result in the cardiovascular prevention and rehabilitation professional having to dispense with their own agenda. It is a question of the marrying of two foci, in order to achieve shared negotiated aims.

It is also worthwhile remembering that evidence suggests that health behaviour change that causes minimal disruption to normal habits and everyday routines results in the most successful outcomes. Significant time during assessment periods may need to be dedicated to this aspect of the rehabilitative process in order that the person themselves sets goals that are meaningful, valued, relevant, and manageable.

4.5.2   Goal-setting as a Process

Goal-setting is not simply an isolated one-off target in rehabilitation, set at the assessment stage and reviewed at the conclusion of the intensive rehabilitation period. Rather, it is a dynamic process that requires review, modification, adaptation, and change. Setting and reviewing goals throughout cardiovascular prevention and rehabilitation is likely to increase commitment and motivation to making behaviour change, as long as the initial goal is owned and valued by the patient.

The process of reviewing, developing, and even resetting goals over time involves checking with people how they have managed in regard to goal attainment, identifying successes, and what the challenges, barriers, and difficulties were in implementation. Barriers might be both practical and emotional in nature. Developing if–then plans to overcome expected barriers is a useful adjunct to such discussions and plans.

When reviewing goal attainment, practitioners are advised to be mindful of issues of low mood and self-esteem amongst participants. In such cases, goals are best advised to be small, achievable, and immediate, rather than complicated and long-term. Empathy is important with such individuals, but practitioners also need to avoid collusion with pessimism and negativity. It is important to help such people to recognise their own success, but care must be taken where practitioners may over-emphasise small gains, especially where they are not readily recognised as achievements by the person, as such responses may be perceived as dismissing the person's difficulties.

4.5.3   Supporting Goal Achievement

Solution-focused approaches to behaviour change suggest that people who own their goals, because they have devised them, are more likely to consider their goals to be important, and with support and guidance are more likely to have the confidence to consider their goals achievable.

A solution-focused approach adopts a particular direction of questioning, focusing on the future, and knowing how solutions can be identified and recognised. Examples of solution-focused questions can be found in the box 'Examples of solution-focused questions'. The advantage of such an approach is that solutions are drawn from the patients who have to carry out those solutions, and helps them to work out how they can recognise when change has been effective. Learning this process is a skill in itself. It can also alter 'stuck' consultations that often happen when patients become too focused on a problem agenda and lose sight of a solution agenda.

Examples of Solution-focused Questions

Opening questions
What are you hoping to achieve from today?
How will you know if it is a good time to make a start?
Have you thought about what you might like to get out of cardiovascular prevention and rehabilitation?

Maintaining future focus
If I met you in a few months' time and you were better, what would you tell me had happened?
If you were better, what would you be doing differently?
If things improved what differences would other people see?

Identifying what works for the person
What has helped in similar situations in the past?
How might you do things differently if you were faced with a similar situation?
What would you not wish to repeat?
What would you say to someone else who was with you?

Scaling questions
On a scale of 1 to 10, where would you say you are now?
What would need to happen for you to move up the scale?
Where would you like to get to on the scale?
How will you know you've made progress?
What do you need to do to achieve this?

Where people may not see the importance of a certain health behaviour, it may be effective to offer some information regarding the advantages of change, without falling into the trap of judging a person for their previously unhealthy choices. Where lack of confidence to carry out the behaviour is the primary issue, focusing on eliciting patient-derived solutions and highlighting previous successes in similar circumstances may be most beneficial. This is in order to increase a sense of self-efficacy for healthful change, and can be done when working one-to-one with a person. It also can be achieved in a group setting, where broader topics like eating more healthily or taking more exercise may be discussed in a similar format. It is important then to focus on what is known, the advantages and disadvantages of change, the degree of importance placed upon making the change, and the degree of confidence within the group to make the change (see the practice example).

Practice Example

Use a flip chart to assess a group's pre-existing knowledge of the benefits and issues in making behaviour changes. The initial task is to take a few minutes to create a picture of a group's understanding of a particular risk factor, whether or not it appears to concur with our own understanding.

What are the pros and cons of trying to eat more healthily?

Pros	Cons
Lose weight	Expensive
Improve health:	Confusing – what is it?
• diabetes	Eating out a problem
• blood pressure	Others do the cooking
• cholesterol	Different meals to family
Look better	Don't like healthy foods
Cheaper	I like chips and chocolate
Reduced chance of another heart attack	Feel hungry/deprived
Gives you more energy	

How important is it that you eat more healthily?

0_____10

Not at all important	Extremely important

How confident are you that you can eat more healthily?

0_____10

Not at all confident	Extremely confident

This example can be developed for a range of behaviour-influenced cardiac risk factors. It highlights in a powerful way the groups' pre-existing knowledge of a particular risk factor. Experience with a wide variety of groups highlights that often there is substantial knowledge about cardiac risk factors within a group, and that participants perceive changes as important, often scoring 8–10 on the importance scale. However, there are usually some misconceptions, and groups often appear to lack a little of the confidence required to establish health behaviour change, frequently scoring 4–7 on the confidence scale.

The information gained from the initial discussion can then be used to tailor the educative part of the session. Recognised advantages to undertaking the behaviour change should be briefly and clearly reinforced. The majority of the session should then be dedicated to addressing any misconceptions and working on solutions to the difficulties and disadvantages that are raised. This reduces the amount of time needed for practitioners to unnecessarily re-teach information that is already known, and allows greater time to focus on possible solutions to the perceived difficulties that often undermine confidence or self-efficacy.

When goals are identified, in addition to patient-derived solutions, formation of implementation intentions can help to increase the likelihood of successful goal achievement. Implementation intentions build upon the idea of an initial goal by working out when, where, and how a goal might be achieved, almost in a contracting way. Asking people to consider when they will start, what exactly they intend to do, with whom they will do it, where they will do it, and for how long can be helpful in building up the goal to be more achievable.

4.5.4   If–Then Plans

This approach advocates asking people to identify particular problem areas, and particular cues to action by developing if–then plans. Examples might be 'If my friend lights up a cigarette at the pub, then I will go for the chat, but will refrain from smoking', or 'If I want a chocolate bar with my lunch, then I will have a piece of fruit instead'. This increases automaticity and habit formation, requiring less effort at the time when things may be forgotten, or where slip-ups might occur in behaviour change.

4.5.5   Maintenance of Goal Achievement

In order to establish new behaviours as routines and habits, significant intensity of input may be required in the early stages of the development of the behaviours. This may be in relation to goal planning, development of cues to action, feedback and monitoring of goal achievement, and frequent review of the goal plans in order to refine them and identify progress. Progress should involve self-monitoring and positive feedback from others, although this must be done with an awareness of self-esteem issues in the person.

Support from important others is an influential factor in the development of health behaviour changes from the point of view of practical help, emotional support, and developing learned responses through processes of conditioning. It is essential that a shared rationale for health behaviour change is developed, as making changes in an unsupportive, or non-understanding environment is considerably harder. Therefore, practitioners are encouraged to include partners or significant others in aspects of rehabilitation, and certainly in the education and exercise sessions, so that a shared understanding of the rationale for health behaviour change is developed.

For short-term health behaviour change to be translated into longer term behavioural habit or routine, patients may well require this support, monitoring, and feedback to continue for a period of time, extending to several months.

4.6   IMPROVING ADHERENCE TO TREATMENT RECOMMENDATIONS

Non-adherence to the use of appropriately prescribed medications can under-mine effectiveness of medical treatments for CVD. In a Cochrane Review of the evidence, Nieuwlaat et al. (2014) report that factors affecting adherence to med-ical regimes are complex and multifactorial, and conclude that 'effective methods to improve adherence must be maintained for as long as the treatment is needed, requiring interventions that can be integrated into the care system in a cost-effective manner'. Given the length of contact that people might have with CPRP services, there is some potential for such services to have a positive impact on adherence.

Any attempt to improve adherence would benefit from taking into account individuals' common-sense beliefs and decision-making (intentional non-adherence) as well as practical barriers that are implicated in non-adherence (unintentional non-adherence). A process of understanding how well the medi-cation regime is understood and 'fits' with a person's beliefs and expectations might help (Horne et al. 2005).

4.7   THE ROLE OF SOCIAL SUPPORT IN HEALTH BEHAVIOUR CHANGE

Although health behaviour change is ultimately an individual issue, the adop-tion of healthy behaviours, for instance physical activity, healthy diet, smoking cessation, and medication adherence, can be influenced by the availability of social support from others.

Lack of social support can have a negative effect on health behaviour change, which in turn may contribute to poor health outcomes. Families and especially partners or spouses often exert powerful effects on patients, influencing their recoveries. However, even with partner support, beneficial health behaviour changes do not necessarily follow (Kiecolt-Glaser and Newton 2001). To out-siders it may appear that someone has an abundance of social support whilst the person actually feels unsupported in meaningful ways. Having others to turn to and satisfaction with the support given appear to be particularly important factors (Sarason et al. 1983). However, support given as positive attention for cardiac symptoms may unwittingly reinforce symptom severity (Itkowitz et al. 2003), thereby increasing the level of disability.

Following a cardiac event, families, especially partners, often feel a responsibility to help patients to improve their health. Unfortunately both patients and partners may hold misconceptions about the exact nature of healthful behaviour changes. At times partners' views of required changes may be detrimental to future health. Partners may on occasion misunderstand the details of what is required to pursue a healthy lifestyle, inadvertently promoting unhealthy behaviours or sometimes imposing undesirable restrictions.

4.7.1   Overprotection

An often-voiced complaint in cardiovascular prevention and rehabilitation is of being overprotected, particularly by partners, often by family members and sometimes even by friends. Twelve months after a first myocardial infarction 58% of men considered they were protected from physical exertion with partners also misunderstanding information, for example, actively seeking to reduce exercise levels, incorrectly believing that exertion might result in further health problems (Wiklund et al. 1984). Some people are actually quite happy about being overprotected, viewing it as an expression of caring, whereas others become quite irritated, finding it restricting and even destructive (Fiske et al. 1991).

4.7.2   Social Control

Some partners may actively seek to exert control over patients' future lifestyles with negative social control often resulting in more health-compromising behaviours (Tucker and Anders 2001). Others may believe that they should even be monitoring and managing patient lifestyle changes (Stewart et al. 2000).

Social control can be employed by partners when they are aware that desirable health behaviour changes are not occurring. Despite often well-meaning attempts of partners to help the other to make changes, social control may lead to decreased patient healthful behaviour (Franks et al. 2006). Spouses may actually engage in both social support and social control to varying degrees, supporting healthy behaviours and seeking to control unhealthy ones. What may superficially be viewed and labelled as social support provided by family members may sometimes lead to, 'unhealthy co-dependency, bullying or manipulation' (NICE 2014, p. 41).

When patients and their partners both participate in CPRPs, with shared commitment to health behaviour change, it may protect against interpretation of support as controlling or overbearing. In those couples whose reported exercise behaviours were similar there was a positive relationship between providing and receiving exercise support from one another (Hong et al. 2005).

4.7.3 The Value of Engaging Others in Cardiovascular Prevention and Rehabilitation

Cardiovascular prevention and rehabilitation group programmes, if structured to facilitate social support amongst participants, can be effective in addressing the lack of a socially supportive network. Using the group to its maximum potential so that participants may share experiences of making health behaviour changes, discussing progress on a weekly basis, often gaining insight into how others overcome obstacles to change can spur them on to enact change. Team members should provide a supportive, caring, and problem-solving environment.

CPRPs vary in the extent to which they accommodate or even welcome the participation of partners, family members, or indeed close friends. Designing programmes to automatically invite partners to attend can be useful. They are able to share information and become more aware of issues related to overprotection and ways in which they themselves might be inadvertently limiting health behaviour change. Also, those people whose partners participated in a CPRP made more positive health behaviour changes, in smoking, eating habits, and physical activity (Elderen-van Kemenade et al. 1994). As some people do not want their partners to participate in group sessions this needs to be explored in a sensitive manner, explaining the potential value of doing so and encouraging attendance.

In couples who have long-standing relationships sharing lifestyle behaviours, often having risk factors in common, the partner may potentially influence the health behaviours of the other, for example, exercise, diet, smoking (Wilson 2002). Attending a CPRP designed to address partners' risk factors as well as those of patients can lead to significant changes in health behaviours for all (Speck et al. 1998).

4.8 EDUCATION IN CARDIOVASCULAR PREVENTION AND REHABILITATION

Historically, people with a long-term condition such as heart disease were simply expected to do as their medical practitioner told them. However, from the 1960s onwards there has been increasing recognition that people are better able to actively manage their condition if they have improved knowledge and understanding about it. Simply giving information to people is not enough for them to be able to take it in and act upon it.

4.8.1   What Do We Mean by 'Patient Education'?

Patient education is defined in many ways, encompassing methods from simple information through to programmes based on counselling or health behaviour change theories. Within the BACPR Standards and Core Components (SCCs), we have used the terms separately in order to ensure that both aspects are covered. However, as is stated in the SCCs, both information in dedicated education sessions and health behaviour change needs to be 'achieved simultaneously and integrated into the whole service' (BACPR 2017b, p. 12). So, for this section of the chapter we will use the following definition for patient education, that it is a:

> *Planned systematic, sequential, and logical process of teaching and learning provided to patients and clients in all clinical settings.* (Dreeben 2010, p. 457)

Patient education has been referred to as 'imparting disease specific education and technical skills', compared to self-management education, which 'teaches problem solving skills' (Bodenheimer et al. 2002). However, simply providing information is not effective without also helping patients to develop the skills and motivation to change their behaviour (Coster and Norman 2009). Systematic reviews of patient education in the management of heart disease found that there was no evidence of effect on mortality or cardiac morbidity and hospitalisation, but that there were some small effects on health-related quality of life (Brown et al. 2013), and that health education was significantly related to behaviour change for activity, diet, and smoking cessation (Ghissi et al. 2014). The findings of this review emphasise that, to be effective, patient education must be delivered within a comprehensive rehabilitation programme incorporating behaviour change techniques.

4.8.2   How Do Adults Learn?

Knowles et al. (2015) proposed that six core principles are considered in order to promote effective adult learning. The core principles are described in Table 4.1.

What Knowles' work demonstrates is that delivery of didactic education sessions, on topics that health professionals believe patients need to understand, is unlikely to be effective or engaging (Clark and Gong 2000). Based on Knowles' core principles, education is increasingly effective where it is tailored to the patient (Coster and Norman 2009).

TABLE 4.1

Knowles' core principle	Meaning
Need to know	Adults will only learn things that they deem important – that they feel they need to know.
Self-concept	As people mature they become more self-directed, and this needs to be recognised by the educator. For example, adults should be involved in assessing what their learning needs are, and how those needs should be met.
Prior experiences	All adults have experiences that influence their current learning, and people attach more meaning to learning that they gain from their experiences.
Readiness to learn	People will be more ready to learn if they perceive that the topics are relevant to their life or work.
Orientation	Adults are more orientated (or drawn) towards problem or performance-centred learning that they can apply to aspects of their lives.
Motivation	As people mature they are more likely to have an internal motivation for learning, such as curiosity, wish to succeed, and self-esteem, rather than an external motivator (such as a reward).

4.8.3 Tips for Group-based Education Sessions

- Planning. As outlined above in the definition (Section 4.8.1), education within cardiovascular prevention and rehabilitation needs to be planned so that participants perceive it to be logical. This seems obvious, but planning is more than simply developing a set of slides about a topic. Each session needs a beginning, middle, and end, and preferably each of these sections to be delivered in different ways. People's concentration span is approximately 20 minutes (with some being able to concentrate for shorter or longer). So, if you change the focus, or ask a question or set a new task after each 20 minutes, you are more likely to hold people's attention.
- Be interesting. Incorporate quizzes, videos, and games into the talks. Set some work in groups, which fosters a more cohesive group environment and may help to promote peer support within the group.
- Appeal to all of the senses. It is hard to beat a nutrition session with simple, healthy, but really appealing tasters – perhaps brought in by the local cardiac patients' group.

- Show it is possible to have a good life afterwards. Invite (hand-picked) graduates from your programmes to come in and discuss how well they got on with cardiovascular prevention and rehabilitation and how it has impacted their lives. If the people are representative of the community that the CPRP is embedded into, this can promote 'modelling' (Bandura 1986), where it is demonstrated to the group that people similar to themselves have successfully achieved and maintained health behaviour change.
- Tailor to your audience. Include topics or information that your needs assessment has shown that participants want. Ensure that the information provided addresses gaps in participants' understanding or knowledge. Although it is important to acknowledge correct understanding there is little gain from subsequently reiterating what is already known.
- Provide the information in more than one format. It is important to cater for the different needs amongst your attendees. Offer them DVDs and CDs as well as books and pamphlets. Visual formats such as DVDs are well suited to people with limited literacy – and, if possible, have them in common languages within your area. As you will probably be aware, the British Heart Foundation has a large catalogue of multimedia information in many different languages. If you do need to develop your own written patient information then please follow the guidance below.
- Trail-blaze the next session in an interesting way to promote people to continue to attend.

4.8.4   Patient Education Materials

With the easy availability of well-designed written or other multimedia information about living with heart disease, the need for cardiovascular prevention and rehabilitation health professionals to develop their own materials is small. The days of the poorly copied sheet which no-one can read should be long gone. However, there may be sections of the communities that you serve for which there are few materials available. Or you may have a novel service available to your attendees that needs written explanation. There are simple principles that should be followed for the development of these education materials.

4.8.5   Principles for Developing Education Materials

- Use simple but engaging language – this is especially important for written materials. For examples of writing for the majority, the tabloid newspapers are excellent in their ability to communicate messages in short sentences and short paragraphs with a lack of jargon. To help to assess whether the language is too technical, within mainstream word processing packages there is an option for the spellchecker to also assess 'readability statistics'. If using these, aim for few passive sentences, a high percentage for reading ease, and a grade level lower than 8. However, it is no good having great readability statistics if what is written is wrong or unintelligible! Ask a service user group to read your materials to check that it is easy to understand.

- Consider how inviting the words look on the paper – use a large font size (Arial 14 or above, or your employer may have specific guidance on this), short paragraphs, and gaps between paragraphs. There should be quite a large proportion of 'white space' so that the words don't look too challenging. Use diagrams/photos if you have them (legally) and they are appropriate (poor clip-art does not improve the look of written information).
- Have different formats (e.g. web-based, apps, DVD, or audio) available for people with different literacy levels. This is particularly important if you are developing materials for people from minority ethnic communities. Develop the information in English (or your native tongue if outside the UK) using best practice (see above) and then use reliable translation services to develop the new material. It is imperative to also undertake a back translation process – where a different person/company translates the newly developed information back into English.

4.9   FLEXIBILITY OF APPROACHES TO CARDIOVASCULAR PREVENTION AND REHABILITATION – WHY DO WE NEED A MENU OF OPTIONS?

Recognition of the individuality of each person recovering from a cardiac event is essential. During assessment it is apparent that people are at varying stages of recovery and have differing needs in relation to health behaviour change. Being mindful of the psychosocial processes underlying change will better inform assessments and planning interventions.

There appear to be widely-held misunderstandings about the precise nature of a menu-driven service. Although respecting patient choice should be of paramount concern it is often mistakenly assumed that the ideal provision for many is a 'deconstructed' approach to cardiovascular prevention and rehabilitation. Although flexibility following an informed patient decision is the most beneficial way forward, participation in group programmes has many benefits that may not be immediately apparent to those recovering from cardiac events. It remains important to promote group programmes but circumstances may dictate the necessity of more flexible programmes for some.

4.10 MAXIMISING GROUP DYNAMICS – TIPS FOR SUCCESSFUL GROUP SUPPORT

Traditional consultations in healthcare are most often undertaken on a one-to-one basis. Although individual sessions may be provided in cardiovascular prevention and rehabilitation settings, particularly before hospital discharge and during the immediate post discharge periods, outpatient groups remain the most frequent method of delivering cardiovascular prevention and rehabilitation. Using groups to their full potential can be invaluable in developing a psychologically informed programme of cardiovascular prevention and rehabilitation.

4.10.1 The Group Experience

Group participants are a diverse range of people, with differing problems and past behaviours, each contributing their unique experience of a cardiac event. No two groups ever function in exactly the same way, with the group climate, or atmosphere, being different dependent on the level and type of participant involvement. Being a member of a well-functioning and supportive group can be an empowering experience.

It is essential to provide a supportive environment within cardiovascular prevention and rehabilitation groups, fostering group cohesion, if people are to be open about their feelings, concerns, and progress. For many recovering from cardiac events being part of a therapeutic or self-help group will be a novel experience. From the outset group guidelines (see box on 'Some examples of group guidelines') should ideally be elicited from the group or failing that stated by group leaders, before any sharing of information is begun.

Some Examples of Group Guidelines

- Agree to keep personal information confidential within the group
- No identifying information to be discussed outside the group
- Bring only relevant information and concerns to the group
- Share experiences that may be helpful to others.
- Listen to what other people are contributing
- Be supportive of each other
- Respect others' viewpoints
- Do not criticise others.

Although many people may be at first unsure about participating, once the group atmosphere has developed, becoming more supportive session by session, those who were initially reluctant to contribute usually find it easier to take part. Group identification may also be an important factor, encouraging session attendance. Visitors to groups should be handled carefully and permission to observe sessions sought from the group members themselves, as new people have the potential to adversely affect group dynamics, even if they do not contribute.

4.10.2   Progress Feedback

Another useful function of the group is to use the setting to encourage individual weekly reporting of progress, reviewing overall goals, re-defining interim goals, and discussing action plans. It is also an opportunity to share numerous concerns, such as emotional aspects of recovery, sleep problems, and challenges of returning to former activities. Participants learn from each other by the process of sharing and their own progress may be viewed differently, often more positively, by comparing with others. A delineated group 'feedback' section of each session provides an opportunistic vehicle for staff to clarify understandings and address potential misunderstandings of various health issues. Individual concerns and anxieties may also emerge during discussion and it is often found that other group members are experiencing similar difficulties, which can help to normalise individual experience.

Some Tips for Successful Group Support

- Start first session with short individual introductions.
- Foster a safe and supportive environment in which people are comfortable to speak (forcing to speak may be counterproductive). Agree group guidelines and discuss boundaries.
- Encourage participants to share information as this is as valuable as that provided by the group leaders, but only when they are comfortable to do this.
- Invite participants to share similar experiences to that disclosed by another group member.
- Explain that participants will benefit from working general principles into their own specific experiences.
- Facilitate focused and productive group interactions, bringing different people into the discussion, not reinforcing the participation of just a few individuals.

- Foster group support by relating patient experience to that previously disclosed by other group members.
- Ensure that each group member receives a similar amount of attention.
- Group leaders should seek to:
  - normalise individual experience
  - demonstrate acceptance
  - not single out individuals as being different
  - promote a warm, caring, and friendly group atmosphere.

4.11   CLOSED VERSUS OPEN GROUPS

CPRPs operate within either closed or open group systems. A closed group is such that an invited set of participants start the programme on the first session and continue together through subsequent sessions. New participants do not join at later sessions. Open or 'rolling' groups operate with a changing mix of people participating in sessions, for example, one individual will start their first session when another is completing their last, whilst others will be participating in a variety of different numbered sessions, as appropriate to their progression through the group.

There are advantages and disadvantages in running both types of group. The most frequently cited advantages for delivering 'rolling' groups are that it is administratively easier to slot people in when a vacancy arises, resulting in shorter waiting times, and having a wealth of role models at varying stages of recovery for newly starting patients to identify with and to learn from. In comparison closed groups benefit from a single starting point with collaboratively developed group guidelines (see box), which may result in a greater shared sense of stage of recovery and ownership of the group. In turn this may foster greater group cohesion, as participants have more chances of getting to know, accept, and trust each other and can identify others with similar problems and those who have already overcome related difficulties. Group leaders are more easily able to develop the skills and understanding of participants over a series of sessions, tailoring information provision accordingly. Consequently, there is less likelihood of falling into the trap of delivering set talks, session by session. Closed groups allow for more flexibility in sessions and tailoring programmes to meet the needs of each groups' unique mix of participants.

Closed groups do need a little more planning in order to ensure a continuous flow of participants, which is actually possible if groups are timetabled to start at regular intervals separated by only a few weeks. However, it may be difficult for some closed programmes to meet BACPR standards (BACPR 2017b) and NICE Guidance (NICE 2013) that advise that cardiovascular rehabilitation should be commenced within 10 working days of discharge or diagnosis. Finding ways in which participants may attend closed groups early after discharge or diagnosis would be ideal, in order to ensure the delivery of more psychologically-minded programmes.

4.12   HOW WILL THE COMPONENT BE ASSESSED AND MONITORED?

The aim of initial assessment must surely be to understand the person better, in order that their rehabilitation can be effectively tailored to their needs and, of course, to develop enough rapport to encourage them back to future planned sessions.

Any attempts to facilitate health behaviour change within the context of cardiovascular prevention and rehabilitation might be advised to avoid focusing entirely on the individual in isolation, but must be informed further by the person's familial, social, economic, and cultural context. It is therefore important to spend appropriate amounts of time asking questions that offer a full picture of the individual during assessment. Practitioners are therefore advised to be mindful of the need for comprehensive psychosocial assessment.

Assessment for this component is also rooted in assessment for all of the modifiable risk factors – to identify each person's unhelpful behaviours. We have shown above techniques that are helpful in assessing motivation for change – including discussion of the pros and cons of change, and of the importance and confidence for the particular behaviour change under discussion. What must always be remembered is that it is up to the patient to identify what they want to change.

Monitoring is achieved by discussion of the goals that each person has set, with supportive feedback, and to identify new or different goals as they progress.

4.12.1   Evaluation of the Intervention

Evaluation of the intervention is also rooted in the evaluation of the unhelpful behaviour. Have they successfully achieved their goals? Has this impacted on their physical activity, their fitness, their diet, their smoking, etc.? However, this is not all that should be evaluated. As part of enabling long-term maintenance of the behaviour changes, the professional should assess how confident the individual is with making changes for the future – has their self-efficacy for self-managing their health improved? Has their motivation to change specific health behaviours altered? This should entail a detailed discussion with each individual, as the programme ends, to promote future changes and to advise on community-based support after completion of the programme.

4.12.2 Consideration for Applications to Other Long-term Conditions

Health behaviour change is obviously not just for people with heart disease – as the growing number of people attending cardiovascular prevention and rehabilitation with multiple co-morbidities can attest. The techniques described here are useful for supporting health behaviour change for any of the long-term conditions.

4.13 CONCLUSION

In this chapter we have defined health behaviour change, and outlined some of the basic principles that are needed to successfully support positive behaviour change within CPRPs. We have introduced reasons why didactic education sessions are sub-optimal, and provided guidance for optimising education sessions and education materials. We also considered ways of improving the effectiveness of health behaviour change and education within cardiovascular rehabilitation interventions, especially in regard to making full use of the potential of group processes.

REFERENCES

Adriaanse, M.A., Vinkers, C.D.W., De Ridder, D.T.D. et al. (2011). Do implementation intentions help to eat a healthy diet? A systematic review and meta-analysis of the empirical evidence. *Appetite* 56 (1): 183–193.

Bandura, A. (1986). *Social Foundations of Thought and Action*. New York: Prentice-Hall.

Bandura, A. (1997). *Self-Efficacy: The Exercise of Control*. New York: Freeman.

Baroletti, S. and Dell'Ofano, H. (2010). Medication adherence in cardiovascular disease. *Circulation* 121 (12): 1455–1458.

Bodenheimer, T., Lorig, K., Holman, H., and Grumbach, K. (2002). Patient self-management of chronic disease in primary care. *The Journal of the American Medical Association* 288 (19): 2469–2475.

British Association for Cardiovascular Prevention and Rehabilitation (2017a). *BACPR Core Competences for the Health Behaviour Change and Education Component of Cardiovascular Rehabilitation Services*. London: BACPR. www.bacpr.com.

British Association for Cardiovascular Prevention and Rehabilitation (2017b). *The BACPR Standards and Core Components for Cardiovascular Disease Prevention and Rehabilitation*, 3e. London: BACPR. www.bacpr.com.

Broadbent, E., Petrie, K.J., Main, J., and Weinman, J. (2006). The brief illness perceptions questionnaire. *Journal of Psychosomatic Research* 60 (6): 631–637.

Brown, J.P., Clark, A.M., Dalal, H. et al. (2013). Effect of patient education in the management of coronary heart disease: a systematic review and meta-analysis of randomized controlled trials. *European Journal of Preventive Cardiology* 20 (4): 701–714.

Clark, N.M. and Gong, M. (2000). Management of chronic disease by practitioner and patients: are we teaching the wrong things? *British Medical Journal* 320 (7234): 572–575.

Conner, M. and Norman, P. (2007). *Predicting Health Behaviour*, 2e. Maidenhead UK: Open University Press.

Coster, S. and Norman, I. (2009). Cochrane reviews of educational and self-management interventions to guide nursing practice: a review. *International Journal of Nursing Studies* 46 (4): 508–528.

deShazer, S. (1985). *Keys to Solutions in Brief Therapy*. New York: Norton.

Dreeben, O. (2010). *Patient Education in Rehabilitation*. Massachusetts, USA: Jones & Bartlett Learning.

van Elderen-van Kemenade, T., Maes, S., and van den Broek, Y. (1994). Effects of a health education programme with telephone follow-up during cardiac rehabilitation. *British Journal of Clinical Psychology* 33 (Part 3): 367–378.

Fiske, V., Coyne, J.C., and Smith, D.A. (1991). Couples coping with myocardial infarction: an empirical reconsideration of the role of overprotectiveness. *Journal of Family Psychology* 5 (1): 4–20.

Franks, M.M., Stephens, M.A.P., Rook, K.S. et al. (2006). Spouses' provision of health-related support and control to patients participating in cardiac rehabilitation. *Journal of Family Psychology* 20 (2): 311–318.

Furze, G., Dumville, J.C., Miles, J. et al. (2009). 'Prehabilitation' prior to CABG surgery improves physical functioning and depression. *International Journal of Cardiology* 132 (1): 51–58.

Furze, G., Lewin, R., Murberg, T.A. et al. (2005). Does it matter what patients think? The relationship between changes in patients' beliefs about angina and their psychological and functional status. *Journal of Psychosomatic Research* 59 (5): 323–329.

Ghissi, G.L.d.M., Abdallah, F., Grace, S.L. et al. (2014). A systematic review of patient education in cardiac patients: do they increase knowledge and promote health behaviour change? *Patient Education and Counseling* 95 (2): 160–174.

Gollwitzer, P.M. (1993). Goal achievement: the role of intentions. In: *European Review of Social Psychology*, vol. 4 (eds. W. Stroebe and M. Hewstone), 141–185. Chichester: Wiley.

Gollwitzer, P.M. and Oettingen, G. (2011). Planning promotes goal striving. In: *Handbook of Self-Regulation: Research, Theory, and Application*, 2e (eds. K.D. Vohs and R.F. Baumeister), 162–185. New York/London: Guilford Press.

Gollwitzer, P.M. and Sheeran, P. (2006). Implementation intentions and goal achieve-ment: a meta-analysis of effects and processes. *Advances in Experimental Social Psychology* 38: 69–119.

Ho, P.M., Magid, D.J., Shetterly, S.M. et al. (2008). Medication nonadherence is asso-ciated with a broad range of adverse outcomes in patients with coronary artery disease. *American Heart Journal* 155 (4): 772–779.

Hong, T.B., Franks, M.M., Gonzalez, R. et al. (2005). A dyadic investigation of exercise support between cardiac patients and their spouses. *Health Psychology* 24 (4): 430–434.

Horne, R., Weinman, J., Barber, N. et al. (2005). *Concordance, Adherence and Compliance in Medicine Taking. Report for the National Co-ordinating Centre for NHS Service Delivery and Organisation R&D*. London: NCCSDO.

Itkowitz, N.I., Kerns, R.D., and Otis, J.D. (2003). Support and CHD: the importance of significant other responses. *Journal of Behavioral Medicine* 26 (1): 19–30.

Kiecolt-Glaser, J.K. and Newton, T.L. (2001). Marriage and health: his and hers. *Psychological Bulletin* 127 (4): 472–503.

Knowles, M.S., Holton, E.F., and Swanson, R.A. (2015). *The Adult Learner: The Definitive Classic in Adult Education and Human Resource Development*, 8e. New York: Routledge.

Lally, P. and Gardner, B. (2013). Promoting habit formation. *Health Psychology Review* 7 (Suppl. 1): S137–S158.

Leventhal, H., Meyer, D., and Nerenz, D.R. (1980). The common sense represen-tation of illness danger. In: *Contributions to Medical Psychology*, vol. 2 (ed. S. Rachman), 17–30. New York: Pergamon Press.

Leventhal, H., Nerenz, D.R., and Steele, D.J. (1984). Illness representations and coping with health threats. In: *Handbook of Psychology and Health*, vol. 4 (eds. A. Baum, S.E. Taylor, and J.E. Singer), 219–252. New Jersey: Lawrence Erlbaum Associates.

Ley, P. (1997). *Communicating with Patients: Improving Communication, Satisfaction, and Compliance*. London: Chapman and Hall.

Luszczynska, A. (2006). An implementation intentions intervention, the use of a planning strategy, and physical activity after myocardial infarction. *Social Science and Medicine* 62 (4): 900–908.

Maeland, J.G. and Havik, O.E. (1989). After the myocardial infarction. A medical and psychological study with special emphasis on perceived illness. *Scandinavian Journal of Rehabilitation Medicine. Supplement* 22: 1–87.

Miller, D., Hubble, A., and Duncan, B. (1996). *Handbook of Solution Focused Brief Therapy: Foundations, Applications and Research*. San Francisco, CA: Jossey-Bass.

Miller, W.R., Rollnick, S., and Conforti, K. (2002). *Motivational Interviewing, Second Edition: Preparing People for Change*, 2e. New York: Guilford Publications.

National Institute for Health and Care Excellence (2013). *CG172 Secondary Prevention Post Myocardial Infarction*. London: NICE.

National Institute for Health and Care Excellence (2014). *Public Health Guidance 49: Behaviour Change: Individual Approaches*. London: NICE.

National Institute for Health and Clinical Excellence (2007). *Public Health Guidance 6: Behaviour Change*. London: NICE.

Nieuwlaat, R., Wilczynski, N., Navarro, T. et al. (2014). Interventions for enhancing medication adherence. *Cochrane Database of Systematic Reviews* (11): CD000011. https://doi.org/10.1002/14651858.CD000011.pub4.

Petrie, K.J. and Weinman, J.A. (1997). Illness representations and recovery from myocardial infarction. In: *Perceptions of Health and Illness* (eds. K.J. Petrie and J.A. Weinman), 441–465. Amsterdam: Harwood Academic Publishers.

Rollnick, S., Mason, P., and Butler, C.C. (1999). *Health Behaviour Change: A Guide for Practitioners*. Edinburgh: Churchill Livingstone.

Sarason, I.G., Levine, H.M., Basham, R.B., and Sarason, B.R. (1983). Assessing social support: the social support questionnaire. *Journal of Personality and Social Psychology* 44: 127–139.

Sheeran, P. (2002). Intention-behaviour relations: a conceptual and empirical view. *European Review of Social Psychology* 12: 1–30.

Speck, L., Jones, D., Jones, C., and Cook, A. (1998). *The HELM (Heart Education for Life, Maesteg) Project: extending the role of the cardiac rehabilitation team*. Paper presented at the British Association for Cardiac Rehabilitation Annual Conference, Cardiff.

Stewart, M., Davidson, K., Meade, D. et al. (2000). Myocardial infarction: survivors' and spouses' stress, coping and support. *Journal of Advanced Nursing* 31 (6): 1351–1360.

Tucker, J.S. and Anders, S.L. (2001). Social control of health behaviours in marriage. *Journal of Applied Social Psychology* 31: 467–485.

Wiklund, I., Sanne, H., Vedin, A., and Wilhelmsson, C. (1984). Psychosocial outcome one year after a first myocardial infarction. *Journal of Psychosomatic Research* 28 (4): 309–321.

Wilson, E. (2002). The health capital of families: an investigation of the inter-spousal correlation in health status. *Social Science and Medicine* 55 (7): 1157–1172.

Wynn, A. (1967). Unwarranted emotional distress in men with ischaemic heart disease. *Medical Journal of Australia* 2 (19): 847–851.

CHAPTER 5

Lifestyle Risk Factor Management

Jennifer Jones[1,2], John Buckley[3], and Gill Furze[4]

[1] National University of Ireland, Galway, Ireland
[2] Department of Clinical Sciences, Brunel University, Uxbridge, UK
[3] Centre for Active Living, University Centre Shrewsbury, Shrewsbury, UK
[4] Faculty of Health and Life Sciences, Coventry University, Coventry, UK

INTRODUCTION

This chapter is made up of the three key areas of lifestyle risk factor management: tobacco cessation, diet and anthropometrics, and physical activity and exercise. Each of these three elements is written as an individual sub-chapter (5a., 5b. and 5c.). It is important to recognise that the common thread running through these three areas is the effective application of behaviour change and education as discussed in Chapter 4. As lifestyle is the cornerstone of any cardiovascular disease (CVD) prevention programme, being mindful of all elements in Chapter 4, is central to the success of long-term, self-managed, well-being following a CVD diagnosis or critical event.

As shown in Chapter 1, at least 80% of acute myocardial infarction is attributable to modifiable risk factors; particularly tobacco use, poor diet and lack of physical activity. Consequently, intensive management to achieve long-term tobacco cessation, adherence to a cardioprotective diet, being sufficiently physically active together with maintaining a healthy weight and shape are recognised as vital to effective cardiovascular prevention and rehabilitation practice.

Not only are these three lifestyle variables most strongly associated with long-term survival, these health behaviours also allow for the reduction in the need for pharmacological intervention and importantly the need for combination therapies that are often associated with more adverse side effects. These key goals in lifestyle risk factor management and how they can be achieved are presented within the three following sub-chapters.

Achieving Long-term Abstinence from Tobacco Use in Patients in a Cardiovascular Prevention and Rehabilitation Setting

Catriona Jennings[1] and Robert West[2]

[1] National Institute for Prevention and Cardiovascular Health, National University of Ireland, Galway, Ireland

[2] Department of Behavioural Science and Health, Institute of Epidemiology and Healthcare, University College London, London, UK

Abstract

This chapter presents a number of considerations for health professionals addressing long-term abstinence from tobacco use in their patients. Whilst an acute cardiac event is a strong predictor of tobacco cessation, relapse is common, and exposure to tobacco is high in people with cardiovascular disease and their families. This chapter suggests strategies to help manage tobacco addiction in patients.

Tobacco cessation is included as a priority and core component in the British Association for Cardiovascular Prevention and Rehabilitation

Cardiovascular Prevention and Rehabilitation in Practice, Second Edition.
Edited by Jennifer Jones, John Buckley, Gill Furze, and Gail Sheppard.

standards. It is expected that tobacco cessation support should be provided as an integral part of comprehensive prevention and rehabilitation. This 'in-house' support for stopping tobacco use, along with all the other core components, facilitates patient- and family-centred care. This kind of care is not only more convenient for patients, but is also likely to be more effective in achieving improved lifestyles and reduced cardiovascular risk.

Keywords: *tobacco cessation, smoking cessation, nicotine dependence, cardiovascular disease (CVD)*

Key Points

- Health professionals working in a cardiovascular prevention and rehabilitation programme (CPRP) should address long-term abstinence from tobacco use in their patients.
- Dependence on tobacco requires a withdrawal-oriented approach to achieve cessation.
- Cessation starts with a comprehensive assessment of tobacco use.
- Behavioural and optimal pharmacological strategies should be employed to support tobacco cessation.
- Opportunities for preventing and managing lapses and relapse to tobacco use should be explored with patients.
- Comprehensive lifestyle approaches used in CPRP provide opportunities to manage weight gain in tobacco cessation.
- It is important to understand the contribution of harm reduction in highly dependent tobacco users who may be unable to make an abrupt quit attempt.

5A.1   RATIONALE AND AIMS

Tobacco use is the second most prominent risk factor worldwide for global disease burden next to hypertension (GBD 2015 Tobacco Collaborators 2017). Cardiovascular disease (CVD) is a common cause of avoidable death in smokers and they are at greater risk of suffering an acute myocardial infarction (Edwards 2004). Smoke-free legislation appears to have had an impact in reducing the risk of myocardial infarction in the general population in countries worldwide (Lin et al. 2013) (Figure 5a.1). In addition, it has had an impact on smoking prevalence in the UK (Figure 5a.2); however, the risk remains higher in the more deprived and less educated areas of the population (Hiscock et al. 2012) (Figure 5a.3).

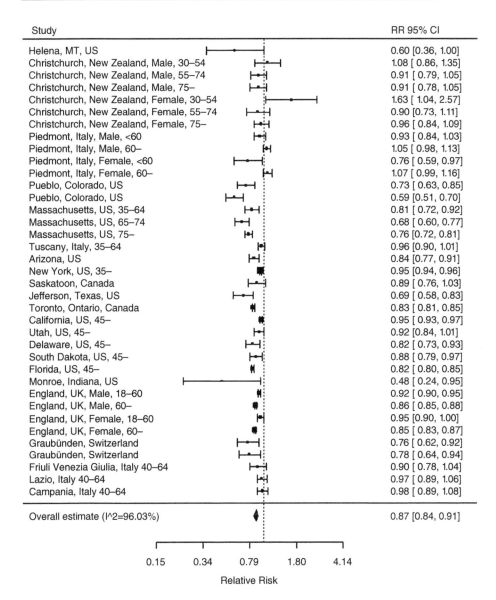

Study		RR 95% CI
Helena, MT, US		0.60 [0.36, 1.00]
Christchurch, New Zealand, Male, 30–54		1.08 [0.86, 1.35]
Christchurch, New Zealand, Male, 55–74		0.91 [0.79, 1.05]
Christchurch, New Zealand, Male, 75–		0.91 [0.78, 1.05]
Christchurch, New Zealand, Female, 30–54		1.63 [1.04, 2.57]
Christchurch, New Zealand, Female, 55–74		0.90 [0.73, 1.11]
Christchurch, New Zealand, Female, 75–		0.96 [0.84, 1.09]
Piedmont, Italy, Male, <60		0.93 [0.84, 1.03]
Piedmont, Italy, Male, 60–		1.05 [0.98, 1.13]
Piedmont, Italy, Female, <60		0.76 [0.59, 0.97]
Piedmont, Italy, Female, 60–		1.07 [0.99, 1.16]
Pueblo, Colorado, US		0.73 [0.63, 0.85]
Pueblo, Colorado, US		0.59 [0.51, 0.70]
Massachusetts, US, 35–64		0.81 [0.72, 0.92]
Massachusetts, US, 65–74		0.68 [0.60, 0.77]
Massachusetts, US, 75–		0.76 [0.72, 0.81]
Tuscany, Italy, 35–64		0.96 [0.90, 1.01]
Arizona, US		0.84 [0.77, 0.91]
New York, US, 35–		0.95 [0.94, 0.96]
Saskatoon, Canada		0.89 [0.76, 1.03]
Jefferson, Texas, US		0.69 [0.58, 0.83]
Toronto, Ontario, Canada		0.83 [0.81, 0.85]
California, US, 45–		0.95 [0.93, 0.97]
Utah, US, 45–		0.92 [0.84, 1.01]
Delaware, US, 45–		0.82 [0.73, 0.93]
South Dakota, US, 45–		0.88 [0.79, 0.97]
Florida, US, 45–		0.82 [0.80, 0.85]
Monroe, Indiana, US		0.48 [0.24, 0.95]
England, UK, Male, 18–60		0.92 [0.90, 0.95]
England, UK, Male, 60–		0.86 [0.85, 0.88]
England, UK, Female, 18–60		0.95 [0.90, 1.00]
England, UK, Female, 60–		0.85 [0.83, 0.87]
Graubünden, Switzerland		0.76 [0.62, 0.92]
Graubünden, Switzerland		0.78 [0.64, 0.94]
Friuli Venezia Giulia, Italy 40–64		0.90 [0.78, 1.04]
Lazio, Italy 40–64		0.97 [0.89, 1.06]
Campania, Italy 40–64		0.98 [0.89, 1.08]
Overall estimate (I^2=96.03%)		0.87 [0.84, 0.91]

0.15   0.34   0.79   1.80   4.14

Relative Risk

FIGURE 5A.1   Effect of smoke-free legislation on the risk of acute myocardial infarction in the general population (Lin et al. 2013).

Smoking prevalence also varies considerably with ethnicity, with Bangladeshi men having the highest smoking prevalence in England, higher than the national average by nearly 20% (Lifestyles Statistics Team, Health and Social Care Information Centre and Niblett 2015). Whilst smoking is low in Bangladeshi women, chewing tobacco is higher in this group than any other in England.

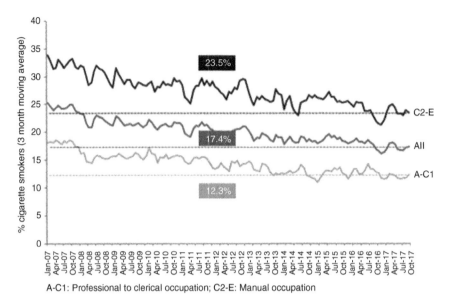

A-C1: Professional to clerical occupation; C2-E: Manual occupation

FIGURE 5A.2   Reduction in smoking prevalence in England since the ban on smoking in public places (Smoking Toolkit Study) (www.smokinginengland.info).

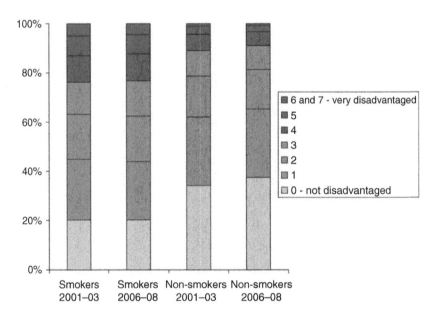

FIGURE 5A.3   Smoking and socioeconomic status in England: the rise of the never smoker and the disadvantaged smoker (Hiscock et al. 2012) (Hiscock et al. 2012).

> **Paan or bidi (originating from India and the Pacific)**
> A psychoactive stimulating preparation of betel leaf, areca nut, and cured tobacco, which is chewed and then either swallowed or spat out.
> **Waterpipe tobacco (originating from Asia and Africa)**
> A way of vapourising and smoking tobacco also known as 'hookah', 'shisha', 'narghile', 'arghila', and 'qalyān'. It is increasingly popular amongst young people in the UK. The misconception is that smoking tobacco which had been passed through water makes it harmless.

FIGURE 5A.4   Alternative ways of using tobacco.

Other ways of taking tobacco (e.g. paan and waterpipe – Figure 5a.4) are also harmful and carry similar risks to smoking tobacco (Akl et al. 2010). All tobacco contains nicotine and is therefore able to induce dependence in its users.

Exposure to environmental tobacco smoke in homes increases cardiovascular risk in spouses and other family members (Law et al. 1997), and reduces the likelihood of a successful quit attempt in coronary patients (Prugger et al. 2014).

A large proportion of smokers with coronary disease or risk factors persist in smoking after diagnosis, although many report an intention to quit in the longer term (Kotseva et al. 2012). Whilst attendance at a prevention and rehabilitation programme is associated with a significantly lower prevalence of smoking, smokers are less likely to attend than non-smokers. In those who spontaneously quit following an acute event, the challenge that health professionals face is prevention of relapse.

5A.2   DEPENDENCE ON TOBACCO

Once tobacco use has become established and regular, addiction to the nicotine in tobacco is commonplace (RCP 2000). After smoke inhalation, nicotine reaches the brain via the lungs within a few seconds, where it binds to nicotinic acetylcholine receptors. This leads to a release of dopamine in the nucleus accumbens, which forms an association between situations in which smoking and the impulse to smoke occur. Thus even non-daily smokers can experience powerful urges to smoke in situations where this would normally occur.

When a smoker is deprived of a cigarette, 'nicotine hunger' occurs, and withdrawal is experienced (after one or two hours) (Figures 5a.5 and 5a.6). This discomfort is relieved by smoking and thus smoking is perceived to have positive effects (West 2009).

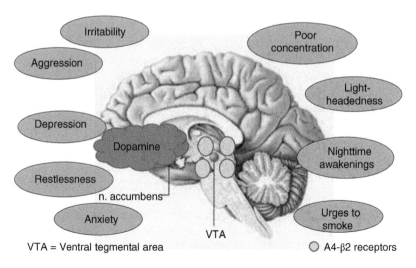

VTA = Ventral tegmental area   ○ A4-β2 receptors

FIGURE 5A.5   Mesolimbic brain reward pathway.

Symptom	Duration
Urges to smoke	Strongest in the first week
Mood disturbance ☐ Irritability ☐ Depression ☐ Anxiety ☐ Restlessness	1 – 4 weeks
Poor concentration	1 – 4 weeks
Increased appetite	12 weeks
Physical symptoms ☐ Increased cough ☐ Constipation ☐ Mouth ulcers	1 – 4 weeks
Nighttime awakenings	1 week

FIGURE 5A.6   Withdrawal symptoms.

5A.3   ASSESSMENT

A comprehensive assessment of tobacco use, which includes status of use (i.e. current user, past user, never user), dependence on nicotine, readiness to quit, psychological co-morbidities, past quit attempts, and tobacco use in the family, is essential in order to provide timely support for patients. Details of the assessment elements are provided below.

5a.3.1 Status of Use

Using interview administered questions (an example can be seen in Figure 5a.7), this assessment will provide information on tobacco habits (current/ex/never) and on lifetime exposure to tobacco by assessing, for example, the number of cigarettes smoked daily over what duration.

Self-reported smoking status should be validated with a biomarker like expired carbon monoxide (CO), which is present in large quantities in tobacco smoke, to increase accuracy. Both Bedfont (Bedfont Scientific Ltd. – Smokerlyzer 2016) and Micromedical (Care Fusion 2016) provide reliable monitors.

Breath CO measurement provides an instant result and is practical in clinical practice. Whilst some exposure to CO may occur in normal day-to-day life, due to environmental pollution, passive smoking, and occupational exposure, the most likely cause of high levels in the breath is tobacco smoking.

Once the CO monitor has been switched on and the countdown initiated, the patient is asked to take in a breath and hold it for 15 s, and then to blow out steadily through the mouthpiece that is attached to the device, emptying the lungs as much as possible. An expired CO level of ≤ 6 ppm is associated with a non-smoking status.

Breath CO levels may be elevated in inflammatory lung diseases, including bronchiectasis, asthma, and COPD with mean values of about 7 ppm being reported. In addition, because of the short half-life of CO, only smoking from the last 12 h will be detected. However, patients seen in a prevention and rehabilitation setting are more likely to be dependent, regular smokers, unable to refrain from smoking for such a long period.

5a.3.2 Measuring Dependence

A measure of 'time of the first cigarette of the day' is a predictor of outcome in cessation (Baker et al. 2007). Those smokers with a higher dependency on nicotine will almost definitely benefit from pharmacological support to aid a quit

Question	Response
1. Have you ever smoked?	Assesses whether there has been any exposure to tobacco
2. How many years have you smoked?	Assesses duration of exposure
3. How long ago did you stop smoking?	Identifies ex-smokers and whether a recent quitter
4. Do you smoke now?	Assesses current smoking

FIGURE 5A.7 Interview administered questions for assessing smoking status.

attempt. The easiest and quickest measure to use is the Heavy Smoking Index (HSI) (Chabrol et al. 2005) (Figure 5a.8), which includes the two most important items from the longer Fagerström Test for Nicotine Dependence (FTND) (Heatherton et al. 1991) (Figure 5a.9).

An additional tool, shown in Figure 5a.10 (Fidler et al. 2011), measures the frequency and strength of the urge an individual feels to smoke over a 24 hour period. This has been found to predict relapse following quit attempts at least as well as the HSI and has the advantage that it is not affected by external conditions that may limit the number of cigarettes people smoke, such as smoke-free environments.

5a.3.3   Assessing Motivation to Quit

Patients who have not quit smoking as a result of their acute event may be ambivalent about stopping smoking. Whilst they will be aware of how smoking compromises their health, addiction creates an enormous barrier to quitting. The confidence of a long-term smoker with 10 or more quit attempts that have ended in relapse can be low. Amongst smokers, the largest group is those who really want to stop but cannot specify when they will do it (Department of Health et al. 2016).

Heavy Smoking Index

1. How many cigarettes does the patient smoke each day?

- ☐ 31 plus   (1.5 pack plus)   = 3 points
- ☐ 21–30   (1–1.5 packs)   = 2 points
- ☐ 11–20   (1/2–1 pack)   = 1 points
- ☐ 1–10   (1/2 pack or less)   = 0 points

2. How soon after waking does the patient smoke the first cigarette?

- ☐ Within 5 minutes   = 3 points
- ☐ From 6–30 minutes   = 2 points
- ☐ From 30 minutes–1 hour   = 1 points
- ☐ More than one (1) hour   = 0 points

Heavy Smoking Index Score (add points 1 & 2 above):

☒ 0–1 = Light Smoker   ☒ 2–3 = Moderate Smoker   ☒ 4–6 = Heavy Smoker

FIGURE 5A.8   The Heavy Smoking Index (HSI) (Chabrol et al. 2005).

Questions		Answers	Points
1.	How soon after you wake up do you smoke your first cigarette?	Within 5 minutes	3
		6–30 minutes	2
		31–60 minutes	1
		After 60 minutes	0
2.	Do you find it difficult to refrain from smoking in places where it is forbidden e.g. in church, at the library, in cinema, etc.?	Yes	1
		No	0
3.	Which cigarette would you hate most to give up?	The first one in the morning	1
		All others	0
4.	How many cigarettes/day do you smoke?	10 or less	0
		11–20	1
		21–30	2
		31 or more	3
5.	Do you smoke more frequently during the first hours after waking than during the rest of the day?	Yes	1
		No	0
6.	Do you smoke if you are so ill that you are in bed most of the day?	Yes	1
		No	0

© Permission to use this scale for other than research purposes should be obtained from K.O. Fagerström

FIGURE 5A.9 Items and scoring for Fagerström Test for Nicotine Dependence (FTND) (Heatherton et al. 1991).

Question	Responses					
How much of the time have you felt the urge to smoke in the past 24 hours?	Not at all	A little of the time	Some of the time	A lot of the time	Almost all of the time	All of the time
In general, how strong have the urges to smoke been?	Slight	Moderate	Strong	Very strong	Extremely strong	

FIGURE 5A.10 Frequency and strength of an individual's urge to smoke over a 24 hour period.

Using motivational techniques (Chapter 4), and proposing effective strategies (promise of support and effective use of pharmacotherapy) may increase self-efficacy and stimulate a new quit attempt.

5a.3.4   Past Quit Attempts

Whilst patients will report failure in previous quit attempts, it is important to establish what strategies have been used in the past, whether they were used optimally, and whether there are any misconceptions. New knowledge and therapies may have emerged and may be available.

Exploring past quit attempts may provide an opportunity to build self-efficacy and confidence. A prolonged past quit attempt can be framed as an example of success even though it ended in an eventual relapse.

5a.3.5   Psychological Co-morbidities

Smokers often believe that smoking helps with mood. Depressed mood is one of the short-term nicotine withdrawal symptoms (Edwards and Kendler 2011). However, it has now been demonstrated that mental health improves after people have stopped smoking (Taylor et al. 2014). Therefore, concern about depressive symptoms emerging should not be seen as a reason for putting off a quit attempt. There are treatment options that may be preferable in such patients, like buproprion (Zyban), which is an antidepressant. In addition, evidence is emerging to suggest that varenicline (Champix) may be equally useful in suppressing depressive symptoms during smoking cessation (Cinciripini et al. 2013) and does not seem to be associated with an increased risk of developing depression or suicidal thoughts (Kotz et al. 2015).

5A.4   PROVIDING SUPPORT

5a.4.1   Opportunities for Smoking Cessation in a CPRP Setting

- Smokers hospitalised with an acute event may benefit from starting nicotine replacement therapy (NRT) or varenicline during hospital admission to help with withdrawal and to maintain their quit attempt after discharge.
- Joined-up care between hospital, CPRP, and general practice will facilitate follow up of patients.
- Patients making a quit attempt can be followed up regularly by the CPRP team, either face to face, by telephone, SMS texting, and/or email.

5a.4.2   Principles of a Withdrawal-oriented Approach

This approach is used in the NHS stop smoking services employing group therapy and adjunctive pharmacological support (Hajek 1989). The principles can be applied to a CPRP setting. Given that relapse following a quit attempt is most likely to occur within the first four weeks success may be improved by ensuring good support during this period.

5a.4.3 Behavioural Support

1. Identify and reinforce personal reasons given for quitting.
2. Build positive but realistic expectations for the quit attempt. Give information about withdrawal symptoms (Figure 5a.6) and the improved chances of success if medication is used to reduce discomfort from withdrawal. Discuss ways of coping (e.g. use of medication during urges, relaxation techniques). Reinforce the benefits of quitting (Figure 5a.11).
3. Elicit commitment to quit. Set a quit date. Recommend complete abstinence after this date – 'not a puff'! and prepare for the date (Figure 5a.12) at home and at work. If the patient prefers not to make a full blown quit attempt in the first instance, advise on reducing with NRT or varenicline (see Sections 5a.5 and 5a.6) for an explanation on how to cut down to stop with NRT or varenicline.
4. Emphasise the seriousness of the quit attempt and the importance of a good start – abstaining in the first week of the quit attempt indicates that they will be 10 times more likely to succeed.
5. Take a baseline CO reading and explain the significance (the CO level will return to normal level within one day of quitting). Repeat the measurement at every subsequent visit, especially in the first few weeks to demonstrate this reduction and check adherence.
6. Help patients to understand their behavioural addiction. Identify 'trigger' situations and record ways to manage them (Figure 5a.13).
7. Emphasise the temporary nature of physical withdrawal and point out that many have succeeded before. Reminders of initial commitment and reasons given for quitting can help.
8. Ensure a good understanding of what the medication can and cannot do. Give information about potential side effects from therapies (see

- HDL-Cholesterol: LDL-Cholesterol ratio will improve.
- Risk of myocardial infarction will halve within a year of quitting.
- Inflammatory markers will return to normal after 5 years.
- Mortality will be reduced.
- Within 15 years of quitting, risk of cardiovascular disease will be reduced to that of never smoker.

FIGURE 5A.11 Benefits of stopping smoking.

- Get rid of ash trays
- Choose the right moment
- Tell people who are important to you about the quit date

FIGURE 5A.12 Preparing to quit smoking.

Smoking trigger	How to deal with it
For example: Coffee in the morning	Have tea instead
1.	
2.	
3.	
4.	

FIGURE 5A.13 Managing smoking triggers.

Section 5a.4.4 on pharmacological agents to support quit attempts below). Encourage adherence and make sure the patient understands correct dosing, special instructions (taking with food, etc.), and duration of treatment. Monitor side effects and advise on how they can be managed.

9. Provide motivational support (encouragement, boosting self-efficacy, affirmation of success). A helpline (or SMS texting) is useful so that you can send a good luck message on the quit day and patients can contact you if they need 'emergency' assistance.

10. Provide guidance and information on how to deal with lapses:
    a. Set a new quit date if the patient continues to smoke daily following the quit date
    b. Encourage the patient to keep in contact even if they lapse or stop using the medication. Remind them that a lapse is not failure
    c. Explore motivation anew and remind patient of initial commitment
    d. Revisit all of the above steps.

5a.4.4 Pharmacological Agents

In the UK, three main types of medicines are used to help people to support quit attempts: nicotine receptor partial agonists (varenicline, known better by its brand name 'Champix'), NRT, and bupropion (Zyban). Medicines are an important adjunct to helping highly dependent smokers to cope with the symptoms of nicotine withdrawal. Unfortunately, these products are underused. Smokers wishing to quit may be unwilling to try them, and also health professionals may be reluctant to prescribe them for fears of safety. All of these medicines have been shown to be effective and are safe for patients with heart disease.

Each product is described below in terms of how the medicine works, how it should be taken, what the possible side effects are and what evidence there is to demonstrate its effectiveness.

5A.5 VARENICLINE

5a.5.1 What Is it?

Varenicline is a non-nicotine treatment developed specifically to aid stop smoking attempts by providing relief from craving and withdrawal symptoms.

5a.5.2 How Does it Work?

Varenicline provides relief from craving and withdrawal by binding to the $\alpha 4 \beta 2$ nicotinic receptor and partially stimulating it. As nicotine levels decline, this partial stimulation provides relief from craving and withdrawal, making it easier to quit smoking.

5a.5.3 How Is it Used?

An initial one week uptitration regime is required and shown in Figure 5a.14. An initiation pack is available, which contains eleven 0.5 mg tablets plus fourteen 1 mg tablets. The maintenance dose is 1 mg twice daily. This gradual increase is necessary to avoid nausea, which is the most commonly experienced side-effect of the drug. The twice daily dose should be taken at the beginning and the end of the day.

Day	Dose
Days 1–3	0.5 mg once daily
Days 4–7	0.5 mg twice daily
From day 8	1 mg twice daily
Quit date 1–2 weeks after starting treatment	

FIGURE 5A.14 Uptitrating varenicline.

5a.5.4 Reducing Smoking with Varenicline

Recent trial evidence suggests that smokers who are not ready to make an abrupt quit attempt in the next month may benefit from using a 24 week course of varenicline to reduce consumption initially by half in the first four weeks, then by three quarters by the end of eight weeks with a view to quitting at 12 weeks (Ebbert et al. 2015).

5a.5.5 Is it Safe?

Varenicline has been shown to be safe in the general population and also in smokers with both stable and acute CVD (Cahill et al. 2013; Eisenberg et al. 2015; Rigotti et al. 2010). Unsubstantiated early reports in the media of violent deaths and suicides in people who were taking varenicline have not been confirmed in large RCTs or comparative studies. In fact, varenicline may even have a protective effect for depression and all-cause mortality.

5a.5.6 Are there any Side Effects?

5a.5.6.1 Nausea

Approximately one third of patients suffer from nausea, often within 30 minutes of taking the medicine. It usually occurs within the first week of the course and sometimes ceases after the quit day. Less than 5% of nausea sufferers experience vomiting. Eating before taking the drug may help and, if necessary, the dose can be reduced from 1 mg twice per day to 0.5 mg twice per day. Many patients will be prepared to tolerate the nausea because of its temporary nature.

5a.5.6.2 Abnormal Dreams

The second most common side effect is abnormal and vivid dreaming. This is also a side effect associated with the 24 hour nicotine patch. The probable explanation for it is the activation of nicotine receptors when a person is asleep, when people do not smoke. Whilst it is important to forewarn people of this side effect, it is not necessarily distressing and may well be tolerated, lasting no more than two or three weeks.

Some people may experience insomnia, although this is also a symptom of withdrawal from nicotine. If it is a result of nicotine withdrawal, it should last for no more than a week.

5a.5.7 Ending Treatment

At the end of the 12 weeks course of varenicline, patients will probably benefit from extending the course for an additional 12 weeks if they quit late or if they relapse during their first course of treatment (Hajek et al. 2009).

5A.6   NICOTINE REPLACEMENT THERAPY

5a.6.1   What Is it?

NRT delivers nicotine into the body more slowly than cigarettes. The method of delivery is either by transdermal patch, or various preparations that are delivered via the buccal route (microtabs, lozenges, mouthspray, inhalator, and gum) or absorbed in the nose (nasal spray). Of these the transdermal patch gives the slowest uptake and the nasal spray the fastest. None of them are as fast as cigarettes.

5a.6.2   How Does it Work?

By replacing the nicotine from cigarettes, this drug aims to reduce the urge to smoke and to reduce the withdrawal symptoms associated with quitting smoking.

5a.6.3   How Is it Used?

- Prescribe a long-acting product (nicotine patch) to deliver a background dose of nicotine throughout the day in the 16 hour preparation, and throughout the day and night in the 24 hour preparation.
- In combination, prescribe short-acting products like nicotine nasal spray, inhalator, gum, lozenges, and microtabs to deliver boosts throughout the course of the day when urges to smoke occur. This combination of slow and faster acting NRT has been demonstrated to be the optimal way to use NRT.
- NRT can be used for prolonged periods of up to and beyond nine months, if necessary, in people who are heavily dependent and still feel vulnerable after quitting.
- Generally start with the highest dose (21 mg) 24 hour patch and reduce if the patient experiences nausea or other untoward symptoms.
- As 16 hour patches are not worn overnight, they are useful for people who suffer from insomnia.
- The nasal spray is very useful in those who are heavily physically dependent (smoking more than 20 per day). The dose ranges from 8 to 64 sprays per day.

5a.6.4   'Cut Down to Stop' with NRT

Some smokers may not be willing to try to quit immediately. A protocol has been proposed by ASH (www.ash.co.uk) to aid gradual reduction of smoking as a prelude to a full quit attempt (Figure 5a.15). Using this protocol could require

Step	When	Goal
1	0–6 weeks	Cut down to 50% of baseline cigarette consumption
2	6 weeks to 6 months	Continue to cut down: stop completely by 6 months
3	6 to 9 months	Stop smoking completely, continue NRT
4	Within 12 months	Stop using NRT by 12 months

FIGURE 5A.15   Using Nicotine Replacement Therapy (NRT) to reduce smoking in the run up to a quit attempt.

treatment for six months or more. Each time you see a patient using this method, it is important to reassess motivation and confidence, assess tolerance of the NRT products and that the correct dose and technique is being used. ASH recommends that prescriptions should be issued two weeks at a time, and no repeat prescriptions should be issued during the cutting down period unless daily reduction is reported (50% by six weeks), validated with breath CO. Once the individual has reached a stage where they want to stop completely, use the baseline smoking consumption level to decide on the dose for NRT during the quit attempt.

Using this method, a third of smokers who reduce their cigarette consumption by half with NRT will be abstinent at one year.

Other regimens have been described for reducing NRT in the run up to a quit attempt. In addition, harm reduction approaches also use NRT to allow reduced intake of tobacco using nicotine.

5a.6.5   Is it Safe?

NRT is no longer contraindicated in patients who have had a myocardial infarction, especially when the danger of continuing to smoke is taken into account. When nicotine is inhaled via a cigarette, it reaches the brain rapidly. NRT does not allow such a rapid entry of nicotine. Since 2005 licensing arrangements for using NRT include the use of NRT in patients with CVD, concurrent use of more than one form of NRT, prolonged use of NRT beyond 12 weeks, and the use of NRT in the context of current smoking with a view to reducing consumption of tobacco.

5a.6.6   Are there any Side Effects?

NRT can cause nausea if it is taken in large doses. It can also cause local skin irritation (patches) and irritation to the mucosa in the mouth and nose (other forms) so rotation of sites is recommended.

5A.7   COMBINING VARENICLINE WITH COMBINATION NRT

A systematic review and meta-analysis of three RCTs from 2015 (Chang et al. 2015), which investigated the combination of varenicline with NRT patch versus placebo showed a significant effect on abstinence. This was especially true when a pre-treatment nicotine patch was used for two weeks prior to the quit date.

5A.8   BUPROPION

As efficacy in varenicline or a combination of long- and short-acting NRT products has been shown to be superior to bupropion, it is now advisable to use bupropion when it is not possible to use the other products.

5a.8.1   What Is It and How Does It Work?

Bupropion is a weak dopamine and nor-epinephrine reuptake inhibitor. Depressive symptoms can occur during smoking cessation. Smoking helps to increase central dopamine levels. Taking bupropion may help to maintain central dopamine in the absence of nicotine. However, the smoking cessation effect of bupropion is independent of the anti-depressant effect.

5a.8.2   How Is It Used?

When prescribing bupropion, the quit date should be set for one to two weeks after the individual has started to take the medication. The dose should be increased from 150 mg every morning for six days to 150 mg twice daily. The treatment should be continued for between seven and nine weeks.

5a.8.3   Safety and Side Effects

Burpropion is contraindicated in people with a history of, or increased risk of, seizures or eating disorders. No increase in cardiovascular or neuropsychiatric events has been reported.

5A.9   EFFICACY AND SAFETY

The evidence for efficacy and safety for all three pharmacological agents is summarised and compared in an overview and network meta-analysis of 12 Cochrane reviews of RCTs (Cahill et al. 2013). The EAGLES trial (Anthenelli et al. 2016), the first and largest RCT to date of approved smoking cessation medicines commissioned by the US Food and Drug Administration (FDA) and the European Medicines Agency (EMA), more recently confirmed the same in both psychiatric and non-psychiatric patients.

In the Cochrane review, the use of network meta-analysis as opposed to a conventional meta-analysis allowed indirect comparisons before high quality direct head to head comparisons like those available in the EAGLES trial were available. It included an assessment of NRT combination short- and long-acting formulations versus single formulations and how they compare with the other drugs, and investigated how well NRT, varenicline, and bupropion compare with placebo and with each other in achieving abstinence beyond six months from tobacco. The review also investigated other therapies that are not used in the UK (e.g. cystisine and nortriptyline) and it also looked at safety. The results of the review are summarised in Figure 5a.16.

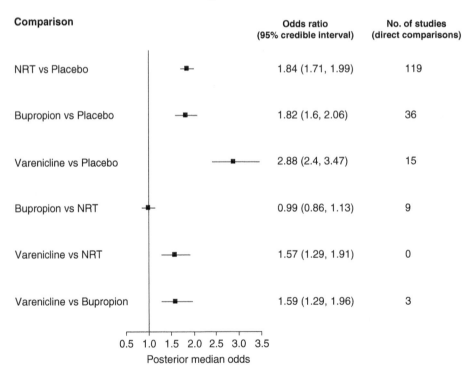

Comparison		Odds ratio (95% credible interval)	No. of studies (direct comparisons)
NRT vs Placebo		1.84 (1.71, 1.99)	119
Bupropion vs Placebo		1.82 (1.6, 2.06)	36
Varenicline vs Placebo		2.88 (2.4, 3.47)	15
Bupropion vs NRT		0.99 (0.86, 1.13)	9
Varenicline vs NRT		1.57 (1.29, 1.91)	0
Varenicline vs Bupropion		1.59 (1.29, 1.96)	3

0.5 1.0 1.5 2.0 2.5 3.0 3.5
Posterior median odds

FIGURE 5A.16   Network meta-analysis of first-line pharmacotherapies versus placebo and versus each other, with Nicotine Replacement Therapy (NRT) split by type (Cahill et al. 2013).

Whilst all three drugs are effective in helping more people to stop than placebo, the most effective agents are varenicline and combination NRT. All three drugs are safe for use in patients with heart disease and do not increase the risk of neuropsychiatric or circulatory problems.

5A.10 ELECTRONIC CIGARETTES

Electronic e-cigarettes [also known as electronic nicotine delivery systems (ENDS) or electronic vaping devices] are becoming increasingly popular in people attempting to quit smoking in England since early 2012 (Figure 5a.17). They have evolved through three generations of product from the early cigarette look-alike to the tank mechanism devices, which are much more effective at delivering nicotine to their users (see Figure 5a.18). Public Health England (https://www.gov.uk/government/collections/electronic-cigarettes) and the Royal College of Physicians (www.rcplondon.ac.uk/news/promote-e-cigarettes-widely-substitute-smoking-says-new-rcp-report) recommend that smoking cessation counsellors support people using e-cigarettes if this is their preferred method to quit. The National Centre for Smoking Cessation Training (NCSCT) issued a briefing for advisers at the beginning of 2016, which is available for download from their website: www.ncsct.co.uk/publication_electronic_cigarette_briefing.php.

Smokers who report that they use nicotine for both temporary abstinence and smoking reduction are more likely than those who use it for either to go on to stop smoking completely.

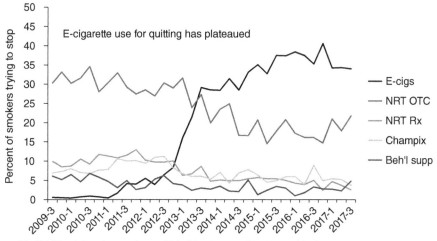

N=13146 adults who smoke and tried to stop or who stopped in the past year; method is coded as any (not exclusive) use

OTC: over the counter

FIGURE 5A.17 Use of e-cigarettes for smoking cessation (www.smokinginengland.info).

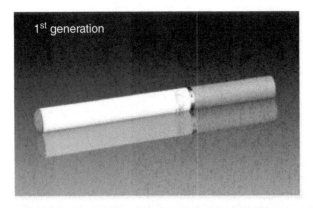

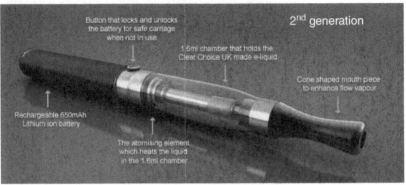

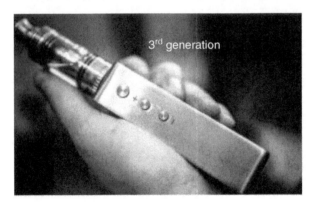

FIGURE 5A.18 Types of e-cigarettes.

Current evidence in relation to e-cigarettes (Hartmann-Boyce et al. 2016; Rahman et al. 2015) concludes that:

- e-cigarettes may be helpful in smoking cessation or in helping smokers who cannot quit safely to reduce their consumption

- Health professionals may consider advising smokers to use e-cigarettes if they have been unsuccessful with conventional therapies
- Regulating e-cigarettes as strictly as cigarettes, or even more strictly as some regulators propose, is not warranted on current evidence
- Smokers who attempt to stop without support are more likely to report continued abstinence using e-cigarettes than those using over the counter NRT or nothing
- We need more high quality research on this topic.

5A.11   CONCLUSION

Tobacco use remains a major risk factor in the UK and takes several years off life expectancy. Nicotine is addictive and a major barrier to tobacco cessation. Smokers suffering an acute cardiovascular event should be offered NRT or varenicline in hospital as they may be suffering acute withdrawal and it may help them to sustain abstinence after hospital discharge. Most smokers want to quit but are lacking in confidence to achieve a successful attempt, so an offer of support should be made in the hope that it will provoke a quit attempt. The most effective pharmacotherapies to support a quit attempt are varenicline and combination long- and short-acting NRT.

5A.12   COMPONENT LEADERS WITHIN A CPRP

Any professional or other health worker who is appropriately trained in smoking cessation strategies can support smokers in a quit attempt. Nurses, pharmacists, and doctors may have an advantage as they are able to prescribe pharmacological aids. However, in the context of this clinical setting, nurses are best placed to lead this component.

5A.13   WEIGHT GAIN AND SMOKING CESSATION

Weight gain after smoking cessation is common with an average increase after 12 months of 4–5 kg (Aubin et al. 2012). It is not usually a reason for relapse, although it can be. Stopping smoking is associated with enormous benefits in terms of life expectancy, which outweigh the risks of weight gain.

Potential opportunities for preventing weight gain present themselves in a CPRP setting because programmes are associated with promoting physical activity and exercise and managing dietary habits. The results of the EUROAC-TION plus varenicline study (Jennings et al. 2014) suggested that weight gain could be mitigated during a programme for vascular and high CVD risk smokers trying to quit, although follow up only extended to 16 weeks. The mean weight gain at this time was 1.63 kg. This compares with between 2.85 and 4.23 kg at 3–6 months in the above referenced meta-analysis of weight gain in the control arms of RCTs testing interventions to prevent weight gain after smoking cessation.

5A.14   HARM REDUCTION

Very dependent smokers may find it difficult and even impossible to stop smoking. Whilst it is best to stop smoking altogether, there may be some benefit in reducing harm by reducing exposure to tobacco in highly dependent smokers. NICE issued guidance in 2013 (NICE 2013) to advise on how best to implement harm reduction strategies. The guiding principle is that in highly dependent individuals, nicotine delivered without tobacco reduces exposure to the dangerous toxins contained in tobacco. Reducing smoking without nicotine leads to compensatory smoking (see Figure 5a.19). The guidance has been written for people who are unable to give up nicotine and achieve an abrupt quit but want to reduce the amount they smoke.

The products that are available for use include both licensed nicotine products like NRT, but also unlicensed products like electronic cigarettes. The NICE guidance does not at present recommend unlicensed products. However, Public Health England and the Royal College of Physicians are supportive of the use of electronic cigarettes for harm reduction. Lifelong exposure to NRT is probably considerably less harmful than smoking; however, evidence is lacking for safety and efficacy of unlicensed products like e-cigarettes. Nevertheless it is quite feasible that they will be less harmful than tobacco.

Barriers to the use of this approach include misconceptions about nicotine with a considerable number of people believing that it is carcinogenic and harmful. In addition both the lay public and health professionals wrongly believe that long-term use is dangerous and reduction using nicotine undermines smoking cessation attempts (Beard et al. 2012).

- When smokers try to reduce their daily consumption, for example from 20 to 10 cigarettes, they will start to draw more heavily on each cigarette they smoke in an attempt to get as much nicotine as possible. They will therefore continue to get just as much of the toxic substances from these cigarettes
- The more the smoker reduces daily consumption, the less they are able to compensate, and the more precious each cigarette becomes
- Reducing the daily consumption rarely leads to complete abstinence
- Reduction should be associated with concomitant use of NRT

FIGURE 5A.19   Reducing cigarette consumption and compensatory smoking.

REFERENCES

Akl, E.A., Gaddam, S., Gunukula, S.K. et al. (2010). The effects of waterpipe tobacco smoking on health outcomes: a systematic review. *International Journal of Epidemiology* 39 (3): 834–857.

Anthenelli, R.M., Benowitz, N.L., West, R. et al. (2016). Neuropsychiatric safety and efficacy of varenicline, bupropion, and nicotine patch in smokers with and without psychiatric disorders (EAGLES): a double-blind, randomised, placebo-controlled clinical trial. *Lancet* 387: 2507–2520.

Aubin, H.J., Farley, A., Lycett, D. et al. (2012). Weight gain in smokers after quitting cigarettes: meta-analysis. *British Medical Journal* 345: e4439.

Baker, T.B., Piper, M.E., McCarthy, D.E. et al. (2007). Time to first cigarette in the morning as an index of ability to quit smoking: implications for nicotine dependence. *Nicotine & Tobacco Research* 9 (4): S555–S570.

Beard, E., Vangeli, E., Michie, S., and West, R. (2012). The use of nicotine replacement therapy for smoking reduction and temporary abstinence: an interview study. *Nicotine & Tobacco Research* 14 (7): 849–856.

Bedfont Scientific Ltd - Smokerlyzer (2016). *Bedfont Scientific Ltd.* http://www.bedfont.com/shop/smokerlyzer (accessed 7 June 2016).

Cahill, K., Stevens, S., Perera, R., and Lancaster, T. (2013). Pharmacological interventions for smoking cessation: an overview and network meta-analysis. *Cochrane Database of Systematic Reviews* 31 (5): CD009329.

Care Fusion (2016). Smoking cessation. Vyaire Medical. http://www.carefusion.co.uk/our-products/respiratory-care/cardio-pulmonary-diagnostics/smoking-cessation (accessed 7 June 2016).

Chabrol, H., Niezborala, M., Chastan, E., and De Leon, J. (2005). Comparison of the heavy smoking index and of the Fagerström test for nicotine dependence in a sample of 749 cigarette smokers. *Addict Behaviours* 30 (7): 1474–1477.

Chang, P., Chiang, C., Ho, W. et al. (2015). Combination therapy of varenicline with nicotine replacement therapy is better than varenicline alone: a systematic review and meta-analysis of randomized controlled trials. *BMC Public Health* 15: 689. https://doi.org/10.1186/s12889-015-2055-0.

Cinciripini, P.M., Robinson, J.D., Karam-Hage, M. et al. (2013). Effects of varenicline and bupropion sustained-release use plus intensive smoking cessation counseling on prolonged abstinence from smoking and on depression, negative affect, and other symptoms of nicotine withdrawal. *Journal of the American Medical Association (JAMA) Psychiatry* 70 (5): 522–533.

Department of Health, Cancer Research UK, Tobacco Research Group and Smoking Tobacco Study (2016). Smoking in England. Cancer Research UK. http://www.smokinginengland.info (accessed 7 June 2016).

Ebbert, J.O., Hughes, J.R., West, R.J. et al. (2015). Effect of Varenicline on smoking cessation through smoking reduction: a randomized clinical trial. *Journal of the American Medical Association* 313 (7): 687–694. https://doi.org/10.1001/jama.2015.280.

Edwards, A.C. and Kendler, K.S. (2011). Nicotine withdrawal-induced negative affect is a function of nicotine dependence and not liability to depression or anxiety. *Nicotine & Tobacco Research* 13 (8): 677–685.

Edwards, R. (2004). The problem of tobacco smoking. *British Medical Journal* 328 (7433): 217–219.

Eisenberg, M.J., Windle, S.B., Roy, N. et al. (2015). Varenicline for smoking cessation in hospitalised patients with acute coronary syndrome. *Circulation* 133: 21–30. https://doi.org/10.1161/CIRCULATIONAHA.115.019634.

Fidler, J.A., Shahab, L., and West, R. (2011). Strength of urges to smoke as a measure of severity of cigarette dependence: comparison with the Fagerström test for nicotine dependence and its components. *Addiction* 106 (3): 631–638.

GBD 2015 Tobacco Collaborators (2017). Smoking prevalence and attributable disease burden in 195 countries and territories, 1990–2015: a systematic analysis from the Global Burden of Disease Study 2015. *Lancet* 389: 1885–1906.

Hajek, P. (1989). Withdrawal-oriented therapy for smokers. *British Journal of Addiction* 84 (6): 591–598.

Hajek, P., Tonnesen, P., Arteaga, C. et al. (2009). Varenicline in prevention of relapse to smoking: effect of quit pattern on response to extended treatment. *Addiction* 104 (9): 1597–1602.

Hartmann-Boyce, J., McRobbie, H., Bullen, C. et al. (2016). Electronic cigarettes for smoking cessation (review). *Cochrane Database of Systematic Reviews* https://doi.org/10.1002/14651858.CD010216.pub3.

Heatherton, T.F., Kozlowski, L.T., Frecker, R.C., and Fagerström, K.O. (1991). The Fagerstrom test for nicotine dependence: a revision of the Fagerström tolerance questionnaire. *British Journal of Addiction* 86 (9): 1119–1127.

Hiscock, R., Bauld, L., Amos, A., and Platt, S. (2012). Smoking and socioeconomic status in England: the rise of the never smoker and the disadvantaged smoker. *Journal of Public Health* 34 (3): 390–396.

Jennings, C., Kotseva, K., De Bacquer, D. et al. (2014). Effectiveness of a preventive cardiology programme for high CVD risk persistent smokers: the EUROACTION PLUS varenicline trial. *European Heart Journal* 35 (21): 1411–1420.

Kotseva, K., Jennings, C.S., Turner, E.L. et al. (2012). ASPIRE-2-PREVENT: a survey of lifestyle, risk factor management and cardioprotective medication in patients with coronary heart disease and people at high risk of developing cardiovascular disease in the UK. *Heart* 98: 865.

Kotz, D., Viechtbauer, W., Simpson, C. et al. (2015). Cardiovascular and neuropsychiatric risks of varenicline: a retrospective cohort study. *The Lancet Respiratory Medicine* 3: 761–768.

Law, M.R., Morris, J.K., and Wald, N.J. (1997). Environmental tobacco smoke exposure and ischaemic heart disease: an evaluation of the evidence. *British Medical Journal* 315 (7114): 973–980.

Lifestyles Statistics Team, Health and Social Care Information Centre; Niblett, P. (2015). Statistics on Smoking, England 2015. NHS Digital. https://files.digital. nhs.uk/publicationimport/pub17xxx/pub17526/stat-smok-eng-2015-rep.pdf (accessed 7 June 2016).

Lin, H., Wang, H., Wu, W. et al. (2013). The effects of smoke-free legislation on acute myocardial infarction: a systematic review and meta-analysis. *BMC Public Health* 13 (529) http://www.biomedcentral.com/1471-2458/13/529.

National Centre for Smoking Cessation and Training (2018). *National Centre for Smoking Cessation and Training* Available at: https://www.ncsct.co.uk/ publication_ncsct-training-standard-learning-outcomes-for-training-stop-smoking-practitioners.php

NICE (2013). Smoking: Harm reduction. National Institute for Health and Care Excellence. www.nice.org.uk/guidance/PH45 (accessed 7 June 2016).

Prugger, C., Wellmann, J., Heidrich, J. et al. (2014). Passive smoking and smoking cessation among patients with coronary heart disease across Europe: results from the EUROASPIRE III survey. *European Heart Journal* 35 (9): 590–598.

Rahman, M.A., Rahman, M.A., Hann, N. et al. (2015). E-cigarettes and smoking cessation: evidence from a systematic review and meta-analysis. *PLoS One* 10 (3): e0122544. https://doi.org/10.1371/journal.pone.0122544.

Rigotti, N.A., Pipe, A.L., Benowitz, N.L. et al. (2010). Efficacy and safety of varenicline for smoking cessation in patients with cardiovascular disease: a randomized trial. *Circulation* 121 (2): 221–229.

Royal College of Physicians (2000). Nicotine addicition in Britain. A report of the Tobacco Advisory Group of the Royal College of Physicians. Royal College of Physicians. Print.

Taylor, G., McNeill, A., Girling, A. et al. (2014). Change in mental health after smoking cessation: systematic review and meta-analysis. *British Medical Journal* 348: g1151. http://dx.doi.org/10.1136/bmj.g1151.

West, R. (2009). The multiple facets of cigarette addiction and what they mean for encouraging and helping smokers to stop. *Journal of Chronic Obstructive Pulmonary Disease* 6 (4): 277–283.

FURTHER READING

West, R. (2013). *The SmokeFree Formula. A revolutionary way to give up smoking.* Croydon, UK: Orion Publishing Group.

Diet and Weight Management

Alison Atrey[1] and Rachel Vine[2]

[1] CVD Management, Toronto, Ontario, Canada
[2] Leeds Community Healthcare NHS Trust, Parkside Community Health Centre, Leeds, UK

Abstract

The aims of this chapter are to investigate the relationship between diet, obesity, and cardiovascular disease (CVD). In meeting these aims, the topics covered include the components of both weight management and helping patients to follow a cardio-protective diet. In relation to weight management, the areas covered are: maintaining weight-loss, avoidance of weight cycling and the role of pharmacological support if required. In applying the concepts from Chapters 2 and 4, diet and weight management support needs to be delivered in an individualised manner. As part of the individualised behaviour change process, helping patients learn self-management skills of food and weight monitoring is key to enabling sustainable eating habits to maintain a healthy weight. An important element of healthy eating includes an understanding of dietary misconceptions that are common within many long term health conditions. At the end of the chapter are several case studies to illustrate how to implement effective dietary and weight management support.

Keywords: *diet, obesity, cardiovascular, Mediterranean diet*

Cardiovascular Prevention and Rehabilitation in Practice, Second Edition.
Edited by Jennifer Jones, John Buckley, Gill Furze, and Gail Sheppard.
© 2020 John Wiley & Sons Ltd. Published 2020 by John Wiley & Sons Ltd.

Key Points

- To ensure trained healthcare professionals are able to support patients effectively with diet and weight issues by accurately assessing diet and body composition, providing tailored 'first line' advice on cardioprotective diets/weight management, and to dispel food myths.
- To provide accurate assessment tools to enable health professionals to identify realistic dietary changes.
- To enable health professionals to understand the influences of dietary intake.

5B.1   RATIONALE AND AIMS

Diet plays an important role in obesity and cardiovascular disease (CVD) management. The relationship between CVD risk factors and abdominal obesity means that many patients referred to prevention and rehabilitation programmes are overweight or obese. The consequence of this is that weight management becomes an integral and essential part of any programme. Using examples of interview techniques, this chapter aims to provide health professionals with tools and techniques to elicit better information from patients. A key factor of dietary assessments is intake and facilitating patients to identify realistic dietary changes. Assessment tools are also used to monitor compliance in the longer term (Gandy 2014).

This section will apply the latest evidence on diet, obesity, and CVD with the aim of providing a 'how to' deliver evidence-based dietary aspects in day-to-day practice.

5B.2   INFLUENCES OF DIETARY INTAKE

For health professionals to complete a detailed and accurate assessment, it is essential that they understand dietary intake has many influences. Factors affecting food choices can be one or a combination of any of the following:

- Cultural background, religious or ethical beliefs
- Psychological (rewarding, punishing, comfort eating)
- Appetite level, taste preferences
- Financial issues/facilities available
- Lifestyle/work hours and commitments (e.g. shift work, business travel)

- Social conventions/how food is eaten (e.g. in front of TV; sat as family at a table; 'on the move')/weekdays and weekend differences/eating out
- Family/peer group pressures or advertising
- Knowledge/beliefs about food and diet
- Previous advice or diet attempts including weight history, e.g. 'yo-yo' dieting.

The dynamic of any household has a strong influence on the dietary habits of the people living within that house. Identification and collaboration with the person who is in charge of the food purchasing and food preparation is essential to improve outcome and long-term dietary change.

All subjects should be assessed for their readiness and motivation to change. Beneficial dietary changes need to be long term. Therefore all suggested changes should be realistic and achievable. For more information see Chapter 4.

5b.2.1   Question Style Influences Accuracy of Dietary Intake Reporting

People are often sensitive about what they consume. This can lead to reluctance and underestimation of what they perceive as 'bad' foods and overestimation of 'good' foods. To reduce this possible error it is important to ask open, indirect, or non-leading questions. To illustrate this last point, compare the following question formats:

'Do you have milk in tea?' (closed question) with 'How do you have your tea?' (open question).

'How much butter do you use?' (direct question) with 'How long does a pack of butter last you?' (indirect question).

'What do you have for breakfast?' (leading question) with 'What would be the first thing you would eat or drink in the morning?' (non-leading question).

5B.3   ASSESSMENT METHODS OF DIETARY INTAKE

In clinical practice there are two methods of assessment: recall and recorded.

5b.3.1   Recall

Recalling dietary intake is interview-led, 24 hours after the patient's last intake. Using this method, the health professional is able to obtain detailed information about usual foods and drinks consumed. Portion sizes, food preparation methods, and food frequency information can also be collected. Using this method multiple days in a row as opposed to a summary interview at the end of several days also improves precision.

The Mediterranean Diet Score (MDS) is another way of using the recall method. It is also interview-led, with the health professional obtaining specific information on the intake of food and alcohol linked with the Mediterranean diet. All aspects of the Mediterranean diet are described and a point is scored for each aspect achieved (see the Mediterranean diet Key Message).

5b.3.2   Recorded Methods

Participants self-record all that is eaten and drunk by writing in diaries. The length of period can vary (three to seven days are most common). The portions are described either in household measures, weighed, in average portions, from photographs, or in pack sizes. This type of method is labour intensive and reliant on subjects having the literacy skills and motivation to complete correctly.

The majority of methods (recall or recorded) are dependent on the estimation of portion sizes. Portions of food are often difficult to quantify. The participant's perception of what an average portion is will vary, especially of those foods that are perceived to be 'bad' or 'good'. The use or taking of photographs showing or recording portion sizes can improve estimation in a non-judgemental manner.

5B.4   ASSESSMENT OF BODY COMPOSITION

Anthropometric measurements provide predictions of body composition, such as body mass, fat stores, and body water. There are a number of different measures. This section focuses on the most common in clinical practice.

5b.4.1   Body Mass Index (BMI)

This is an index of 'weight for height'.

$$BMI = weight(kg) / (height(m))^2$$

It is commonly used to classify underweight, overweight, and obesity in adults. This WHO classification is primarily based on the association between body mass index (BMI) and mortality. The Asian population's risk for CVD develops at lower BMI levels and therefore the BMI classification differs (Figure 5b.1).

White European Population	Asian Population	Description
<18.5	< 18.5	Underweight
18.5–24.9	18.5–23	Increasing but acceptable risk
25–29.9	23–27.5	Increased risk
30 or higher	27.5 or higher	High risk

FIGURE 5B.1   Body Mass Index (BMI) public health action points for White European and Asian populations (NICE 2013a).

European	Men	≥ 94cm (37 inches)
	Women	≥ 80cm (31.5 inches)
South Asian	Men	≥ 90cm (35 inches)
	Women	≥ 80cm (31.5 inches)
Chinese	Men	≥ 90cm (35 inches)
	Women	≥ 80cm (31.5 inches)
Japanese	Men	≥ 90cm (35 inches)
	Women	≥ 80cm (31.5 inches)
Ethnic South and Central Americans	Use South Asian until more specific recommendations are available	
Sub Saharan Africans, Eastern Mediterranean, and Middle East (Arab)	Use European until more specific recommendations are available	

FIGURE 5B.2   Waist circumference (WC) thresholds as a measure of central obesity (NICE 2013a).

5b.4.2   Waist Circumference

Waist circumference (WC) measures abdominal obesity and is a useful anthropometric predictor of cardiovascular risk. A 1 cm increase in WC is associated with a 2% increase in risk of future CVD (Despres et al. 2001). Figure 5b.2 shows classifications for WC (NICE 2013a).

How to measure:

- Sit in front of the individual.
- Ensure the individual is standing straight with both feet together (supporting themselves on a piece of furniture if they cannot balance) looking straight ahead.
- Measure next to the skin or over one piece of light clothing.

To measure waist:

- Measure midway between the lower rib margin and the iliac crest (approx. 2.5 cm above the naval).
- Mark the level of the lowest rib margin and iliac crest in the mid-axillary line.
- Pass the tape horizontally around the subject's circumference midway between the marked points.
- The tape should be taut. Ensure individual is relaxed and breathing normally. Take measurement on expiration.

Technology is providing a variety of ways to monitor and assess diet and weight.

Online tools:

- Dietary intake – http://dapa-toolkit.mrc.ac.uk/dietary-assessment
- Weight – http://www.bdaweightwise.com
- Example of photographic portion size resource: http://www.carbsandcals.com/hcp/hcp

Smartphone applications:

- NHS Choices – http://www.nhs.uk/conditions/nhs-health-check/pages/tools-and-technology-that-can-help.aspx

Tools to measure outcomes:

- MDS
- **S**pecific, **M**easurable, **A**ttainable, **R**elevant, and **T**ime-bound (SMART) goals
- Target weight and/or WC
- Dietary targets set.

5B.5   COMPONENTS OF CARDIOPROTECTIVE DIETARY ADVICE

5b.5.1   Mediterranean Diet

- The composition of the Mediterranean diet pattern can be established by looking at the MDS. Each question highlights a different aspect of this dietary pattern.

- Mediterranean diet comes from epidemiology research and trial data, e.g.:
  - Sofi et al. (2008) showed a two-point change in the 9-point MDS, equivalent to a 9% reduction in CVD risk.
  - PREDIMED (Estruch et al. 2013) used a 14-point MDS for people following a Mediterranean dietary pattern supplemented with either extra virgin oil or mixed nuts, experienced a 30% reduction in CVD risk.

Key Message

Emphasise that the Mediterranean diet is a 'whole' diet approach. The MDS captures numerically the overall quality of the dietary pattern. It can be used as both an audit tool and as part of a dietary assessment. During any intervention the score should ideally rise. MDS is now part of NACR and a tool to facilitate use for non-dietitians is available through the National Audit of Cardiac Rehabilitation (NACR 2013).

5b.5.2   Fats

It is often misconceived that a cardioprotective diet is low in fat. However, a modified fat diet, where saturated fat content is reduced and replaced with unsaturated fat is associated with a 17% reduction in CVD risk (Hooper et al. 2015).

- Fat is normally divided into three main types depending on their structure. Figure 5b.3 shows their sources and effect on CVD factors.
- Guidelines may sometimes appear to provide conflicting messages on which unsaturated fat is best to eat. For instance, NICE guidance post myocardial infarction (MI) (NICE 2013b) recommends swapping saturated fatty acids (SFA) with monounsaturated fatty acids (MUFA) as part of a Mediterranean diet. Whereas the latest JBS3 Board (2014) recommendations for the whole CVD prevention continuum (people at risk +/− with CVD) highlight that the wealth of evidence resides with research promoting SFA be swapped with polyunsaturated fatty acids (PUFA) rather then MUFA due to the lack of data on MUFA. Due to recent media, public, and scientific debate on saturated fats, the UK Scientific Advisory Committee on Nutrition (SACN) has set up a working group to examine the evidence linking saturated fats and health outcomes.

Type of Fat (Fatty Acid)	Where it is found	Effect on CVD risk factors
Saturated Fatty Acids (SFA) *(Palmitic acid Stearic acid)*	**Animal Products** – Meat fat, cheese, cream, butter, dripping, pastry, ghee **Plant Products** – Coconut, palm oil	▪ **Increases LDL and HDL cholesterol** ▪ **Enhances atherosclerosis development**
Monounsaturated Fatty Acids (MFA) **Omega-9** *(Oleic acid)*	▪ Olive oil ▪ Rapeseed oil ▪ Groundnut (peanut) oil ▪ Nuts & Seeds (almonds, hazelnuts, pecan, macadamia) ▪ Avocado	▪ **Reduces total & LDL cholesterol when substituting SFA** ▪ **Small change in HDL cholesterol** ▪ **Less risk of lipid peroxidation than PUFA**
Polyunsaturated Fatty Acids (PFA) Omega-3 *(Alpha-linoleic acid ALA EPA DHA)*	**Oily fish**–mackerel, salmon, sardines, trout, pilchards, herrings **Oils**–Canola/rapeseed & flaxseed **Enriched products** – eggs, milk, yoghurt which contain ALA sources	▪ **Minimal effect on blood cholesterol** ▪ **Very high doses via supplementation reduces triglycerides** ▪ **Anti-thrombotic, anti-arrhythmic & anti-inflammatory effect**
Polyunsaturated Fatty Acids Omega-6 (PFA – Omega 6) *(Linoleic acid Arahidonic acid)*	**Oils**–sunflower, safflower, corn, walnut and soybean	▪ **Reduces LDL & total cholesterol** ▪ **Increases HDL cholesterol slightly,** ▪ **Enhance lipid peroxidation & free radical production.**
Trans Fatty Acids (TFA) *(Partially hydrogenated fatty acids)*	Artificially created through a chemical process of the hydrogenation of oils and found in: – Dairy products, cakes, biscuits, processed foods, deep fried fast foods	▪ **Increases LDL and total cholesterol** ▪ **Reduces HDL cholesterol** ▪ **Enhances atherosclerosis development**

FIGURE 5B.3   Different types of fat, sources, and effect on CVD.

- Latest guidelines are consistent on not advising omega-3 supplementation when people are unable to eat oily fish. This recent change is due to the fact that more recent studies have not been able to replicate the largely protective effect previously seen when medical treatment is optimised.
- There is no evidence of harm and oily fish is still part of a cardioprotective diet so should be included but the higher intake emphasised in previous guidelines has now changed.

Key Message

Replace SFA with PUFA or MUFA where possible and promote practical tips to improve fat intake (BDA 2015a). Such tips may include:

- Avoid very high sources of SFA and trans fatty acids (TFA)
- Increase the use of unsaturated fats – nuts/seeds as a healthy snack
- Instead of frying – steam, boil, microwave, or bake
- Limit fat added to cooking by measuring it out
- Choose leaner meats and leaner cuts of meat, remove skin from poultry
- Choose lower fat options
- Change the proportions on your plate so you have more vegetables than protein or carbohydrate.

Recommendations relating to intake of omega-3 can be:

- Do not routinely recommend eating oily fish for the sole purpose of preventing another MI. If people choose to consume oily fish, health-care professionals should be aware that there is no evidence of harm of a high intake, and fish may form part of a Mediterranean-style diet, i.e. three servings a week.
- Do not offer or advise people to use omega-3 fatty acid capsules or omega-3 fatty acid supplemented foods to prevent another MI.

To reduce the intake of TFA, recommend patients to limit food where the ingredients state they are made with hydrogenated or partially hydrogenated fat, e.g. found in margarines, bought cakes/pastries/biscuits, processed foods, and deep fat fried fast food (BDA 2014a).

The results of changing eating habits can be measured using the MDS (NACR 2013).

5b.5.3   Fruit and Vegetables

Fruit and vegetables are a key component of a cardioprotective diet due to their beneficial properties:

- High in soluble fibre and therefore have a low glycaemic index (GI)
- High in antioxidants, folic acid, and potassium
- Low in fat and calories.

They improve CV risk by:

- Reducing cholesterol levels, blood pressure, homocysteine levels
- Protecting against formation of oxidised LDL and free radicals
- Helping with weight management
- Improving gut transit time and glycaemic control.

Key Message

Work towards achieving the United Kingdom's '5 A DAY' message. However, a Mediterranean diet should be equivalent to $8 \times 80\,g$ UK portions per day (five from vegetables and three from fruit). Portion size should also be clarified. A rough guide for portion control is to use the palm of your hand. When counting fruit portions, fresh, frozen, tinned, dried, or fruit juice can be counted. Limit fruit juice and smoothies to 150 ml per day as one portion (SACN 2015). Potatoes do not count towards the vegetable portion (BDA 2014; NHS Choices 2016a).

Different coloured fruit and vegetables should be encouraged to maximise vitamin and mineral content. There is no need to take vitamin and mineral supplements if a balanced diet is consumed. High doses of supplements have been associated with harmful effects.

5b.5.4   Whole Grains and Fibre

There is an inverse relationship between fibre intake and CVD risk. Soluble rather than insoluble fibre appears to have a greater benefit by reducing LDL cholesterol. Ideal intake is 25–30 g of total dietary fibre, of which 7–13 g should be soluble fibre (fibre from oat bran, β-glucan, and psyllium) (Threpleton et al. 2013). Those with a high fibre diet also tend to have healthier lifestyles, e.g. low saturated fat intake, more exercise, and are non-smokers, and consequently a lower BMI, blood pressure, and triglyceride levels.

The glucose spikes after meals adversely affect vascular function and structure via multiple mechanisms (oxidative stress, inflammation, LDL oxidation, protein glycation, and procoagulant activity). The GI is a measure of the blood glucose raising potential of foods. Therefore, promoting low GI foods as part of a cardioprotective diet is beneficial (Kelly et al. 2004).

Key Message

Encourage people to choose and incorporate wholegrains and high fibre foods where possible (SACN 2015). Examples of low GI foods to incorporate into their diet include fruit, vegetables, barley, basmati rice, beans, lentils, pasta, noodles, yam, sweet potatoes, porridge, oat-based cereals, wholegrain/granary bread (BDA 2013; NHS Choices 2016b).

5b.5.5   Nuts

A frequent nut intake (>1 serving/week) is associated with a reduced risk of CHD mortality (Luo et al. 2014). The complex nature of nuts makes it hard to establish which component influences the cardioprotective effect observed in the studies. They have a good fat profile, are high in fibre, phytosterols, folate, magnesium, vitamin E, and arginine. Possible mechanisms include decreasing lipoprotein oxidation, inhibition of inflammation, decreased insulin resistance, improved endothelial function, and improve lipid profiles. Peanuts are the most commonly studied nut but other nuts that have been studied are almonds, pistachios, pecans, and macadamia nuts.

> **Key Message**
> Nuts are high in calories so portion size must be strictly monitored. 1 portion = 30 g. The intake of coated nuts should be discouraged.

5b.5.6   Salt

The intake of sodium in the UK ($8.1\,g\,d^{-1}$), principally from common salt (mostly hidden in breakfast cereals and other processed foods), exceeds that required to meet metabolic needs. The recommended intake is $<6\,g\,d^{-1}$ although the greater the salt reduction the greater the blood pressure reduction (He et al. 2004). NICE has recommended a reduction in salt to $3\,g\,d^{-1}$ by 2025 (NICE 2010).

> **Key Message**
> There are various strategies to reduce salt intake. These include:
>
> - Discouraging the use of salt at the table or in cooking
> - Avoiding 'LoSalt' due to high potassium levels
> - Encouraging the use of alternative ingredients to flavour foods such as herbs, spices, lemon juice, garlic, pepper, vinegar, and chilli
> - Discouraging consumption of foods with a high salt content, such as ready-made meals, cheese, tinned or packet soups and sauces, sausages, pies, pâté, smoked products, stock cubes, meat and vegetable extracts, soya sauce, and Marmite™.
>
> Providing support and information on how to read food labels will help to identify healthier food choices (NHS Choices 2016c).

5b.5.7 Sugar

Sugar has very little nutritional value and is often described as being 'empty calories'. The intake of sugar has increased globally from changes in processed food formulation to reduce fat and to ensure the product remains palatable. The other major contributor to this increased sugar intake is the increased intake of sugar sweetened beverages (SSB). This is up to 10% of total energy in some countries. This increased intake of SSB tracks the rising rates of obesity (Huang et al. 2014).

SSBs have a very high GI and therefore may contribute to a high dietary glycaemic load. This could lead to inflammation, insulin resistance, impaired beta cell function, and raised blood pressure, as well as increased visceral fat and an impaired lipid profile.

Key Message

The SACN (2015) recommends that the average intake, across the UK population, of free sugars should not exceed 5% of total dietary energy intake.

Tips to achieve this recommendation are:

- Avoid sweetened drinks as much as possible and swap to water, lower-fat milk, unsweetened tea and coffee, and 'no-calorie', 'sugar-free', or 'no-added' sugar carbonated drinks or squashes.

- Free sugars are also naturally found in fruit juices and smoothies – limit to 150 ml only per day.

- Other free sugars to reduce are those added to food (e.g. sucrose [table sugar], glucose) or those naturally present in honey and syrups, but excludes lactose in milk and milk products (BDA 2015b; NHS Choices 2016d).

5b.5.8 Alcohol

Observation studies have shown a protective effect with a daily consumption of 1–2 units and CVD compared to abstainers. Possible mechanisms for the protective effect of alcohol are the effect on lipid levels (increases HDL), the inhibition of clotting promoters including platelet aggregation, and fibrinogen levels.

A high alcohol intake, >3 units/day, is associated with many diseases, e.g. alcoholism, liver disease, cancer, and with higher levels of blood pressure and triglycerides. The pattern of alcohol consumption is important. Binge drinking and infrequent drinking is associated with greater risk compared to frequent drinking of small quantities (Klatsky 2010; Mukamal et al. 2003). The type of alcohol does **not** appear to have a significant effect on total CVD risk, however wine drinkers often have better risk factor profiles than beer or spirit drinkers (Rimm et al. 1996).

National UK guidance on alcohol has been revised (DH 2016), as the Chief Medical Officer found that there is significant new evidence on the effects of alcohol relating to the risk of cancers, especially breast cancer.

> **Key Message**
>
> Many people underestimate their alcohol intake. It is important to assess the pattern of alcohol consumption as well as the total units and type of alcohol being ingested. There is still not enough robust evidence to pressure abstainers for religious, cultural, or personal reasons to start to drink alcohol.
>
> The new recommended maximum intake (DH 2016) is 14 units a week:
>
> - Men and women two to three units per day with two alcohol free days
>
> Guidance is available for those calculating and amending their alcohol intake (Drinkaware 2016; NHS Choices 2016e, 2016f).

5B.6   WEIGHT LOSS, MAINTENANCE, AND AVOIDANCE OF CYCLING, INCLUDING PHARMACOLOGICAL SUPPORT

Obesity management requires an effective multi-component lifestyle approach, which addresses dietary intake, physical activity, and behavioural change to achieve realistic targets of 3–5% loss of body weight (NICE 2014).

5b.6.1   Avoidance of Weight Cycling

It is the health professional's duty of care to ensure patients' expectations are realistic and explain that small changes over time can make significant improvements in CVD risk. This is especially true in relation to weight targets to avoid weight cycling. Unrealistic expectations often lead to repeated loss and regain of weight. There are harmful associations between weight fluctuations and CVD mortality/morbidity.

5b.6.2   How Is Realistic Weight Loss Achieved?

Body weight is based on the energy equation shown in Figure 5b.4. Typically this can explain that changes in lifestyle such as becoming less active but habitually still eating the same amount of food causes a weight gain pattern.

5b.6.3   Weight Maintenance

Strategies to prevent weight regain should be core components of supporting people to lose weight. To prevent 'relapse' discuss high-risk situations and encourage patients to problem solve how to manage them better, e.g. family/time/social pressures, living alone, comfort eating, less active job.

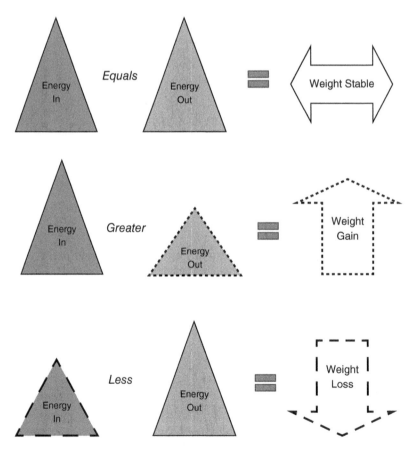

FIGURE 5B.4   Energy Equation – key message for maintenance or weight changes.

5b.6.4   Pharmacotherapy Input

Orlistat is currently the only medication prescribed to support weight loss. It reduces fat absorption and with lifestyle interventions can achieve 5% weight loss (Avenell et al. 2004). Gastric side effects can occur if the diet is too high in fat. Fat soluble vitamin intake should be monitored during prolonged use. Orlistat is available on prescription from a GP or a lower dose is also available to buy over the counter in pharmacies with guidelines, e.g. BMI ≥ 28. The pharmacist should provide dietary advice and/or signpost patients to the Orlistat website.

Key Message

When discussing dietary strategies for weight loss/maintenance with patients it is essential that physical activity (Chapter 5c) and behaviour modification (Chapter 4) are incorporated. It is important to set realistic and SMART goals for weight loss and lifestyle changes to achieve a negative energy balance. Monitor the motivation levels of the patient and use appropriate individualised diet strategies to account for relapse, unplanned eating/drinking, and social occasions. If the patient is struggling it is recommended to refer them to NHS specialist weight management programmes.

Support for weight management can be found on a variety of online sources (BDA 2013a; NHS Choices 2016g). The average male and female energy requirements are between 2500 and 2000 calories per day respectively. Calculate a patient's tailored energy requirements using the NHS BMI calculator (NHS Choices 2016h) and NHS Calorie Counter (NHS Choices 2016i).

The outcomes of dietary strategies can be measured by comparing the target weight and WC with the SMART goals and dietary targets set.

5b.6.5   Tailored Advice

Tailoring dietary advice needs to be facilitated in a 'discursive rather than a didactic fashion' (BACPR 2012). The Eatwell plate (Figure 5b.5) should be used as a framework for any dietary discussions. It should be conveyed that 'healthy eating' is not just a list of 'foods to avoid' and 'foods to eat' but about getting the balance right. Realistic/SMART targets may be agreed around upsizing/downsizing portions or swapping or reducing frequency of food items or changing cooking techniques.

Tailoring dietary advice requires an integrated approach. By referring to Chapter 4 and the Key Messages contained throughout this chapter, a holistic approach to dietary advice can be provided.

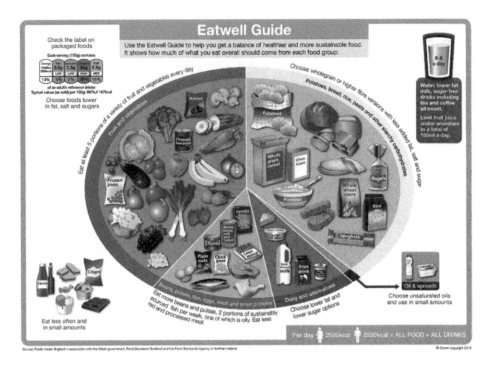

FIGURE 5B.5   The Eatwell Guide (NHS Choices 2016j).

5B.7   COMMON MISCONCEPTIONS AND FREQUENTLY ASKED QUESTIONS

The British Association for Cardiovascular Prevention and Rehabilitation (BACPR 2012) states that all patients should have opportunity to discuss and be corrected on any misconceptions about diet.

5b.7.1   Is Chocolate Good for the Heart?

Although coco/flavonoids have been linked to CVD prevention, the research quality is poor. Commercial chocolate is high in fat and sugar and should only be consumed in moderation.

5b.7.2   Are any Supplements Useful?

- Garlic to lower cholesterol:
  - The effect is too small to recommend. However, garlic in cooking is a good replacement for salt when flavouring food.

- Cod liver oil:
  - No as there is no substantial evidence to show the benefits of taking cod liver oil (with/out added omega-3) for either joint mobility or cholesterol-lowering effects.
- Vitamin D and CoEnzyme Q10:
  - No, as there is no substantial evidence to show the benefits of taking either supplement, although it is unlikely to cause harm. A few studies have shown reduction in statin side effects for CoEnzyme Q10 but it is not conclusive.

5b.7.3 Can I Still Eat Fruit and Vegetables Now I Take Warfarin?

Yes – patients should keep their intake consistent, as any changes in fruit/vegetables (containing vitamin K) can reduce the anti-coagulant effects of warfarin. When patients increase their fruit/vegetable intake, this should be done gradually with INR monitoring.

5b.7.4 Is Coffee Bad for the Heart?

There is no clear pattern from research. Nevertheless, heavy coffee drinking should be avoided as it is related to high homocysteine levels.

5b.7.5 Can Soya Lower Cholesterol?

Soya research suggests that 25–48 g soya a day may help in providing a small reduction in LDL cholesterol levels. Thus, eating soya products is a matter of individual dietary preferences.

5b.7.6 How Many Eggs Can I Eat a Week?

Up to one egg a day, with occasional consumption of other foods containing dietary cholesterol, such as prawns or offal, all cooked in a healthy way.

5b.7.7 Do I Need to Buy Plant Stanol/Sterol Enriched Margarine?

Plant stanol/sterols do not reduce CVD outcomes. Plant stanol/sterols can reduce LDL cholesterol by 10–15% if taken in the correct doses (BDA 2015c).

5b.7.8   If I Heat my Oil Too High when Cooking, Will it Become Harmful?

Heating any type of unsaturated oil at high temperatures can result in unfavourable changes. However, temperatures in home cooking as opposed to commercial frying provide no concern, provided the oil is used only once.

5b.7.9   Are Artificial Sweeteners Safe?

Yes - reassure patients that current intakes fall below 'safe limits' (NHS Choices 2016k). Artificial sweeteners can be a useful strategy for diabetes/weight management; but avoid sugar alcohols, i.e. sorbital and xylitol as they are not calorie free.

5b.7.10   I Read in the Newspaper that Eating XYZ Is Bad for my Heart, Is that True?

Food stories are very popular in the media. To check out the evidence behind a media story and clarify any misconceptions with your patients, look up 'NHS Choices – Behind the Headlines' (NHS Choices 2015l).

5b.7.11   I Don't Understand Food Labelling

A new style of voluntary food labelling in the UK has been agreed from 2014 (see Figure 5b.6).

It is useful to have some spare food packaging to discuss food labelling with your patients (British Heart Foundation 2015; NHS Choices 2016c).

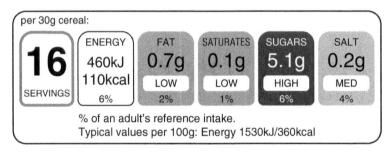

FIGURE 5B.6   New Style of Voluntary Food Labelling.

5b.7.12 Can I Drink Grapefruit Juice?

People taking statins, such as simvastatin, should avoid grapefruit juice – check with your local pharmacist. (NHS Choices 2015m).

5B.8 RELATIONSHIP WITH OTHER LONG-TERM CONDITIONS

5b.8.1 Heart Failure

Heart failure is the inability of the heart to pump effectively and efficiently to adequately support circulation. All patients are advised to weigh themselves daily to check for any fluid retention. Trends in weight changes can help to identify if the variation is fluid only or 'dry' body weight changes. The Butler (2016) review on heart failure has highlighted that dietary manipulation needs to progress further than simple recommendation of salt and fluid restriction.

Heart failure is classified into categories:

- Classes I and II (mild) – dietary treatment is a cardioprotective diet as all patients will have underlying CVD. Weight management is important to relieve dyspnoea.
- Class III (moderate) – during periods when symptoms of fatigue, palpitation, and dyspnoea are exacerbated appetite *may* reduce and cause unexplained 'dry' body weight loss. See post-surgery advice below.
- Class IV (severe) – all the above symptoms are severe. At risk of malnutrition and cardiac cachexia. See post-surgery advice below.

5b.8.2 Post-Surgery

People should be encouraged to follow a cardioprotective diet post-surgery. However, inadequate nutritional intake may hinder wound healing and delay recovery. Nutritional screening in hospitals will identify and treat people who are malnourished/at risk of malnutrition, e.g. oral nutritional sip feeds. On discharge, a 'food first' approach will be advised:

- Eat three small meals a day and three nourishing snacks
- Fortify foods with full fat products such as milk/yoghurts and spreading fats.

Clarify to patients that this advice is only appropriate in the short term whilst appetite is poor and they are at risk of malnutrition (BDA 2015d).

5b.8.3   Chronic Kidney Disease

Chronic kidney disease (CKD) is described in different stages:

- Stages 1–3 (mild–moderate) – dietary management encompasses tailoring advice for blood pressure, hyperlipidaemia, weight management, and diabetes (Figure 5b.7).
- Stages 4–5 (severe and very severe) – requires referral to a specialist renal dietitian.

Disease/Condition	Special Considerations
Dyslipidaemia	**Reduction of LDL:** ▪ Decrease saturated fatty acids and trans fatty acids ▪ Choose MUFA, PUFA and soluble fibre ▪ Weight loss in the overweight/obese **Increasing HDL:** ▪ Increase physical activity ▪ Weight loss in the overweight/obese ▪ Improve glycaemic control in diabetics **Reduction of Triglycerides:** ▪ Increase physical activity ▪ Weight loss in the overweight/obese ▪ Improve glycaemic control ▪ Reduce alcohol and sugar consumption ▪ Increase oily fish consumption
Blood Pressure	▪ Reduction of salt and alcohol intake ▪ Increase potassium and calcium intake from fruit and vegetables ▪ Weight loss in the overweight/obese ▪ Increase physical activity
Obesity	▪ Reduce total calorie intake ▪ Increase physical activity ▪ Set realistic weight loss target (3–5% in 3 months)
Diabetes & Impaired Glucose Tolerance	▪ Glycaemic control – referral to dietitian if poorly controlled (hyper or hypo) ▪ Ensure regular intake of low glycaemic index foods ▪ Weight loss in the overweight/obese

FIGURE 5B.7   Summary of dietary strategies for long-term conditions.

Support and information relating to CKD is offered by the British Kidney Patient Association (Kidney Care UK 2015).

5b.8.4 Diabetes

The goals for nutrition therapy are optimal metabolic outcomes for blood glucose, lipids, and blood pressure (Figure 5b.7). To support people with diabetes, dietitians and front line staff need appropriate competencies (Deakin 2011). Diabetes UK is a registered charity that provides support and information to those patients suffering from diabetes (Diabetes UK 2016).

5B.9 CONCLUSION

Ideally patients should be assessed by a dietitian with a special interest in CVD, especially when supporting patients with multiple long-term conditions. If dietetic cover is not available, then another health professional could assess the patient and give first line advice as long as they receive some additional training (BACPR 2012).

Health professionals should also be able to identify when the patient requires more in-depth support and hence a referral on to a dietetic department, weight management group, or diabetes, or renal specialist team.

REFERENCES

Avenell, A., Brown, T.J., McGee, M.A. et al. (2004). What interventions should we add to weight reducing diets in adults with obesity? A systematic review of randomized controlled trials of adding drug therapy, exercise, behaviour therapy or combinations of these interventions. *Journal of Human Nutrition and Dietetics* 17 (4): 293–316.

BACPR (2012). British Association for Cardiovascular Prevention and Rehabilitation Standards and Core Components for Cardiovascular Disease Prevention and Rehabilitation (2e). BACPR. http://www.bacpr.com/pages/page_box_contents. asp?pageid=791 (accessed 7 July 2016).

BDA (2013). Food Fact Sheet – Glycaemic Index. The British Dietetic Association. http://www.bda.uk.com/foodfacts/GIDiet.pdf (accessed 14 June 2016).

BDA (2013a). Weight wise – struggling to lose weight? The British Dietetic Association. http://www.bdaweightwise.com/support/support_struggling.html (accessed 14 June 2016).

BDA (2014). Food Fact Sheet – Fruit and Vegetables. The British Dietetic Association. http://www.bda.uk.com/foodfacts/FruitVeg.pdf (accessed 14 June 2016).

BDA (2014a). Food Fact Sheet – Trans Fats. The British Dietetic Association. http://www.bda.uk.com/foodfacts/TransFats.pdf (accessed 14 June 2016).

BDA (2015a). Food Fact Sheet – Fats. The British Dietetic Association. http://www.bda.uk.com/foodfacts/FatFacts.pdf (accessed 14 June 2016).

BDA (2015b). Food Fact Sheet – Sugar. The British Dietetic Association. http://www.bda.uk.com/foodfacts/Sugar.pdf (accessed 7 July 2016).

BDA (2015c). Food Fact Sheet – Stanols and Sterols. The British Dietetic Association. http://www.bda.uk.com/foodfacts/PlantStanolsAndSterols.pdf (accessed 14 June 2016).

BDA (2015d). Food Fact Sheet – Malnutrition. The British Dietetic Association. http://www.bda.uk.com/foodfacts/MalnutritionFactSheet.pdf (accessed 14 June 2016).

British Heart Foundation (2015). This label could change your life. British Heart Foundation. http://www.bhf.org.uk/publications/view-publication.aspx?ps=1000110 (accessed 14 June 2016).

Butler, T. (2016). Dietary management of heart failure: room for improvement? *British Journal of Nutrition*. https://doi.org/10.1017/S00071145100553X.

Deakin, T. (2011). *An integrated career and competency framework for dietitians and frontline staff*. [Online]. Diabetes UK. https://diabetes-resources-production.s3-eu-west-1.amazonaws.com/diabetes-storage/migration/pdf/Dietetic%2520Competency%2520Framework_amendment%2520July%25202016.pdf.

Department of Health (2016). UK Chief Medical Officers' Alcohol Guidelines Review: summary of the proposed new guidelines. Department of Health. https://www.gov.uk/government/uploads/system/uploads/attachment_data/file/489795/summary.pdf (accessed 7 July 2016).

Despres, J.P., Lemieux, I., and Prud'homme, D. (2001). Treatment of obesity: need to focus on high risk abdominally obese patients. *British Medical Journal* 322 (7288): 716–720.

Diabetes UK (2016). *Diabetes UK – Care. Connect. Campaign.* Diabetes UK. www.diabetes.org.uk (accessed 14 June 2016).

Drinkaware (2016). *Drink Aware*. Drinkaware. www.drinkaware.co.uk (accessed 14 June 2016).

Estruch, R., Ros, E., Salas-Salvado, J. et al. (2013). Primary prevention of cardiovascular disease with a Mediterranean diet. *The New England Journal of Medicine* 368: 1279–1290.

Gandy, J. (2014). *Manual of Dietetic Practice*, 5e. Wiley-Blackwell on behalf of the British Dietetic Association.

He, F.J., Li, J., and Macgregor, G.A. (2004). Effect of longer-term modest salt reduction on blood pressure: Cochrane database of systematic reviews. *British Medical Journal* 346 (f1325) https://doi.org/10.1136/bmj.f1325.

Hooper, L., Martin, N., Abdelhamid, A., and Davey-Smith, G. (2015). Reduced in saturated fat for cardiovascular disease. *Cochrane Database of Systematic Reviews* (6): CD011737. https://doi.org/10.1002/14651858.CD011737.

Huang, C., Huang, J., Tian, Y. et al. (2014). Sugar sweetened beverages consumption and risk of coronary heart disease: a meta-analysis of prospective studies. *Atherosclerosis* 234 (1): 11–16.

JBS3 Board (2014). Joint British Societies' consensus recommendations for the prevention of cardiovascular disease (JBS3). *Heart* 100: ii1–ii1167. https://doi.org/10.1136/heartjnl-2014-305693.

Kelly, S., Frost, G., Whittaker, V., and Summerbell, C. (2004). Low glycaemic index diets for coronary heart disease. *The Cochrane Database of Systematic Reviews* 18 (4): CD004467.

Kidney Care UK (2015). Kidney Care UK: About Kidney Health. Kidney Care UK. https://www.kidneycareuk.org/about-kidney-health (accessed 28 August 2019).

Klatsky, A.L. (2010). Alcohol and cardiovascular health. *Physiological Behaviour* 100 (1): 76–81.

Luo, C., Zhang, Y., Ding, Y. et al. (2014). Nut consumption and risk of type 2 diabetes, cardiovascular disease, and all-cause mortality: a systematic review and meta-analysis. *The Amerian Journal of Clinical Nutrition* 100: 256–269.

Mukamal, K.J., Conigrave, K.M., Mittleman, M.A. et al. (2003). Roles of drinking pattern and type of alcohol consumed in coronary heart disease in men. *New England Journal of Medicine* 348: 109–118.

NACR (2013). Mediterranean Diet Score Tool. NHS Digital. http://www.cardiacrehabilitation.org.uk/docs/Mediterranean-Diet-Score.pdf (accessed 14 June 2016).

NHS Choices (2016a). 5 A DAY. NHS. http://www.nhs.uk/livewell/5ADAY/Pages/5ADAYhome.aspx (accessed 14 June 2016).

NHS Choices (2016b). Starchy foods and carbohydrates. NHS. http://www.nhs.uk/Livewell/Goodfood/Pages/starchy-foods.aspx (accessed 14 June 2016).

NHS Choices (2016c). Food labels. NHS. http://www.nhs.uk/Livewell/Goodfood/Pages/food-labelling.aspx (accessed 14 June 2016).

NHS Choices (2016d). How does sugar in our diet affect our health? NHS. http://www.nhs.uk/Livewell/Goodfood/Pages/sugars.aspx (accessed 14 June 2016).

NHS Choices (2016e). Cutting down on alcohol. NHS. http://www.nhs.uk/change4life/Pages/cutting-down-alcohol.aspx (accessed 14 June 2016).

NHS Choices (2016f). Alcohol units. NHS. http://www.nhs.uk/Livewell/alcohol/Pages/alcohol-units.aspx (accessed 14 June 2016).

NHS Choices (2016g). Weight loss guide. NHS. http://www.nhs.uk/Livewell/weight-loss-guide/Pages/weight-loss-guide.aspx (accessed 14 June 2016).

NHS Choices (2016h). BMI healthy weight calculator - health tools - NHS choices. NHS. http://www.nhs.uk/Tools/Pages/Healthyweightcalculator.aspx (accessed 14 June 2016).

NHS Choices (2016i). Calorie checker. NHS. http://www.nhs.uk/Livewell/weight-loss-guide/Pages/calorie-counting.aspx (accessed 14 June 2016).

NHS Choices (2016j). The Eatwell guide. NHS. http://www.nhs.uk/Livewell/Goodfood/Pages/the-eatwell-guide.aspx (accessed 14 June 2016).

NHS Choices (2016k). The truth about sweeteners. NHS. http://www.nhs.uk/livewell/goodfood/pages/the-truth-about-artificial-sweeteners.aspx (accessed 14 June 2016).

NHS Choices (2015l). Behind the headlines. NHS. http://www.nhs.uk/news/Pages/NewsIndex.aspx (accessed 14 June 2016).

NHS Choices (2015m). Does grapefruit affect my medicine? NHS. http://www.nhs.uk/chq/Pages/2474.aspx?CategoryID=73 (accessed 14 June 2016).

NICE (2010). Guidance on the Prevention of Cardiovascular Disease at the Population Level. National Institute for Health and Clinical Excellence.

NICE (2013a). Assessing body mass index and waist circumference thresholds for intervening to prevent ill health and premature death among adults from black, Asian and other minority ethnic groups in the UK. BMI: preventing ill health and premature death in black, Asian and other minority ethnic groups. National Institute for Health and Clinical Excellence.

NICE (2013b). MI – secondary prevention: Secondary prevention in primary and secondary care for patients following a myocardial infarction. *National Institute for Health and Care Excellence*: NICE Clinical Guideline 141. National Institute for Health and Clinical Excellence.

NICE (2014). Managing overweight and obesity in adults – lifestyle weight management services. National Institute for Health and Clinical Excellence.

Rimm, E.B., Klatsky, A., Grobbee, D., and Stampfer, M.J. (1996). Review of moderate alcohol consumption and reduced risk of coronary heart disease: is the effect due to beer, wine, or spirits? *British Medical Journal* 312 (7033): 731–736.

SACN (2015). Carbohydrates and Health Report. London: TSO. https://www.gov.uk/government/uploads/system/uploads/attachment_data/file/445503/SACN_Carbohydrates_and_Health.pdf (accessed 7 July 2016).

SofiI, F., Cesari, F., Abbate, R. et al. (2008). Adherence to Mediterranean diet and health status: meta-analysis. *British Medical Journal* 337: a1344.

Threpleton, D.E., Greenwood, D.C., Evans, C.E. et al. (2013). Dietary fibre intake and risk of cardiovascular disease: systematic review and meta-analysis. *British Medical Journal* 347: f6879.

CHAPTER 5C

Physical Activity and Exercise

John Buckley[1], Tim Grove[2], Sally Turner[3], and Samantha Breen[4]

[1] Centre for Active Living, University Centre Shrewsbury, Shrewsbury, UK
[2] Department of Clinical Sciences, Brunel University, Uxbridge, UK
[3] Basingstoke & Alton Cardiac Rehabilitation Charity Ltd, Alton, UK
[4] Manchester Royal Infirmary and St Mary's Hospital, Manchester University NHS Foundation Trust, Manchester, UK

Abstract

This chapter focuses on the current practicalities of providing the exercise component of cardiac rehabilitation in contemporary settings (hospital, community, or home-based) and the scientific rationale that supports delivery of an exercise service. The text includes references to both the primary and secondary prevention of cardiovascular disease, with signposting to many additional resources. It stresses the value of 'early' commencement of exercise programming following diagnosis, intervention, and procedures as well as discussing the role of 'prehabilitation' for surgical patients.

One of the key messages emphasises the importance of reducing levels of physical inactivity in the general population as well as in those with cardiovascular disease and how this may be achieved through behaviour change and education. The guidance is clear: more activity starts with

Cardiovascular Prevention and Rehabilitation in Practice, Second Edition.
Edited by Jennifer Jones, John Buckley, Gill Furze, and Gail Sheppard.
© 2020 John Wiley & Sons Ltd. Published 2020 by John Wiley & Sons Ltd.

simply promoting that people spend less time seated and even regular light activity throughout the day confers many additional benefits to performing 75–150 minutes of moderate to vigorous activity per week.

The chapter ends with an example of a typical patient as a case study: a young male with Type II diabetes who has recently undergone a primary percutaneous coronary intervention to his left anterior descending artery following a diagnosis of acute anterior myocardial infarction (MI). It includes a clear description of best practice in assessment (with psycho-social and co-morbid considerations), treatment plan, and the provision of an appropriate individually tailored exercise programme.

Keywords: *exercise, cardiac rehabilitation, risk factor management*

Key Points

- The role of physical activity in preventing cardiovascular disease.
- The role of physical activity, including structured exercise, in the rehabilitation and secondary prevention of coronary artery disease.
- The modes and volumes of physical activity from regular avoidance of sitting to expending in excess of 1000 kcal of energy per week through moderate to vigorous activity.
- The role of strength training in risk factor management, physical functioning in work and in leisure, and quality of life
- The earliest commencement of physical activity following diagnosis and treatment.
- Considerations for more contemporary means of exercise including interval training that involves high intensity activity.
- Considerations for similarities and differences between key groups (angina and MI treated either by percutaneous coronary intervention [PCI] or coronary artery by-pass surgery [CABG], and heart failure).

5C.1   RATIONALE AND AIMS

In this chapter we aim to highlight the key elements that provide both the scientific rationale and the practical elements that need considering when offering/delivering the physical activity component to clients and patients. In keeping with the most recent NICE guidelines (NICE 2013) and BACPR Standards and Core Components (BACPR et al. 2013), the physical activity and exercise component should be delivered with a patient-centred approach. The programme should aim to maximise the chances of early uptake and long-term adherence towards a physically active lifestyle by being sensitive to the individual patient's psychological, social, and physical health needs.

With the BACPR and others already providing numerous detailed publications and educational resources for the exercise component, this chapter will signpost the reader to these other resources. Much of the detailed information can be accessed through these three key organisations:

- British Association for Cardiovascular Prevention and Rehabilitation
- The Association of Chartered Physiotherapists in Cardiac Rehabilitation
- American Heart Association.

This chapter will therefore make a critical overview of the requirements for contemporary physical activity programming, especially in relation to participation behaviour, education, uptake, adherence, and long-term changes.

5C.2   CONSISTENCY IN COMMUNICATING CONCEPTS TO PATIENTS

It is important that all members of the multidisciplinary team understand and communicate consistently to the patients the underpinning concepts of what is meant by physical activity, exercise, and fitness. The messaging given to patients must be clear in terms of the benefits and the challenges to achieving cardiovascular health gains from being more physically active.

'Physical activity' is any human movement that is created by the contraction of skeletal muscle.

'Sedentary behaviour' is a more recent area being linked with physical (in) activity, which has attracted much attention on the ills of prolonged bouts of sitting. Independent of physical activity, the time one spends sitting is now accepted as a significant risk factor for cardiometabolic diseases.

Exercise or exercise training is also considered physical activity but performed in an organised structured manner, with an aim or a goal (e.g. fitness, health, performance, rehabilitation).

Physical fitness is the ability or set of attributes required to perform any given physical activity/task and is reliant upon a combination of factors, including: aerobic capacity and endurance, muscular strength and endurance, joint mobility/flexibility and balance, and coordination and skill.

5C.3   PHYSICAL ACTIVITY WITHIN THE CONTEXT OF CARDIOVASCULAR HEALTH

5c.3.1   Preventing Cardiovascular Disease

Although records of the potential health benefits of exercise date back over 2500 years to the time of Hippocrates, the scientific link between physical activity and cardiovascular health was only first demonstrated in the 1950s and 1960s (Morris et al. 1953; Morris and Crawford 1958; Paffenbarger et al. 1970). This is not to disrespect that, in 1772, Heberden did note in a patient case of angina that the regular sawing of wood for 30 minutes per day did resolve symptoms of chest pain (Payne 1802). In reflecting on the studies led by Morris and by Paffenbarger, and in fact Heberden's single case in 1772, it is important to note that the modes of physical activity were in fact occupational work and not exercise or sport. All too often exercise and sport can tend to be a main focus of politically driven health promotion schemes. Twentieth century ground breaking scientific studies reported the lower incidence of heart disease and mortality in the following occupations: bus conductors versus drivers, active versus sedentary postal workers and active versus sedentary dock workers (longshoremen). The important fact of these studies was the loss of activity in occupational settings and not due to lack of sport or exercise as the key agents to (ill) health. It is interesting to note that Hippocrates did recognise this value of health-related activity coming from both 'natural exercise' (that which occurs in daily life) and 'artificial exercise' (sport and recreation) (Berryman 2010).

Emerging evidence is now beginning to show that it is not just how much activity one performs per week that should be a cause for concern, it is the act of sitting for extended periods (e.g. the bus driver, the office worker, the television viewer), independent of physical activity, which is also a significant culprit of cardiometabolic disease (Healy et al. 2011; Thorp et al. 2011). Recent evidence shows that people who sit for most of their day at work have a 15% greater risk of premature mortality, compared with those who have a job that requires standing most of the day (Katzmarzyk 2013; Katzmarzyk and Lee 2012; Torbeyns et al. 2014). It is therefore possible that the relative higher risk in Morris' bus drivers and Paffenbarger's office-based workers could have been greatly affected by them sitting all day, as opposed to the more recognised benefits of the active bus conductors, postal workers, or dock workers. Sensibly, the most recent evidence would suggest that the relative risk gap is probably a function of both prolonged sitting of the drivers or the seated postal workers or the office workers compared to the regular prolonged standing, walking, or cycling of the bus conductors and postal delivery workers.

The British Heart Foundation (BHF) has reported that the average person in the UK spends more than 60% of waking hours sitting, where only 20–30% is spent in standing or performing light physical activity and with less than 10% of the day (<20 minutes) spent performing any type of moderate to vigorous physical activity (BHF 2017; Townsend et al. 2012b). Moreover, the greatest shift in physical activity patterns over the past 50 years have been from people engaging in less 'light' activity towards more sedentary behaviours, whereas the numbers engaged in moderate-to-vigorous activity are actually unchanged and, in some cases, have increased in the past 15 years (BHF 2017; Townsend et al. 2012b). Emerging evidence for cardiac rehabilitation participants has shown that the participation in exercise does not influence sedentary behaviour (Biswas 2018; Ter Hoeve 2017). In one study of patients who completed a full programme of exercise, those who were less sedentary had greater improvement in their cardiometabolic health status (Prince et al. 2015). Therefore, the total loss of energy expenditure in occupational and domestic life continues to far outweigh what many people feel may be counteracted by participating in sport, exercise, and other leisure pursuits. It is therefore not surprising that in the most recent targets for the World Health Organization, they have described one of their goals as globally 'reducing physical inactivity' by 10% (WHO 2012). Globally, physical inactivity prevails in 40% of individuals with cardiovascular disease (CVD) but more alarming is that in the UK this figure rises to 70% of individuals (Hallal et al. 2012).

The UK's Joint Chief Medical Officers' (CMOs') Report, *Start Active Stay Active* (CMOS 2011) highlights the independent role that physical activity plays in reducing the risk of CVD by up to 35%. The scientific evidence underpinning this report is based on people achieving activity energy expenditure in excess of 1000 kcal per week. This has been translated into the following public health messages: 150 minutes of moderate-intensity aerobic activity each week or 75 minutes of vigorous-intensity aerobic activity per week, or equivalent combinations. There is a reported greater benefit to preventing all-cause mortality from activity that leads to improved cardiorespiratory fitness, when measured from an exercise test, compared to self-reported physical activity in leisure time (Lee et al. 2011). It however continues to be problematic to make these comparisons knowing the inaccuracies of self-reported data, which often do not capture very well the non-exercise activity (occupational and domestic) (Troiano et al. 2008). The CMOs' report also provides specific recommendations for children and older or frail adults and importantly the need to avoid sitting too much. The recommended doses of aerobic activity can be performed in multiple bouts of at least 10 minutes. With regard to strength training, it has beneficial effects on CVD risk factors, including blood glucose, insulin control, and resting metabolic rate, along with better functionality and quality of life for older frailer individuals (Williams et al. 2007).

5c.3.2   Physical Activity Within Rehabilitation and Secondary Prevention

One of the strengths of the exercise evidence base in CVD rehabilitation and secondary prevention is that it is mainly from interventional randomised controlled trials (Heran et al. 2011). Whereas for primary prevention (noted above), much of the evidence base is epidemiological. This is not to say there are no practical confounders in the cardiac rehabilitation evidence. With respect to the lower than ideal uptake of cardiac rehabilitation nationally and globally (Grace et al. 2013; NACR 2014; Turk-Adawi et al. 2014) it means there is a likely 'selection bias' of patients entered into research trials; usually those that have a keener willingness and more educated approach to participation. Education and socio-economic status are strong key risk factors in themselves for CVD (Aiello and Kaplan 2009). One of the challenges that most front-line cardiac rehabilitation professionals face is to offer a service that reflects the research trials; in many ways the research trials are tightly controlled, with a high ratio of staff supervision, and often excluding the types of participants (e.g. older, lower socio-demographic levels, and those with many co-morbidities) who are most in need of rehabilitation and secondary prevention guidance (Heran et al. 2011; Taylor et al. 2014). Furthermore, the modes of exercise used in these trials are often limited to just cycle ergometer and treadmill. Encouragingly, there are an increasing number of trials and guidelines that recommend combining aerobic and strength training, which leads to better outcomes compared to just aerobic exercise (Mandic et al. 2011; Marzolini et al. 2014). Rehabilitation programmes must, however, always aim to provide an evidence-based programme as best as possible to support the case for an appropriately 'dosed' exercise component (Almodhy et al. 2016; Sandercock et al. 2013). The exercise dose is noted below in terms of the frequency, duration, and intensity, and it would seem frequency of activity is the likely main culprit for people not attaining the correct 'dose'.

The Cochrane Reviews of randomised controlled trials have clearly defined a relationship between aerobic training and cardiac mortality in patients with established coronary heart disease (CHD) (Heran et al. 2011). The typical dose of activity reported in this review's evidence provides for the following recommendations, upon which current BACPR recommendations have been made:

- A frequency of three to five sessions per week,
- An accumulated duration of sessions performed for 20–60 minutes
- An intensity of moderate to vigorous effort (in the range 40–75% VO_2max or for more precision set to a level near or at the ventilatory threshold) (Conraads et al. 2015; Hansen et al. 2012; Swain and Franklin 2002a; Swain and Franklin 2002b). Associated target heart rates (40–70% heart

rate reserve; HRR), and ratings of perceived exertion (RPE; Borg ratings 11–14) are typically used in practical settings to represent these ranges or thresholds of intensity.

- Inclusion of resistance/strength training for 8–10 major muscle groups, performing 10–15 repetitions at an intensity of up to 70% of a one-repetition maximum.

Key Message

The specific details for setting up an exercise session and practically determining/monitoring intensity are set out by the BACPR's course manual (2014) and the Association of Chartered Physiotherapists in Cardiovascular Rehabilitation (ACPICR) standards (2015). In the absence of a maximal exercise test for establishing a target HRR for CHD patients without heart failure, the maximal heart rate is to be estimated by the following equation (Franklin et al. 2003; Inbar et al. 1994; Karvonen et al. 1957; Robergs and Landwehr 2002; Swain and Franklin 2002a):

$$HR_{max} = 206 - (0.7 \times age).$$

The relationships between relative exercise intensity (%VO$_2$ max; %HRR) and RPE are summarised in Table 5c.1.

TABLE 5C.1   Relationship between heart rate reserve (HRR), oxygen uptake (VO$_2$; metabolic equivalents; METs) and ratings of perceived exertion (RPE) using Borg's 6–20 and CR10 scales.

% VO$_2$ max % METs max % HRR max	Perceived exertion descriptor	Borg RPE (6–20)	Borg CR10
28	Very light	9	1
42	Light	11	2
56	Somewhat light	12–13	3.0–3.5
70	Somewhat hard	13–14	3.5–4.5
83	Hard	15–16	5.5–6.5
100	Extremely Hard to Maximal	19	10

Source: Adapted from ACSM 2013, Borg 1998, Brubaker et al. 1994, Buckley 2006, Buckley et al. 2009, Eston and Connolly 1996, Eston and Thompson 1997, Garber et al. 2011, Gutmann et al. 1981, Head et al. 1997, Robergs and Landwehr 2002.

The combined outcomes from the evidence for exercise-based rehabilitation have the greatest impact in reducing cardiovascular mortality and hospital readmissions, improved functional capacity, and self-perceived quality of life (Anderson 2016; Lam et al. 2011; Lawler et al. 2011; Taylor et al. 2014; Yohannes et al. 2010). These findings underpin the exercise component of internationally respected secondary prevention guidelines (NICE 2013). In addition to patients achieving the traditionally recommended exercise training goals, cardiovascular health and rehabilitation specialists need to place equal value on patients being as active as possible throughout their day, even if it includes lighter intensity activity and avoiding prolonged periods of sitting (ACRA 2004; Deanfield and Board 2014).

5c.3.3   The Evidence Base Used in Educating Healthcare Professionals and Patients

In relation to Chapter 4 on behaviour change and education, this next section refers to some of the key patient learning points that must be included as part of the education and behaviour change process of all rehabilitation programmes. The key is how to put these known physiological benefits into meaningful words for easy patient understanding (see boxes).

Key Message

Being more physically active and aerobically physically fitter is independently associated with reduced morbidity and mortality. Even in the presence of diagnosed CVD, when other key co-morbidities and CVD risk factors remain unchanged such as obesity, diabetes, high lipids, hypertension, and smoking, those who are more active and fitter will still gain significant health benefits and live longer. Ideally, when exercise is combined with medical and other lifestyle risk factor management programmes (diet and smoking cessation), it further contributes to a powerful means of improving health and reducing morbidity and premature mortality.

5c.3.4   Plain Language Guidance and Education Points for Patients

Being more active has many benefits for your heart and circulation; for your muscles and joints; for your stamina, strength, balance, and coordination; and above all how you feel mentally in managing your life.

Being active and fitter reduces your chances of going to hospital in the future and allows you to cope with life's stresses and strains; helping you get the most out of life. Not only does it help with your blood pressure, cholesterol, blood sugar levels, and your weight, it literally helps the blood flow more freely to your heart, your brain, and key organs like your kidneys. The inside walls of all your blood vessels, not just the ones the cardiologist or surgeon have fixed, become healthier and fitter. Being more active means you should generally find it easier to move during any activity; all of which reduces the 'all-round' strain on your heart, lungs, and joints as well as your ability to burn more calories every day. The great benefit of being more active is it helps improve more than just your heart and circulation – it affects all parts of your health, physical and mental, which can literally add years to your life or life to your years.

The formal exercise sessions offered (at the hospital, community or leisure centre, or at home) are mainly designed to help you become physically fitter and for you to learn about your physical limits so as to not over-stress your heart when you're at home or at work. The exercise sessions also provide an in-built assessment of how you are progressing, especially if you have specific health or physical fitness requirements for your work or hobbies. Physical exertion can be risky sometimes but if you know how to manage it (at work or at home) then heart and circulation problems can be prevented. In addition to the more formal types of activity and advice for activity that we provide you with, it is key that you reduce spending too much time sitting, even if you are doing regular exercise. Even small amounts of movement for short but regular periods throughout the day help to keep your arteries, veins, and blood cleaner and healthier, including lowered levels of blood fat and sugars.

If you find that particular activities make you breathless or you are getting general feelings of tiredness, aching muscles and joints, or general feelings of being 'run-down', then inform your heart health/rehabilitation specialists. It is often only when you are active that you can tell if your physical health is improving or if your health could be changing (for better or worse), which can then trigger you to seek a check-up from your doctor.

The causal relationship between physical activity and the reduction of CVD has been attributed to multiple biological, psychological, and social changes, which favourably alter a number of established atherogenic risk factors, including the integrity of both the coronary and systemic arterial endothelia, and factors affecting or improving myocardial function (Franklin and Gordon 2009). Risk factors benefitting from physical activity include high blood pressure, dyslipidaemia, and insulin resistance (Cornelissen and Fagard 2004; Fagard 2011; Fagard and Cornelissen 2007; Kodama et al. 2007). Whilst it can be argued that many of these risk factors can be managed medically, exercise has proven to have its own independent benefits on cardiovascular health in both primary and secondary prevention including arterial endothelial integrity as influenced by an enhanced vasodilatory responsiveness to exertion/stress, a reduction in the potential of atheromatous plaques to rupture, and reduced inflammatory markers associated with the development of atheroma (Franklin and Gordon 2009; Hamer et al. 2012; Hambrecht et al. 1993, 2000a, 2000b, 2004; Myers et al. 2002). In one trial in stable angina patients, 12 months of exercise proved more medically effective than angioplasty with a 10% greater 'event free' survival rate (Hambrecht et al. 2004).

As highlighted in the BACPR's Standards and Core Components (BACPR et al. 2013; BACPR 2017), the earliest possible commencement to exercise following a coronary event or intervention is also an important factor in preventing subsequent negative myocardial remodelling (Hassmén et al. 2000; Haykowsky et al. 2011). In addition, further benefits from physical activity that are linked to reducing CVD risk/progression include a number of psychological factors, including stress, anxiety, and depression (Hassmén et al. 2000).

Figure 5c.1 summarises the benefits of increasing physical activity and aerobic fitness in people with or at high risk of developing CVD. The risk factor benefits are seen as correlated benefits, whereas the arterial and myocardial integrity benefits are direct and independent benefits resulting from increased physical activity and/or aerobic fitness. It is the latter that is likely to be linked to exercise capacity as being one of the strongest independent prognostic indicators of cardiovascular health and reduced risk of early mortality (Myers et al. 2002). In those with and without CVD, each one metabolic equivalent (MET) increase in exercise capacity is associated with a 12% reduction in all-cause mortality and 15% reduction in CVD events (Kodama et al. 2007, Kodama et al. 2009; Myers et al. 2002). Furthermore, 65–70% of individuals with a low exercise capacity were usually inactive; thus if one has an exercise capacity less than

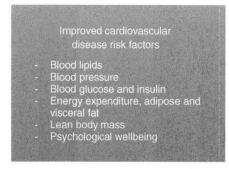
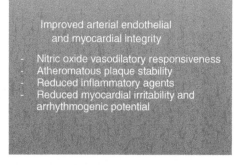

FIGURE 5C.1   CVD risk factors and myocardial function elements, which are affected by physical activity and exercise training (adapted from Myers et al. 2002, 2004; Franklin and Gordon 2009).

8 METs, inactivity is a likely significant contributing factor to this lower capacity (Myers et al. 2002, 2004; Gordon and Franklin 2009).

5C.4   MOVING FROM TRADITIONAL TO CONTEMPORARY MODELS OF PHYSICAL ACTIVITY AND REHABILITATION

Historically, physical activity following a cardiac event has always been included in early mobilisation and subsequent therapeutic and preventative exercise training (Bethell 2000; Coats et al. 1995). This goal remains essentially unchanged; however exercise has often been regarded as the central component to rehabilitation. Without demeaning the value of exercise, since 2007 the BACPR have aimed to give all components (discussed within this book) equal value and put behaviour change and education as the central integrating and underpinning element to all these components (BACPR 2012, 2017; BACPR et al. 2013). Within a comprehensive model of cardiac rehabilitation, it has been estimated that half of the benefit comes from the contribution of exercise training and the other half to reductions in the major risk factors (medical, psychological, and lifestyle interventions), especially smoking cessation (Taylor et al. 2006). However, the value of exercise in the longer term is an area that needs more attention. Programmes delivered for 12 weeks have reported maintenance of exercise capacity up to 1.5 years (Blum et al. 2013), but few studies have provided data for periods longer than this. One study, which followed up patients for 14 years (Beauchamp et al. 2013), reported that those who attended more sessions within a four-month rehabilitation period had greater survival at 14 years but much of the influence was affected by smoking status. Questions thus arise on how long-term sustainability of physical activity and exercise capacity can be achieved, when most programmes only last 12 weeks. Factors related to developing patient's self-management skills and long-term maintenance are covered in Chapters 4 and 8 respectively.

5c.4.1   Traditional Provision

Based on the UK's national audit data (NACR 2017) and information collected from over 2000 case-studies submitted for the BACPR exercise instructor qualification since 1999, many current programmes offer exercise as part of a traditional standard outpatient (phase III) process; commencing no earlier than 6 weeks after event/diagnosis and lasting for 6–12 weeks. These programmes have typically included: a pre-participation screening and risk stratification for exertion-related events; risk factor profiling that can be influenced by exercise (blood pressure, lipids, body composition, physical activity levels, aerobic fitness, mental health, and wellbeing); an assessment of functional capacity; and an exercise programme. Although all of these elements should continue to exist, in looking to the future there needs to be a broadening of provision for when, how, and where the physical activity component is delivered so as to best influence uptake, adherence, completion, and long-term maintenance of an active lifestyle (BACPR 2017).

5c.4.2 The Future Provision and Need for Early Commencement

The BACPR emphasises the earliest commencement of all components of reha-bilitation, including physical activity and exercise training (BACPR 2017). In meeting the patient's widest physical needs, this involves more than just the structured exercise sessions. It requires the encapsulation of all the patient's mobility/exertion needs and physical daily demands. This approach applies the Department of Health's 2010 Commissioning Pack guide (DoH 2010), which illustrates a flexible seven stage pathway and the NICE recommendations for commencing rehabilitation within 10 days of discharge (NICE 2013). It is under-pinned by an assessment-based care continuum from a defined point of diag-nosis or identification of significant future risk, through to long-term self-management, which should include support from the patient's own primary care team (Chapter 8). The physical activity component should therefore com-mence with an inpatient assessment of current mobilisation and daily func-tioning needs with relevant advice for being safely active within daily life. This should be followed up within 10 days by an outpatient assessment and com-mencement of the rehabilitation exercise programme. The outpatient physical activity plan should be commenced following risk stratification and an assessment of functional capacity, which also becomes part of the risk stratifica-tion (see Section 5c.7 on exercise assessment). The evidence for early commence-ment and related strategies for increasing patient uptake of rehabilitation is robust but more evidence is required on the most effective ways to influence adherence (BACPR 2013; BACPR 2017; Davies et al. 2010; NICE 2013). With the advancement of new 'personalised' and electronic technologies for managing and measuring daily activity and exercise (Reid et al. 2011), it will be of interest for future investigators to evaluate their role in long-term adherence as part of or following a programme of rehabilitation.

5C.5 KEY ISSUES FOR EARLY COMMENCEMENT OF EXERCISE

It is not unexpected that within the BACPR aims for 'early' commencement of exercise, there could be concern for some patient groups, especially those who have either recently undergone coronary artery bypass surgery (CABG), had a diagnosis of congestive heart failure, suffered a MI, received a heart transplant, or therapy and/or implantation of a device for controlling arrhythmias. Establishing the physical activity plan and exercise programme for some of these groups should, however, be thought of as no different an approach to how patients with heart failure are prescribed beta-blocker medication. If the full 'recommended dose' were to be given at the outset it could put the patient at risk. However, if the prescription and administration of the dose is titrated over weeks up to an optimised level, which works in concert with the expected adaptation/healing processes, it gives the body time to adapt and adjust in a safe and effective way. For physical activity, this managed up-titration model should also be seen as a psychological and social process (Acevado and Ekkikakis 2006; Buckley 2006). As noted in this chapter and others within this text, there is good evidence for key psychological and behavioural benefits to support the vital aim of early engagement of the patient in becoming mobile and active (to whatever appropriate degree).

A whole chapter or even a book could be devoted to providing guidance on 'early' rehabilitation exercise in all the above noted groups. In light of national data on the most represented groups of patients attending cardiac rehabilitation (NACR 2017), the greatest amount of evidence relates mainly to those with coronary artery disease (post-MI, post-revascularisation) and heart failure. For the specific details to exercise programming in these conditions and other specialised groups, the BACPR education course resources (BACPR 2014) and the ACPICR Standards (ACPICR 2015) provide such condition specific guidance along with recommendations for those with key co-morbidities (e.g. diabetes, peripheral vascular disease, implanted devices and arrhythmias, pulmonary disease, etc.).

5c.5.1   Reducing Risk of Exertion-related Events

For whatever cardiovascular condition(s) a patient has, the BACPR and ACPICR have set out a clear set of factors for reducing the risk of provoking an exertion-related event. This is of particular importance with starting rehabilitation early, which coincides with periods of healing and physiological stabilisation following an acute event, treatment, and/or surgery. There are three factors needing consideration:

- Assessment and risk stratification
- Pre-activity screening and monitoring patient status or contraindications to physical activity
- Monitoring intensity and related levels of supervision (see later section on staffing)
- All moderate to vigorous exercise sessions should be preceded by a graduated warm-up (up to $<40\%VO_2$ max or $<40\%$ HRR or $<$RPE 11) and

proceeded by a graduated cool-down. Pragmatically to cover all the activities required for an effective warm-up and cool-down and to ensure necessary physiological processes have occurred to best prevent any adverse events of ischaemia, dyspnoea, syncope, or arrhythmia, 15 and 10 minutes are required, respectively (ACPICR 2015; BACPR 2014).

These above elements have different parameters dependent on the context in which physical activity is being performed, including:

- Exercise tests and assessments (submaximal or maximal)
- Light to moderate intensity activity that is part of normal daily functioning at home, at work, or as part of transport
- Non-supervised moderate-to-vigorous activity (structured sessions or as part of work or leisure pursuits and transport)
- Supervised structured moderate-to-vigorous activity.

Many guidelines and standards are written with the assumption of risk stratification and contraindications being set for individuals undergoing a maximal exercise test or moderate-to-vigorous supervised activity (see Australian model in Section 5c.5.6 on post-MI exercise).

5c.5.2 Post-Surgery and Early Rehabilitation

This sub-section aims to provide guidance on how physical activity can and should be included in early rehabilitation for those following CABG (also applicable to valve surgery) alongside other key components: education and risk factor management, developing self-management skills, and psychosocial wellbeing.

Since the NACR data was first collected in 2007 the greatest relative uptake (>70%) for any group participating in rehabilitation has consistently been patients who have undergone CABG. This is likely to be a result of the pathway of treatment and care for CABG being very predictable, timed, and structured. Along with the overt visual reminder to the patient of the seriousness of their disease and the surgical procedure, these facts seem to conspire towards patients more easily adopting and achieving the goals of rehabilitation compared with other groups. This structure includes designated pre-surgery preparations and education (see prehabilitation Section 5c.5.5), an inpatient phase of five to seven days in hospital, and up to six weeks required convalescence (NHS Choices 2015).

Structured moderate-to-more-vigorous aerobic exercise training has been recommended to commence no earlier than two weeks post hospital discharge and more ideally at four weeks (Carrel and Mohacsi 1998; Hillis et al. 2011). Dubach et al. (1998) demonstrated that in the first four to eight weeks post-surgery, improvement in aerobic fitness was as much a function of spontaneous healing/recovery as it was to exercise training. They did however acknowledge that they did not assess whether delayed rehabilitation would impact negatively on psychosocial aspects of health and wellbeing.

5c.5.3 Post-Surgery, Early Aerobic Activity, and Strength Training

In keeping with current BACPR (2013) recommendations and relevant to the above and follow-on evidence, commencing post-CABG rehabilitation early (~10 days post-discharge) should involve light intensity aerobic activity, upper body mobility, and lower limb strength training. There is now good evidence, which includes older people (>75 years), that it is safe and effective to commence normal resistance strength training of the lower limbs (e.g. 10–15 repetitions at 60% one repetition maximum) at two weeks post-CABG discharge (Adams et al. 2006; Busch et al. 2012). Parker and Adams (2008) and Adams et al. (2014) have even demonstrated that performing upper body exercise with moderate weights soon after CABG surgery can be performed safely with far less stress on the sternum than a forceful sneeze. As a precaution, sternal stress can be greatly reduced if arm exercises are performed with the humerus/shoulder held in adduction (elbows kept near to the thorax). The key assumptions of all the above elements assume the patient has recovered without complication, is feeling well, and the surgical wounds in both the chest and the leg are healing well without infection.

5c.5.4 Typical Post-Surgical Complications

Transient atrial fibrillation (AF) may be found in 25–30% of patients in the early post-operative period, but can be present in up to 60% for those following more complex surgery (e.g. addition of valve surgery). AF is usually self-limited and the vast majority of cases will revert to sinus rhythm within 24 hours. However, in a smaller proportion of patients it can persist up to many weeks before spontaneously resolving (Banach et al. 2010; Hillis et al. 2011; Mariscalco et al. 2013; Siribaddana 2012). These reviews revealed that predisposing factors to AF normally include: advancing age, presence of heart failure, peripheral vascular disease, pulmonary disease, pre-operative tachyarrhythmias, or pericarditis. Pre-exercise risk stratification, screening, medical management, and programme adaptation should therefore include all the above factors and heart rate/symptom reporting should be routinely documented on a regular basis during the whole period of rehabilitation. The need to ensure participants with AF can use RPE effectively is important and also to document the METs at which they are observably comfortable or struggling. This can be determined either during an exercise assessment or during activities where METs can be best and accurately estimated (e.g. cycle ergometer, treadmill walking, stepping height, and rate) (Buckley 2006).

For more detailed guidance on the management of transient or persistent AF, refer to NICE clinical guidance 180 (NICE 2014).

5c.5.5 'Prehabilitation' Exercise for Surgical Patients

The evaluation of pre-surgical cardiorespiratory fitness and exercise training for many conditions is increasingly becoming a common practice aimed at reducing surgical and post-surgical complications along with improving post-surgical health outcomes (Santa Mina et al. 2014). In a Scottish prospective randomised controlled trial of pre-rehabilitation for CABG, 12-year follow-up survival rates were significantly favourable for those who received pre-surgery exercise training (Rideout et al. 2011). It was also noted that pre-surgery anxiety and depression were predictors of increased mortality, again raising important matters of psychological aspects of rehabilitation and the potential contributions that exercise may have, along with targeted pre-surgery psychological interventions (Furze et al. 2009). Furthermore, prehabilitation can influence post-surgery uptake and the benefits of rehabilitation (Arthur et al. 2000; Furze et al. 2009). Inspiratory muscle training has also received some attention pre- and post-surgery but larger trials or datasets are required to increase confidence in their validity (Padula and Yeaw 2007). In this systematic review, favourable short-term outcomes in pulmonary function recovery were reported in CABG, heart failure, and asthma patients, which could potentially help accelerate the time to which the exercise part of their rehabilitation could commence.

5c.5.6 Post-Angioplasty and Post-MI

Compared to the >70% uptake in CABG groups, exercise-based rehabilitation uptake in post-angioplasty and post-MI patients is ~40 and ~50%, respectively (NACR 2017). Following treatment for MI and ischaemic heart disease, the soonest contact and making of an appointment to commence rehabilitation has shown some favourable influences to increasing uptake of exercise (BACPR et al. 2013; Karmali et al. 2014; Pack et al. 2013).

Unlike CABG, hospital stays for those having coronary angioplasty (PCI) following either elective treatment or MI, are now very short. This reduces the time available for 'inpatient' rehabilitation and secondary prevention preparations. Furthermore, many patients will return to normal aspects of their social and work life within a few weeks (NHS Choices 2016). Such achievements in medicine seem impressive but this does reduce the amount of time to engage with patients to encourage and support participation in exercise sessions and provide advice on becoming more physically active in daily life. From this perspective alone, it highlights the value of commencing rehabilitation as soon as possible and offering patients choices to where and when (time of day) they can participate.

The NACR (2014) reported that in one third of patients who do not attend outpatient exercise sessions, it is due to a lack of interest/belief, which corresponds to trialled research evidence within other state-run health systems (Redfern et al. 2007). It is, however, interesting to note that from the NACR data, neither an early return to work nor available transport to rehabilitation were found to be non-significant reasons for taking up rehabilitation.

In stable patients, early exercise rehabilitation following MI, which begins within one-week of discharge and lasts for 12 weeks provides beneficial effects on left ventricular (LV) remodelling (Haykowsky et al. 2011). This review reported a gradient effect, where with every one-week delay in commencement, it was calculated that an extra month of exercise training would be required to achieve the same ventricular remodelling benefit. In all the 12 studies (647 patients) from this review, the exercise intensity was >60% VO_2 peak, which is within the target intensity range recommended by the BACPR (40–70% VO_2 max); an appropriate level for early commencement of exercise. Of note from a review of key evidence, Swain and Franklin (2002a, 2002b) found it difficult to define a 'minimum' beneficial threshold of intensity in cardiac patients due to a number of other competing factors at baseline (e.g. baseline fitness and previous activity levels) but there was confidence in outcomes when the exercise intensity exceeded 40% of VO_2 max. In promoting the BACPR's flexible model for the provision of exercise, which must be adapted to the psychological, sociological, and geographical (clinic, community, or home-based) needs of the patient, this intensity range also encompasses the effective lower supervision, lower intensity, and lower risk Australian model pioneered by Goble and Worcester (ACRA 2004). This model was designed to suit the needs for achieving the widest delivery of safe and beneficial rehabilitation in the disparate low population density make-up of Australia.

5c.5.7 Post-angioplasty Complications

An obvious cause for concern with early rehabilitation following angioplasty is that some patients may be in a vulnerable period for complications, which can lead to re-hospitalisation within 30–60 days (Khawaja et al. 2012; Moretti et al. 2014). Between 10 and 20% of post-angioplasty patients will be readmitted to hospital within 30 days (BCIS 2013; Lam et al. 2011). These patients tend to be either older, female, or with existing heart failure or chronic kidney disease (Wasfy et al. 2013). Rehabilitation practitioners should therefore include these factors in their risk stratification and ensure symptom assessments are frequent, which includes encouraging patient self-monitoring.

Presenting symptoms of post-angioplasty complications include recurrent angina (BCIS 2013; Izzo et al. 2012), which can be caused by a number of factors, including:

- Incomplete revascularization
- In-stent restenosis
- In-stent thrombosis
- Progression of atherosclerosis
- Epicardial coronary spasm
- Arterial 'stretch pain' caused by the stent over-stretching or irritating the coronary adventitia
- Microvascular dysfunction.

A recent study (Iliou et al. 2015) reported that the event rate between early ($n = 1821$) and late ($n = 1311$) rehabilitation commencement (<1 month versus >1 month post-angioplasty) showed no difference in subsequent coronary events. In offering early exercise-based rehabilitation, which includes standardised pre-activity screening by trained clinical staff, the chances of early detection of such complications may be enhanced and is known to reduce costly 60 day re-hospitalisation rates by up to 58% of the predicted rates (BACPR et al. 2013; Lam et al. 2011). Compared with more sedentary individuals, patients who are regularly physically active, as part of a dedicated self-management programme, are likely to better detect and/or manage symptoms and recognise the onset of disease progression (McGillion et al. 2014).

With the promotion of early rehabilitation, it is of interest for the future to see if evidence emerges to evaluate whether exercise can contribute, like statins (Prasad 2013), to similar acute endothelial function and antithrombotic benefits. As noted earlier, exercise has proven to give some significant benefits in the longer-term effects of endothelial function and prevention of atheromatic events following rehabilitation, but usually with the commencement of exercise after four weeks post-event (Hambrecht et al. 2004; Lam et al. 2011). The independent effect of exercise in more recent times is less clear because it is usually delivered as part of a lifestyle and risk factor management package (BACPR et al. 2013; Franklin et al. 2003; Lee et al. 2014). Future evaluation of the acute ameliorating effects of exercise soon after angioplasty may help to better highlight its independent benefits singularly or collectively in reducing endothelial dysfunction, thrombosis, and restenosis.

5c.5.8 Heart Failure

Exercise-based rehabilitation for chronic or congestive heart failure (CHF) improves health-related quality of life, reduces CHF-related hospitalisation in people with systolic dysfunction, and a trend towards reduced mortality in those surviving beyond one year from the point of diagnosis (Taylor et al. 2014). All the trials in this Cochrane review, which also consisted of more recent evidence for those with HFPEF (heart failure with preserved ejection fraction), included aerobic exercise training and some with strength training. Participants were mainly NYHA II and III, male Caucasian and with an average age of 62 years. Only three studies ($n = 279$) specifically recruited participants over age 70 years, where in the UK, 77 years is the average age of diagnosis for CHF (BSH 2013).

Due to the older age group of people with CHF, lower absolute exercise capacity and co-morbidities (musculoskeletal and neurological) are more likely. Typical symptoms from CHF of dyspnoea and muscle fatigue along with low functional capacity, are very similar characteristics to those with chronic pulmonary disease, chronic kidney disease, and those at risk of falls (Gosker et al. 2000; Moinuddin and Leehey 2008; Skalska et al. 2014). For the exercise component of rehabilitation, it has been reported as beneficial to combine CHF patients' exercise with these other groups with similar functionally limiting symptoms (Evans 2011; Evans et al. 2010). With current cardiac rehabilitation programmes often unable to include CHF patients due to factors of capacity (NACR 2014), this could be a pragmatic means to significantly increase provision and uptake of rehabilitation for this group. With groups of individuals over age 75, exercise that enhances both function and health-related quality of life proves a more robust outcome than simply morbidity and mortality (Taylor et al. 2014).

Similar to a group of elite athletes compared with each other, for individuals with heart failure, their exercise capacity (VO_2 max or peak) is not necessarily the most defining element linked to practical physical function (performance) (Beckers et al. 2008; Foster and Lucia 2007; Hagberg and Coyle 1983). This evidence demonstrates that exercise training (endurance and strength/resistance training), which leads to the ability to sustain/endure activity at a given submaximal level along with improvements in 'movement economy', can often prove a more vital outcome to the participant/patient than simply aiming to increase aerobic capacity/fitness.

The BACPR (2014) and ACPICR (2015) recommend an exercise dose that continues to reflect the elements reported in the Cochrane review, including:

- A median frequency of three to four sessions per week.
- A median duration of 30–50 minutes (range 15–120 minutes).
- An intensity range between 30 and 70% VO_2 max or HRR.

- The inclusion of strength, balance, and coordination training, especially for those with very limited capacity who rely more on muscular strength/endurance and anaerobic metabolism for performing basic daily activities.
- All moderate to vigorous exercise sessions should be preceded by a graduated warm-up (up to <40%VO$_2$ max or <40% HRR or <RPE 11) and proceeded by a de-graduating cool-down. Pragmatically to cover all the activities required for an effective warm-up and cool-down and to ensure necessary physiological processes have occurred to best prevent any adverse events of ischaemia, dyspnoea, syncope, or arrhythmia, 15 and 10 minutes are normally required, respectively (ACPICR 2015; BACPR 2014). Low-functioning patients may however find any activity moderate-to-vigorous and the warm-up and cool-down may need adapting (see ACPICR 2015).

5c.5.9   Heart Rate and Perceived Exertion Use in Heart Failure

The use of heart rate as a means of monitoring exercise intensity in CHF can be problematic for two reasons:

1. ~25% of people with CHF have atrial fibrillation, with an increasing prevalence with age (Heck et al. 2013).
2. Heart rate response to physical exertion is usually sympathetically dampened (often termed chronotropic incompetence) and therefore is less well correlated with changes in oxygen uptake or aerobic metabolism (Brubaker and Kitzman 2011; Witte and Clark 2009). The maximal heart rate is also lower in CHF and lowered further due to most patients being on beta-blocker medication (Keteyian et al. 2012). In the event that patients have a regular heart rhythm, their maximal heart rate can be estimated by this formula:

$$119 + (0.5 \times \text{resting HR}) - (0.5 \times \text{age}).$$

As with any estimation for maximal heart rate this formula has an error of estimation of up to ±18 beats per minute (Keteyian et al. 2012). It is recommended that in the absence of a maximal exercise test, the estimated maximum value from the above formula is then included in Karvonen's method for determining 30–70% of HRR (ACPICR 2015; BACPR 2014; Carvalho and Mezzani 2011; Karvonen et al. 1957).

The obvious alternative or adjunct to heart rate is to use RPE as a means of measuring or monitoring intensity. It has been used widely in both research and many guidelines for exercise in CHF; however there are very few studies that have validated RPE for use in CHF (Carvalho et al. 2009; Iellamo et al. 2014;

Levinger et al. 2004). An important element for its effective use is to respect the key 'psychophysical components' and physical symptoms in CHF compared to other populations. Specifically, in CHF patients have very distinct sensations of breathlessness and muscle fatigue, which can occur at relatively low absolute exercise intensities. In healthy individuals there is usually good congruency between these two key sensory elements and exercise intensity (Borg 1990, 1998; Borg et al. 2010) but for those with dyspnoea or muscle fatigue (CHF or chronic obstructive pulmonary disease [COPD]) this may not hold true. In keeping with Borg's recommendations, it would be best to assess differentiated ratings of breathlessness and muscle fatigue plus the usual overall rating of exertion using Borg's CR10 scale (Borg 1990, 1998; Stendardi et al. 2005). This would be more appropriate than using Borg's RPE 6–20 scale, which was designed to correspond to the linear response nature of overall sensations of exertion related to predominantly aerobic activity (Borg 1990).

5c.5.10   Commencing Rehabilitation Prior to Optimisation of Heart Failure Medication

As part of the BACPR aims for commencing 'early' rehabilitation after diagnosis or primary treatment, heart failure too has the challenge that patients require a number of weeks (2–5) to optimise their medications and attain an expected stable condition (NICE 2010b). Few studies have reported on this, but one UK study that did commence rehabilitation exercise within four weeks showed it was safe (Houchen et al. 2012). The key element is to ensure patients' symptoms (breathlessness, body-weight fluctuations, oedema, blood pressure, and heart rate) are stable (ACPICR 2015). Encouragingly for those UK programmes that offer CHF rehabilitation, the median commencement date is approaching this 'early' commencement criteria at 35 days (5 weeks) from diagnosis and primary treatment (NACR 2017).

5C.6   EMERGING AREAS RELATED TO ACTIVITY INTENSITY – FROM SEDENTARY BEHAVIOUR, LIGHT MOBILITY, AND MODERATE INTENSITY TO HIGH INTENSITY INTERVAL TRAINING

Encouraging patients to be more active in all aspects of life is important and beneficial, whether this be avoiding too much sitting, more active domestic activities, transport, and leisure, through to specific moderate to vigorous intensity exercise training. Simply standing more has shown to benefit CVD risk and risk factors of blood glucose/insulin and energy expenditure (Crichton and Alkerwi 2014; Dempsey et al. 2014). Furthermore, for older aged individuals, avoiding sedentary behaviour decreases risk of falls by preserving balance, strength, and bone density (Chastin and Skelton 2012; Skelton 2001). Regular lower intensity walking in stable angina patients, though not necessarily leading to improvements in aerobic capacity, has been shown to reduce angina symptoms and use of GTN, and improved self-perceived physical functioning (Lewin et al. 2002). For very low-functioning patients benefits in physical functioning, though not clear influences on morbidity and mortality, Tai Chi can be either a starting point or adjunctive mode of activity to more traditional aerobic and muscular strength exercises (Lan et al. 2008). Most of the evidence for cardiac rehabilitation has used moderate-to-vigorous intensity aerobic exercise (Heran et al. 2011; Taylor et al. 2014). The combination of both aerobic and muscular strength exercise has also shown to be better than aerobic exercise alone (Mandic et al. 2011; Meka et al. 2008). More recently there has been much attention around high intensity interval training (HIIT) in both CHD and CHF (Guiraud et al. 2012; Haykowsky et al. 2013).

The physiological benefits from HIIT in the research trials (<12 months) have proven to be superior to moderate intensity interval or continuous exercise training; however, the BACPR has not yet moved to recommending HIIT for the following reasons:

- The trials mostly involved younger aged participants (<65 years) who were free of many typical co-morbidities of the CR population in the UK (NACR 2014).
- All the trials used maximal cardiopulmonary exercise testing to screen participants for trial inclusion and then for setting precisely prescribed programmes.
- The trials involved closely monitored and individually supervised exercise training sessions.
- The trials used a variety of different ways for determining a HIIT protocol (e.g. a number of variations in the durations of the training and rest intervals and variation in what constituted high intensity).
- There is a lack of trials performing a more comprehensive evaluation of participation behaviour and related rationale; e.g. was the HIIT programme aimed at something to be used for shorter-term rehabilitation to 'get people on their feet again' or was it to be the type of activity expected to be performed longer term?
- There is still the need for evidence on longer-term health outcomes for HIIT (>12 months relating to morbidity, mortality, physical or psychological, or social functioning and quality of life).

5C.7   ASSESSING FUNCTIONAL CAPACITY AND PHYSICAL ACTIVITY – GUIDANCE, PRESCRIPTION, AND RISK STRATIFICATION OUTCOMES EVALUATION AND AUDIT

With regard to audit and evaluation of the exercise component of CR it is ideal to measure both changes in the volume (frequency, duration, and intensity) of physical activity and changes in physical fitness. The NACR database aims to capture these as well. Audit normally reflects the collective overall changes or improvements in these two parameters for groups of patients starting and completing rehabilitation, and compares these with expected changes related to health outcomes. Evaluation tends to look at the more individual nature of assessment results in order to determine baseline levels, exercise guidance and prescription, programme progression, and changes in physical activity levels and fitness following a programme. These are aimed at supporting individual patient care.

The BACPR (2014) and the ACPICR (2015) outline clearly the types of assessment to measure both physical activity participation levels and practical measures of physical fitness. The gold standard for functional aerobic fitness is a maximal test (usually treadmill or cycle ergometer), which employs direct measures of cardiopulmonary function (ECG, pulmonary responses, and derived metabolic or physiologic markers, representing integrated muscular, circulatory, cardiac, and pulmonary functions). Since 2010 NICE, in its clinical guidance (CG95) (NICE 2010a), have removed the use of exercise ECGs in the diagnosis of suspect stable coronary artery disease (typically presented as angina) due to its moderate level of sensitivity and specificity (~65–70%). This, however, does not mean it is not of value for assessing baseline functional capacity and outcomes, evaluating ECG and haemodynamic changes in individuals with known coronary disease, arrhythmia, or heart failure.

In the UK, cardiac rehabilitation resources are limited and maximal exercise testing, using either full cardiopulmonary assessments or just ECG, are limited to specialist treatment and/or research centres. The BACPR have therefore recommended the use of field-based assessments including the six-minute walk test, the incremental shuttle walk test, the Chester Step Test (or similar protocol), or an adapted Astrand cycle ergometer test (ACPICR 2015; BACPR 2014). Online resources are available for these as well.

The guidelines within these practice standards have demonstrated the value of how such tests can be used to assess individual patient's functional capacity and risk stratification as an aid to exercise prescription and instruction, along with programme evaluation required as an auditable outcome measure. In order for practitioners to effectively employ these various applications, a clear understanding and working knowledge of the relationship between heart rate, RPE, and METs is required. In relation to METs, practitioners must also have a working knowledge of how these relate to the intensity of various modes of exercise (walking speed, exercise ergometer workrates, outdoor leisure activities, and activities in daily living).

5C.8   STAFFING, CORE, AND QUALITY STANDARDS

To ensure the individualised safety and effectiveness of the exercise component for each patient, the exercise staff should be suitably qualified to:

- Evaluate the physical, psychological, and social needs of the patient
- Provide patient-centred consultations towards goal-setting
- Accurately risk stratify patients that will be reflected in levels of exercise intensity and related supervision/instruction
- Agree with the patient an appropriate exercise prescription
- Instruct and provide adequate induction programmes for all patients
- Determine and provide pre-participation screening (either from specialist staff or guide patients to self-assess) prior to the commencement of every exercise session
- Perform basic life support and use an Automatic External Defibrillator (AED), and assess the need for when to call for advanced life support services (please refer to the national policy statement on cardiopulmonary resuscitation, 2013 [Resuscitation Council (UK) 2014]).

Resource links are provided below regarding the specialist knowledge, skills, and competences of CR staff. These are underpinned by the pursuance of local protocols for health and safety as the mainstay for providing the safe and effective delivery of exercise in cardiac populations. There are several important documents available to guide managers and CR practitioners in meeting the required criteria for professional supervision of the exercise component of CR programmes independent of the venue (see ACPICR and BACPR websites).

The minimum recommendations for staffing a structured, moderate-to-vigorous exercise intensity session in early rehabilitation include:

- One appropriately qualified exercise professional to lead and take overall responsibility for the delivery of the exercise component
- Supporting staff made up of trained health or exercise professionals, where to provide a staff-to-patient ratio of 1:5, with this increasing to at least 1:3 for higher risk or complex patients.

Upon completion of early CR, one qualified BACPR exercise professional or equivalent is usually adequate for leading and supervising exercise in long-term maintenance programmes.

Standard policies, procedures, and algorithms for managing medical emergencies should be in place, displayed in the exercise area and reviewed regularly. Emergency equipment must be readily available at all times and staff should undergo regular training to maintain competency in responding to potential life-threatening events, such as diabetic hyper- or hypoglycaemia, arrhythmias, a suspected MI, or cardiac arrest. Adverse clinical events during exercise sessions are far less likely to occur if programmes adhere to standards at all times of the BACPR, ACPICR, National Occupational frameworks for exercise professionals, or the British Association of Sport and Exercise Sciences (BASES).

5c.8.1   Location of Prevention and Rehabilitation Programmes

The location of where (hospital, community leisure centre, home) and how (circuit classes, gym equipment, or home-based individual adaptations) formal sessions are delivered can have an impact on the chances of longer-term adherence and prevention of hospital readmission (BACPR et al. 2013; Canyon and Meshgin 2008; Davies et al. 2010). The patients' early initial assessment must therefore include discussing the best possible location of their activity and exercise along with appreciating the level of supervision required and individual social and psychological needs. Current evidence demonstrates that equal outcomes can be achieved from hospital, community, or home-based programmes and thus the most important element is the patient's choice (BACPR et al. 2013; Dent et al. 2011).

The BACPR is very supportive of the increasing number of services around the UK who provide the 'outpatient' exercise component within community settings, where clinical and community staff are integrated into working together. By engaging community exercise professionals within the outpatient service, a more seamless pathway for patients is provided from early rehabilitation through to long-term management. The UK (led by BACPR) is one of the few if any countries in the World that currently offers an exercise instructor qualification, which was specifically designed for keeping people active once discharged from a formal rehabilitation programme.

The environment and setting for exercise sessions is also important and the following are considerations:

- Size of the exercise room ($1.8-2.3 \times 6\,m^2$ of space per individual)
- Room temperature maintained between 18 and 23 °C
- Regular maintenance of equipment
- Drinking water available
- Infection control measures in place.

5C.9   FUTURE CHALLENGES FOR EXERCISE IN CARDIOVASCULAR DISEASE PREVENTION AND REHABILITATION

The BACPR (2017) have highlighted that the profile of morbidity and mortality due to CVD could change in the future. Over the past three decades there has been a steady decline in the incidence of mortality of MI in those under 75 years of age but there has been little change in the number of people living with CVD (Townsend et al. 2012a), and often with some degree of disablement. This coupled with an ageing population who are likely to have at least one other co-morbidity, will require the adoption of a chronic disease management approach, which engenders long-term adherence to a physically active lifestyle and the related self-management skills. Programmes will need adapting for these co-morbidities, and in some cases it may be both clinically and cost effective to combine rehabilitation and prevention with other key chronic diseases, which manifest similar levels of reduced function and symptoms (e.g. pulmonary diseases, metabolic disorders, and some cancers).

Case Study

Mr S

Patient Background

Male: South Asian, Age 52
Occupation: Bank Clerk
Family status: Married with three teenage children

Current Cardiac Event and Diagnosis
Anterior ST-segment elevation MI

> *Investigations*
> Angiogram: left main stem (LMS) unobstructed, left anterior descending (LAD) artery occluded proximally, left circumflex (LCx) artery moderate atheromatous disease distally (non-flow limiting), and right coronary mild atheromatous disease (unobstructed).
>
> *Intervention and treatments*
> Primary percutaneous coronary intervention with drug-eluting stent to the left anterior descending coronary artery; left circumflex and right coronary artery medically managed.
>
> *Post treatment investigations*
> Echocardiogram: moderate LV systolic impairment, ejection fraction 45%

Resting Blood Pressure: 130/70 mmHg
Resting Heart Rate: 50 bpm
Height: 172 cm **Weight:** 88 kg
Body mass index: 29.7
Waist: 102 cm

Current Medication
Aspirin, Prasugrel, Ramipril, Bisoprolol, Atorvastatin, Metformin, Gliclazide, Nicotine replacement therapy.

Past Medical History
Hypertension
Hypercholesterolaemia
Smoker
Type II diabetes
Family history, father died of an MI at 55 years of age

Initial Risk Stratification for Event on Exertion:
Moderate
Rationale based on American Association of Cardiovascular and Pulmonary Rehabilitation (AACVPR) criteria (ACPICR 2015; BACPR 2014): Ejection fraction <50%; no previous MI; uncomplicated recovery; no previous cardiac history, no cardiac arrest, no complex arrhythmias or residual myocardial ischaemia; estimated maximal exercise capacity 7.1 METs (Table 5c.2; achieved 5 METs at 70% of HRR, RPE 14).

Rehabilitation Programme
Mr S was referred to a community-based CPRP. Seven days following his cardiac event, Mr S was assessed by the cardiovascular health team, including: a specialist nurse, a dietitian, and a physical activity specialist.

Physical Activity Considerations
Prior to Mr S's cardiac event he participated in badminton once per week (>5 METs) and was able to easily perform several domestic activities around his home including hoovering and general cleaning (<5 METs) (Ainsworth et al. 2011). Mr S works as a Bank Clerk and spends most of his day sitting at a desk and he commutes to work by bus. At present, Mr S is fearful of returning back to playing badminton as he is worried about 'overworking his heart' and causing another cardiac event.

His blood pressure and diabetes are well managed and he reported no previous complications on exertion either in domestic physical activities or when playing badminton.

TABLE 5C.2   Exercise capacity assessment results (Chester step test).

LEVEL 2 min stages	Steps per min	METs 15 cm step	Initial Assessment		12 week reassessment	
			HR (%HRR)[a]	RPE	HR (%HRR)[a]	RPE
1	15	3.0	79 (33%)	9	74 (<30%)	8
			86 (40%)	11	79 (33%)	10
2	20	4.0	93 (47%)	12	82 (35%)	11
			98 (53%)	12	87 (40%)	11
3	25	5.0	108 (65%)	13	94 (48%)	12
			113 (70%)	14	99 (54%)	12
4	30	6.0			110 (66%)	13
					115 (73%)	14
5	35	7.0				

METs=metabolic equivalents; HR=heart rate; %HRR=%heart rate reserve; RPE=rating of perceived exertion.
[a] HRR calculated using Karvonen formula (BACPR 2014, ACPICR 2015).

5C.10   OVERARCHING GUIDANCE

It is important for Mr S to at least maintain his current exercise capacity, if not increase it. A capacity of <7 METs is distinctly linked to increases in both the risk of an exertion-related event and a longer-term prognosis for premature mortality (ACSM 2013; Myers et al. 2002, 2005). He has a very sedentary job and should aim to avoid prolonged periods of sitting. More physical activity can be added to his day by increasing more walking as a part of his daily transport to work, and performing moderate-to-vigorous intensity exercise on at least three days per week. In performing any activities at an intensity of >4 METs (e.g. including brisk walking, cutting the lawn, and badminton), will require 55–70% of his exercise capacity and if performed/accumulated for >20 minutes on any given day, will be at a level to confer some potential fitness gain.

5C.11   SPECIFIC PHYSICAL ACTIVITY AND EXERCISE GOALS AND GUIDANCE

Returning to badminton is as important (if not more) for his psychosocial wellbeing as it is for his physical health. In the long term it could be a key part of his weekly physical activity requirements. In respect to his fear of returning to play, the goal of building his confidence needs to include learning to know the sensations of exertion during his supervised exercise sessions. His estimated maximal capacity is 7.1 METs and, depending upon the type and intensity of badminton (singles, doubles, highly competitive), it has an intensity range of 5.5 to 7 METs (Ainsworth et al. 2011). His current level of fitness (Table 5c.2) shows that moderate intensity activity is in the range of 3–5 METs (RPE 11–14; 40–70% HRR; 40–70% of maximal capacity), which means he can be reassured to certainly return to recommencing badminton of at least doubles and in practice sessions, where he should feel less compelled to over-exert; more competitive environments do elicit greater levels of adrenaline (Krahenbuhl 1975). Helping Mr S realise the goal of a full return to badminton is seen as a key rationale for him needing to improve his aerobic fitness.

5C.12   SPECIFIC EXERCISE SESSIONS

In keeping with the BACPR standards (BACPR et al. 2013), Mr S was assessed and commenced exercise within two weeks of discharge. The programme was for 12 weeks. It included pre-activity checks of blood pressure, blood glucose, medication changes or problems, and a review of symptoms (see ACPICR 2015; BACPR 2014 for detailed processes). On the first three sessions post-exercise blood-sugar levels were also recorded to assess any notable changes and review with Mr S the normal values that should be expected before, during, and after exercise, and if he needs any carbohydrate supplements. He participated in the group circuit classes and post-class educational sessions covering various topics on: smoking cessation, cardiovascular medication, healthy heart diet, maintaining behaviour change, stress management, and the benefits of physical activity. Sessions were supervised by three members of staff (physical activity specialist, nurse, and dietitian), which provided a staff:patient ratio of 1:5 patients (ACPICR 2015) and led by a physical activity specialist in keeping with BACPR standards (BACPR et al. 2013).

Each session provided the recommended 15 minute warm-up and 10 minute cool-down and the circuit involved six stations, which included a choice of two levels of exercises at each station. The circuit at week one alternated between cardiorespiratory conditioning and active recovery exercise stations. Mr S commenced his programme performing each station for two minutes and the circuit of exercises was completed twice, totalling 24 minutes, where 12 minutes targeted cardiorespiratory training. The active recovery exercises were lower intensity and used smaller muscle groups. During the circuit of exercises, Mr S was carefully monitored and encouraged to work within a heart rate zone of 86–113 beats per minute (40–70% HRR; Table 5c.2) and to relate the effort sensations to an RPE range of 11–14. He was reminded to focus on his RPE so that eventually he would not need to rely on the heart rate monitor to guide his pacing. This would work towards him being able to more naturally and independently monitor activity whenever he was on his own, whether in activities of daily life or during sport and exercise.

The shuttle walk (pace) and the stepping (height and rate) stations would allow the staff to more easily and specifically check the estimated MET values at which he was working as part of checking progress and improvement over the course of the programme (Ainsworth et al. 2011; BACPR 2014).

Once Mr S had attended three sessions, he demonstrated a clearer understanding of RPE, was able to regulate his exercise intensity more independently, and was thus encouraged to perform more activity at home on a regular basis including 20–30 minutes of walking per day at paces similar to that in the class sessions.

5C.13   PROGRAMME OUTCOMES

By the 12th week Mr S had progressed to a level where he was performing 24 minutes of continuous cardiorespiratory conditioning exercises (no active recovery stations), which now equated to exercise levels of up to 6 METs (start of programme up to 5 METs). He was encouraged to return to his badminton as one of his three exercise sessions per week. If he wanted, he could borrow a heart rate monitor to check what his heart rates were during the badminton and compare these with his perceived effort sensations.

His follow-up step-test confirmed that he had improved his exercise capacity (Table 5c.2), where for the same heart rate (70%HRR) and RPE (14) he was working at one MET greater. At 5 METs of exertion his heart rate was 14 beats per minute lower. His estimated maximal capacity thus increased 16% from 7.1 to 8.2 METs, which relates to a 12% reduction in risk of premature mortality (Myers et al. 2002). Additionally, his weight decreased by 3 kg and a corresponding decrease in waist circumference of 2 cm. Throughout the programme, with each visit, the rehabilitation team reviewed with Mr S his progress of physical functioning, symptoms, and CVD risk factors. In respecting his personal and social circumstances, encouragement and behaviour change processes were pursued so he could independently achieve and maintain healthy levels of physical activity (e.g. walking at >5 METs for 20–30 minute per day) and the confidence to play badminton.

5C.14 CONCLUSION

Increased physical activity performed regularly, whether from light intensity activities used to break up sedentary behaviour right through to higher intensity structured exercise, collectively have an impact on cardiovascular health and psychosocial wellbeing. For those without diagnosed cardiovascular disease or at high risk of developing disease, being more active and fitter is protective against the development of significant disease and premature mortality. In those with established disease, being more active and fitter is associated with improvements in physiological, cardiometabolic and psychosocial recovery, improved risk factor profile, early mortality, and reduced costly hospital readmissions. Practitioners guiding participants to be more active should not only focus on regular moderate vigorous intensity aerobic endurance activity but also muscular strength and endurance activity, and preventing prolonged periods of daily sedentary behaviour.

REFERENCES

Acevado, E.O. and Ekkikakis, P.E. (2006). *The Psychobiology of Physical Activity*. Champaign, Illinois: Human Kinetics.

ACPICR (2015). *Standards for Physical Activity and Exercise in the Cardiac Population*. London: Association of Chartered Physiotherapists in Cardiac Rehabilitation.

ACRA (2004). Recommended Framework for Cardiac '04. Canberra: National Heart Foundation of Australia and the Australian Cardiac Rehabilitation Association.

ACSM (2013). *ACSM's Guidelines for Exercise Testing and Prescription*. Lippincott, Williams and Wilkins: Baltimore.

Adams, J., Cline, M., Reed, M. et al. (2006). Importance of resistance training for patients after a cardiac event. *Proceedings (Bayloyr University Medical Centre)* 19 (3): 246–248.

Adams, J., Schmid, J., Parker, R.D. et al. (2014). Comparison of force exerted on the sternum during a sneeze versus during low-, moderate-, and high-intensity bench press resistance exercise with and without the valsalva maneuver in healthy volunteers. *The American Journal of Cardiology* 113 (6): 1045–1048.

Aiello, A.E. and Kaplan, G.A. (2009). Socioeconomic position and inflammatory and immune biomarkers of cardiovascular disease: applications to the panel study of income dynamics. *Biodemography and Social Biology* 55 (2): 178–205.

Ainsworth, B.E., Haskell, W.L., Herrmann, S.D. et al. (2011). 2011 compendium of physical activities: a second update of codes and MET values. *Medicine and Science in Sports and Exercise* 43 (8): 1575–1581.

Almodhy, M., Ingle, L., and Sandercock, G.R. (2016). Effects of exercise-based cardiac rehabilitation on cardiorespiratory fitness: a meta-analysis of UK studies. *International Journal of Cardiology* 221: 644–651.

Arthur, H.M., Daniels, C., McKelvie, R. et al. (2000). Effect of a preoperative intervention on preoperative and postoperative outcomes in low-risk patients awaiting elective coronary artery bypass graft surgery. A randomized, controlled trial. *Annals of Internal Medicine* 133 (4): 253–262.

BACPR (2014). *A Practical Approach to Exercise and Physical Activity in the Prevention and Management of Cardiovascular Disease*. London: British Association for Cardiovascular Prevention and Rehabilitation.

BACPR, Buckley, J.P., Furze, G. et al. (2013). BACPR scientific statement: British standards and core components for cardiovascular disease prevention and rehabilitation. *Heart* 99 (15): 1069–1071.

Banach, M., Kourliouros, A., Reinhart, K.M. et al. (2010). Postoperative atrial fibrillation - what do we really know? *Current Vascular Pharmacology* 8 (4): 553–572.

BCIS (2013). *British Cardiovascular Intervention Society (BCIS) Audit Returns Adult Intervention Procedures* (ed. F. Ludman). London: British Cardiovascular Society.

Beauchamp, A., Worcester, M., Ng, A. et al. (2013). Attendance at cardiac rehabilitation is associated with lower all-cause mortality after 14 years of follow-up. *Heart* 99: 620–625.

Beckers, P.J., Denollet, J., Possemiers, N.M. et al. (2008). Combined endurance-resistance training vs. endurance training in patients with chronic heart failure: a prospective randomized study. *European Heart Journal* 29 (15): 1858–1866.

Berryman, J.W. (2010). Exercise is medicine: a historical perspective. *Current Sports Medicine Reports* 9 (4): 195–201.

Bethell, H.J. (2000). Cardiac rehabilitation: from Hellerstein to the millennium. *International Journal of Clinical Practice* 54 (2): 92–97.

Blum, M.R., Schmid, J.P., Eser, P., and Saner, H. (2013). Long-term results of a 12-week comprehensive ambulatory cardiac rehabilitation program. *Journal of Cardiopulmonary Rehabilitation and Prevention* 33 (2): 84–90.

Borg, E., Borg, G., Larsson, K. et al. (2010). An index for breathlessness and leg fatigue. *Scandinavian Journal of Medicine and Science in Sports* 20 (4): 644–650.

Borg, G. (1990). Psychophysical scaling with applications in physical work and the perception of exertion. *Scandinavian Journal of Work, Environment & Health* 16 (Suppl 1): 55–58.

Borg, G. (1998). *Borg's Perceived Exertion and Pain Scales*. Human Kinetics: Champaign, Illinois.

Brubaker, P.H. and Kitzman, D.W. (2011). Chronotropic incompetence: causes, consequences, and management. *Circulation* 123 (9): 1010–1020.

Brubaker, P.H., Rejeski, J.W., Law, H.C. et al. (1994). 'Cardiac patients' perception of work intensity during graded exercise testing. *Journal of Cardiopulmonary Rehabilitation* 4 (2): 127–133.

BSH (2013). *National Heart Failure Audit of the British Society of Heart Failure.* London: National Institute for Cardiovascular Outcomes Research.

Buckley, J.P. (2006). Exercise physiology and monitoring of exercise in cardiac rehabilitation. In: *Exercise Leadership in Cardiac Rehabilitation for High-Risk Groups: An Evidence-Based Approach* (ed. M.K. Thow). United Kingdom: Wiley-Blackwell (an imprint of John Wiley & Sons Ltd).

Buckley, J.P., Sim, J., and Eston, R.G. (2009). Reproducibility of ratings of perceived exertion soon after myocardial infarction: responses in the stress-testing clinic and the rehabilitation gymnasium. *Ergonomics* 52 (4): 421–427.

Busch, J.C., Lillou, D., Wittig, G. et al. (2012). Resistance and balance training improves functional capacity in very old participants attending cardiac rehabilitation after coronary bypass surgery. *Journal of the American Geriatrics Society* 60 (12): 2270–2276. https://doi.org/10.1111/jgs.12030.

Canyon, S. and Meshgin, N. (2008). Cardiac rehabilitation - reducing hospital readmissions through community-based programs. *Australian Family Physician* 37 (7): 575–577.

Carrel, T. and Mohacsi, P. (1998). Optimal timing of rehabilitation after cardiac surgery: the surgeon's view. *European Heart Journal* 19 (Suppl O): O38–O41.

Carvalho, V.O., Bocchi, E.A., and Guimarães, G.V. (2009). The Borg scale as an important tool of self-monitoring and self-regulation of exercise prescription in heart failure patients during hydrotherapy. *Circulation Journal* 73 (10): 1871–1876. https://doi.org/10.1253/circj.cj-09-0333.

Carvalho, V.O. and Mezzani, A. (2011). Aerobic exercise training intensity in patients with chronic heart failure: principles of assessment and prescription. *European Journal of Cardiovascular Prevention and Rehabilitation* 18 (1): 5–14.

Chastin, S.F.M. and Skelton, D.A. (2012). Minimise sedentary behaviour at all ages for healthy ageing. *British Medical Journal* 344: e2451–e2451. https://doi.org/10.1136/bmj.e2451.

CMOS (2011). Start Active Stay Active, a report of the UK's Chief Medical Officers. Department of Health and Social Care.

Coats, A.J., McGee, H., Stokes, S., and Thompson, D.R. (eds.) (1995). *BACR Guidelines for Cardiac Rehabilitation.* Oxford: Blackwell Science.

Conraads, V.M., Pattyn, N., De Maeyer, C. et al. (2015). Aerobic interval training and continuous training equally improve aerobic exercise capacity in patients with coronary artery disease: the SAINTEX-CAD study. *International Journal of Cardiology* 179: 203–210.

Cornelissen, V.A. and Fagard, R.H. (2004). Exercise intensity and postexercise hypotension. *Journal of Hypertension* 22 (10): 1859–1861. https://doi.org/10.1097/00004872-200410000-00004.

Crichton, G.E. and Alkerwi, A. (2014). Association of sedentary behavior time with ideal cardiovascular health: the ORISCAV-LUX study. *Public Library of Science ONE* 9 (6): e99829. https://doi.org/10.1371/journal.pone.0099829.

Davies, P., Taylor, F., Beswick, A. et al. (2010). Promoting patient uptake and adherence in cardiac rehabilitation. *The Cochrane Database of Systemic Reviews* 7 (7): CD007131. https://doi.org/10.1002/14651858.CD007131.pub2.

Deanfield, J. and Board, J. (2014). Joint British Societies' consensus recommendations for the prevention of cardiovascular disease (JBS3). *Heart* 100: 1–67.

Dempsey, P.C., Owen, N., Biddle, S.J., and Dunstan, D.W. (2014). Managing sedentary behavior to reduce the risk of diabetes and cardiovascular disease. *Current Diabetes Reports* 14: 522.

Dent, L., Taylor, R., Jolly, K., and Raftery, J. (2011). 'Flogging dead horses': evaluating when have clinical trials achieved sufficiency and stability? A case study in cardiac rehabilitation. *Trials* 12 (1): 83. https://doi.org/10.1186/1745-6215-12-83.

DOH (2010). Commissioning pack for Cardiac rehabilitation. NHS Digital http://www.cardiacrehabilitation.org.uk/resources.htm#dhc.

Dubach, P., Myers, J., and Wagner, D. (1998). Optimal timing of phase II rehabilitation after cardiac surgery - the cardiologist's view. *European Heart Journal* 19 (Suppl O): O35–O37.

Eston, R. and Connolly, D. (1996). The use of ratings of perceived exertion for exercise prescription in patients receiving beta-blocker therapy. *Sports Medicine* 21 (3): 176–190.

Eston, R.G. and Thompson, M. (1997). Use of ratings of perceived exertion for predicting maximal work rate and prescribing exercise intensity in patients taking atenolol. *British Journal of Sports Medicine* 31 (2): 114–119.

Evans, R., Singh, S., Collier, R. et al. (2010). Generic, symptom-based, exercise rehabilitation; integrating patients with COPD and heart failure. *Respiratory Medicine* 104 (10): 1473–1481.

Evans, R.A. (2011). Developing the model of pulmonary rehabilitation for chronic heart failure. *Chronic Respiratory Disease* 8: 259–269.

Fagard, R.H. (2011). Exercise therapy in hypertensive cardiovascular disease. *Progress in Cardiovascular Diseases* 53 (6): 404–411.

Fagard, R.H. and Cornelissen, V.A. (2007). Effect of exercise on blood pressure control in hypertensive patients. *European Journal of Cardiovascular Prevention and Rehabilitation* 14 (1): 12–17.

Foster, C. and Lucia, A. (2007). Running economy: the forgotten factor in elite performance. *Sports Medicine* 37 (4–5): 316–319.

Franklin, B., Swain, D., and Shephard, R. (2003). New insights in the prescription of exercise for coronary patients. *The Journal of Cardiovascular Nursing* 18 (2): 116–123.

Furze, G., Dumville, J., Miles, J. et al. (2009). 'Prehabilitation' prior to CABG surgery improves physical functioning and depression. *International Journal of Cardiology* 132 (1): 51–58.

Garber, C., Blissmer, B., Deschenes, M. et al. (2011). American College of Sports Medicine position stand. Quantity and quality of exercise for developing and maintaining cardiorespiratory, musculoskeletal, and neuromotor fitness in apparently healthy adults: guidance for prescribing exercise. *Medicine and Science in Sports and Exercise* 43 (7): 1334–1359.

Franklin, B.A. and Gordon, N.F. (2009). *Contemporary Diagnosis and Management in Cardiovascular Exercise*. United States: Assocs in Medical Marketing Co.

Gosker, H., Wouters, E., van der Vusse, G., and Schols, A. (2000). Skeletal muscle dysfunction in chronic obstructive pulmonary disease and chronic heart failure: underlying mechanisms and therapy perspectives. *The American Journal of Clinical Nutrition* 71 (5): 1033–1047.

Grace, S., Warburton, D., Stone, J. et al. (2013). International charter on cardiovascular prevention and rehabilitation: a call for action. *Journal of Cardiopulmonary Rehabilitation and Prevention* 33 (2): 128–131.

Guiraud, T., Nigam, A., Gremeaux, V. et al. (2012). High-intensity interval training in cardiac rehabilitation. *Sports Medicine* 42 (7): 587–605.

Gutmann, M.C., Squires, R.W., Pollock, M.L., and Al, E. (1981). Perceived exertion-heart rate relationship during exercise testing and training in cardiac patients. *Journal of Cardiac Rehabilitation* 1: 52–61.

Hagberg, J. and Coyle, E. (1983). Physiological determinants of endurance performance as studied in competitive racewalkers. *Medicine and Science in Sports and Exercise* 15 (4): 287–289.

Hallal, P.C., Andersen, L.B., Bull, F.C. et al. (2012). Global physical activity levels: surveillance progress, pitfalls, and prospects. *Lancet* 380 (9838): 247–257.

Hambrecht, R., Gielen, S., Linke, A. et al. (2000a). Effects of exercise training on left ventricular function and peripheral resistance in patients with chronic heart failure: a randomized trial. *The Journal of the American Medical Association (JAMA)*. 283 (23): 3095–3101.

Hambrecht, R., Hilbrich, L., Erbs, S. et al. (2000b). Correction of endothelial dysfunction in chronic heart failure: additional effects of exercise training and oral L-arginine supplementation. *Journal of the American College of Cardiology* 35 (3): 706–713.

Hambrecht, R., Niebauer, J., Marburger, C. et al. (1993). Various intensities of leisure time physical activity in patients with coronary artery disease: effects on cardiorespiratory fitness and progression of coronary atherosclerotic lesions. *Journal of the American College of Cardiology* 22 (2): 468–477.

Hambrecht, R., Walther, C., Möbius-Winkler, S. et al. (2004). Percutaneous coronary angioplasty compared with exercise training in patients with stable coronary artery disease: a randomized trial. *Circulation* 109 (11): 1371–1378.

Hamer, M., Sabia, S., Batty, G. et al. (2012). Physical activity and inflammatory markers over 10 years: follow-up in men and women from the Whitehall II cohort study. *Circulation* 126 (8): 928–933.

Hansen, D., Stevens, A., Eijnde, B., and Dendale, P. (2012). Endurance exercise intensity determination in the rehabilitation of coronary artery disease patients: a critical re-appraisal of current evidence. *Sports Medicine* 42 (1): 11–30.

Hassmén, P., Koivula, N., and Uutela, A. (2000). Physical exercise and psychological well-being: a population study in Finland. *Preventive Medicine* 30 (1): 17–25.

Haykowsky, M., Scott, J., Esch, B. et al. (2011). A meta-analysis of the effects of exercise training on left ventricular remodeling following myocardial infarction: start early and go longer for greatest exercise benefits on remodeling. *Trials* 12: 92.

Haykowsky, M., Timmons, M., Kruger, C. et al. (2013). Meta-analysis of aerobic interval training on exercise capacity and systolic function in patients with heart failure and reduced ejection fractions. *The American Journal of Cardiology* 111 (10): 1466–1469.

Head, A., Maxwell, S., and Kendall, M. (1997). Exercise metabolism in healthy volunteers taking celiprolol, atenolol, and placebo. *British Journal of Sports Medicine* 31 (2): 120–125.

Healy, G., Matthews, C., Dunstan, D. et al. (2011). Sedentary time and cardiometabolic biomarkers in US adults: NHANES 2003–06. *European Heart Journal* 32 (5): 590–597.

Heck, P., Lee, J., and Kistler, P. (2013). Atrial fibrillation in heart failure in the older population. *Heart Failure Clinics* 9 (4): 451–459. viii–ix.

Heran, B., Chen, J., Ebrahim, S. et al. (2011). Exercise-based cardiac rehabilitation for coronary heart disease. *The Cochrane Database of Systematic Reviews* 6 (7): CD001800. https://doi.org/10.1002/14651858.CD001800.pub2.

Hillis, L., Smith, P., Anderson, J. et al. (2011). 2011 ACCF/AHA guideline for coronary artery bypass graft surgery: executive summary: a report of the American College of Cardiology Foundation/American Heart Association task force on practice guidelines. *Circulation* 124 (23): 2610–2642.

Houchen, L., Watt, A., Boyce, S., and Singh, S. (2012). A pilot study to explore the effectiveness of "early" rehabilitation after a hospital admission for chronic heart failure. *Physiotherapy Theory and Practice* 28: 355–358.

Iellamo, F., Manzi, V., Caminiti, G. et al. (2014). Validation of rate of perceived exertion-based exercise training in patients with heart failure: insights from autonomic nervous system adaptations. *International Journal of Cardiology* 176 (2): 394–398.

Iliou, M., Pavy, B., Martinez, J. et al. (2015). Exercise training is safe after coronary stenting: a prospective multicentre study. *European Journal of Preventive Cardiology* 22 (1): 27–34.

Inbar, O., Oren, A., Scheinowitz, M. et al. (1994). Normal cardiopulmonary responses during incremental exercise in 20- to 70-yr-old men. *Medicine and Science in Sports and Exercise* 26 (5): 538–546.

Izzo, P., Macchi, A., Gennaro, D. et al. (2012). Recurrent angina after coronary angioplasty: mechanisms, diagnostic and therapeutic options. *European Heart Journal Acute Cardiovascular Care* 1 (2): 158–169.

Karvonen, M., Kentala, E., and Mustala, O. (1957). The effects of training on heart rate; a longitudinal study. *Annales Medicinae Experimentalis et Biologiae Fenniae* 35 (3): 307–315.

Katzmarzyk, P. (2013). Standing and mortality in a prospective cohort of Canadian adults. *Medicine and Science in Sports and Exercise* 46 (5): 940–946.

Katzmarzyk, P.T. and Lee, I.-M. (2012). Sedentary behaviour and life expectancy in the USA: a cause-deleted life table analysis. *British Medical Journal Open* 2 (4): 828. https://doi.org/10.1136/bmjopen-2012-000828.

Keteyian, S.J., Kitzman, D., Zannad, F. et al. (2012). Predicting maximal heart rate in heart failure patients receiving beta-blockade therapy. *Medicine and Science in Sports and Exercise* 44 (3): 371–376.

Khawaja, F., Shah, N., Lennon, R. et al. (2012). Factors associated with 30-day readmission rates after percutaneous coronary intervention. *Archives of Internal Medicine* 172 (2): 112–117.

Kodama, S., Tanaka, S., Saito, K. et al. (2007). Effect of aerobic exercise training on serum levels of high-density lipoprotein cholesterol: a meta-analysis. *Archives of Internal Medicine* 167 (10): 999–1008.

Krahenbuhl, G. (1975). Adrenaline, arousal and sport. *The Journal of Sports Medicine* 3 (3): 117–121.

Lam, G., Snow, R., Shaffer, L. et al. (2011). The effect of a comprehensive cardiac rehabilitation program on 60-day hospital readmissions after an acute myocardial infarction. *Journal of the American College of Cardiology* 57 (14): e597. https://doi.org/10.1016/S0735-1097(11)60597-4.

Lan, C., Chen, S., Wong, M., and Lai, J. (2008). Tai Chi training for patients with coronary heart disease. *Medicine and Sport Science* 52: 182–194.

Lawler, P., Filion, K., and Eisenberg, M. (2011). Efficacy of exercise-based cardiac rehabilitation post-myocardial infarction: a systematic review and meta-analysis of randomized controlled trials. *American Heart Journal* 162 (4): 571–584.

Lee, D., Sui, X., Ortega, F. et al. (2011). Comparisons of leisure-time physical activity and cardiorespiratory fitness as predictors of all-cause mortality in men and women. *British Journal of Sports Medicine* 45 (6): 504–510.

Lee, J., Yun, S., Ahn, J. et al. (2014). Impact of cardiac rehabilitation on angiographic outcomes after drug-eluting stents in patients with de novo long coronary artery lesions. *The American Journal of Cardiology* 113 (12): 1977–1985.

Levinger, I., Bronks, R., Cody, D. et al. (2004). Perceived exertion as an exercise intensity indicator in chronic heart failure patients on Beta-blockers. *Journal of Sports Science and Medicine* 3: 23–27.

Lewin, R.J.P., Furze, G., Robinson, J. et al. (2002). A randomised controlled trial of a self-management plan for patients with newly diagnosed angina. *British Journal of General Practice* 52 (476): 194–196. 199–201.

Mandic, S., Myers, J., Selig, S., and Levinger, I. (2011). Resistance versus aerobic exercise training in chronic heart failure. *Current Heart Failure Reports* 9 (1): 57–64.

Mariscalco, G., Musumeci, F., and Banach, M. (2013). Factors influencing post-coronary artery bypass grafting atrial fibrillation episodes. *Kardiologia Polska* 71 (11): 1115–1120.

Marzolini, S., Swardfager, W., Alter, D. et al. (2014). Quality of life and psychosocial measures influenced by exercise modality in patients with coronary artery disease. *European Journal of Physical and Rehabilitation Medicine* 51 (3): 291–299.

McGillion, M., O'Keefe-McCarthy, S., Carroll, S. et al. (2014). Impact of self-management interventions on stable angina symptoms and health-related quality of life: a meta-analysis. *BMC Cardiovascular Disorders* 14: 14.

Meka, N., Katragadda, S., Cherian, B., and Arora, R. (2008). Endurance exercise and resistance training in cardiovascular disease. *Therapeutic Advances in Cardiovascular Disease* 2 (2): 115–121.

Moinuddin, I. and Leehey, D. (2008). A comparison of aerobic exercise and resistance training in patients with and without chronic kidney disease. *Advances in Chronic Kidney Disease* 15 (1): 83–96.

Moretti, C., D'Ascenzo, F., Omedè, P. et al. (2014). Thirty-day readmission rates after PCI in a metropolitan center in Europe: incidence and impact on prognosis. *Journal of Cardiovascular Medicine (Hagerstown, MD.)* 16 (3): 238–245.

Morris, J. and Crawford, M. (1958). Coronary heart disease and physical activity of work; evidence of a national necropsy survey. *British Medical Journal* 2 (5111): 1485–1496.

Morris, J.N., Heady, J.A., Raffle, P.A.B. et al. (1953). Coronary heart disease and physical activity of work. *The Lancet* 262 (6795): 1053–1057. https://doi.org/10.1016/S0140-6736(53)90665-5.

Myers, J., Kaykha, A., George, S. et al. (2004). Fitness versus physical activity patterns in predicting mortality in men. *The American Journal of Medicine* 117 (12): 912–918.

Myers, J., Prakash, M., Froelicher, V. et al. (2002). Exercise capacity and mortality among men referred for exercise testing. *New England Journal of Medicine* 346 (11): 793–801. https://doi.org/10.1056/nejmoa011858.

NACR (2017). *National Audit for Cardiac Rehabilitation*. British Heart Foundation, York University.

NHS Choices (2015). Coronary artery bypass graft. NHS. http://www.nhs.uk/conditions/Coronary-artery-bypass (accessed 20 June 2016).

NHS Choices (2016). Heart attack - recovery. NHS. http://www.nhs.uk/Conditions/Heart-attack/Pages/Recovery.aspx (accessed 18 June 2016).

NICE (2010a). *Chest Pain of Recent Onset: Assessment and Diagnosis of Recent Onset Chest Pain or Discomfort of Suspected Cardiac Origin*. London: National Institute for Health Care Excellence, Department of Health.

NICE (2010b). *NICE CG108, Chronic Heart Failure: Management of Chronic Heart Failure in Adults in Primary and Secondary Care*. London: National Institute of Health Care Excellence, Department of Health.

NICE (2013). *Cardiac Rehabilitation Services; Guide for Commissioners CMG40*. London: National Institute for Health Care Excellence, Department of Health.

NICE (2014). Atrial Fibrillation: Management. London: National Institute for Health Care Excellence, Department of Health. www.nice.org.uk/guidance/CG180 (accessed 20 June 2016).

Pack, Q., Goel, K., Lahr, B. et al. (2013). Participation in cardiac rehabilitation and survival after coronary artery bypass graft surgery: A community-based study. *Circulation* 128 (6): 590–597.

Padula, C. and Yeaw, E. (2007). Inspiratory muscle training: integrative review of use in conditions other than COPD. *Research and Theory for Nursing Practice* 21 (2): 98–118.

Paffenbarger, R., Laughlin, M., Gima, A., and Black, R. (1970). Work activity of long-shoremen as related to death from coronary heart disease and stroke. *The New England Journal of Medicine* 282 (20): 1109–1114.

Parker, R.D. and Adams, J. (2008). Activity restrictions and recovery after open chest surgery: understanding the patient's perspective. *Proceedings (Baylor University Medical Centre)* 21 (4): 421–425.

Heberden, W. (1802). *Commentaries on the History and Cure of Diseases*, 161. London: Payne and Foss.

Prasad, K. (2013). Do statins have a role in reduction/prevention of post-pCI restenosis? *Cardiovascular Therapeutics* 31 (1): 12–26.

Prince, S.A., Blanchard, C.M., Grace, S.L., and Reid, R.D. (2015). Objectively-measured sedentary time and its association with markers of cardiometabolic health and fitness among cardiac rehabilitation graduates. *European Journal of Preventive Cardiology* 23 (8): 818–825.

Redfern, J., Ellis, E., Briffa, T., and Freedman, S. (2007). High risk-factor level and low risk-factor knowledge in patients not accessing cardiac rehabilitation after acute coronary syndrome. *The Medical Journal of Australia* 186 (1): 21–25.

Reid, R., Morrin, L., Beaton, L. et al. (2011). Randomized trial of an internet-based computer-tailored expert system for physical activity in patients with heart disease. *European Journal of Preventive Cardiology* 19 (6): 1357–1364.

Resuscitation Council (UK) (2014). Adult life support. Resuscitation Council (UK). www.resus.org.uk/dnacpr/decisions-relating-to-cpr (accessed 20 June 2016).

Rideout, A., Lindsay, G., and Godwin, J. (2011). Patient mortality in the 12 years following enrolment into a pre-surgical cardiac rehabilitation programme. *Clinical Rehabilitation* 26 (7): 642–647.

Robergs, R.A. and Landwehr, R. (2002). The surprising history of the 'HRmax=220-age' equation. *Journal of Exercise Physiology online* 5 (2): 1–10.

Sandercock, G., Cardoso, F., Almodhy, M., and Pepera, G. (2013). Cardiorespiratory fitness changes in patients receiving comprehensive outpatient cardiac rehabilitation in the UK: A multicentre study. *Heart* 99 (11): 785–790.

Santa Mina, D., Clarke, H., Ritvo, P. et al. (2014). Effect of total-body prehabilitation on postoperative outcomes: a systematic review and meta-analysis. *Physiotherapy* 100 (3): 196–207. https://doi.org/10.1016/j.physio.2013.08.008.

Siribaddana, S. (2012). Cardiac dysfunction in the CABG patient. *Current Opinion in Pharmacology* 12 (2): 166–171.

Skalska, A., Wizner, B., Więcek, A. et al. (2014). Reduced functionality in everyday activities of patients with self-reported heart failure hospitalization – population-based study results. *International Journal of Cardiology* 176 (2): 423–429.

Skelton, D. (2001). Effects of physical activity on postural stability. *Age and Ageing* 30 (Suppl 4): 33–39.

Stendardi, L., Grazzini, M., Gigliotti, F. et al. (2005). Dyspnea and leg effort during exercise. *Respiratory Medicine* 99 (8): 933–942.

Swain, D. and Franklin, B. (2002a). Is there a threshold intensity for aerobic training in cardiac patients? *Medicine and Science in Sports and Exercise* 34 (7): 1071–1075.

Swain, D. and Franklin, B. (2002b). VO(2) reserve and the minimal intensity for improving cardiorespiratory fitness. *Medicine and Science in Sports and Exercise* 34 (1): 152–157.

Taylor, R., Sagar, V., Davies, E. et al. (2014). Exercise-based rehabilitation for heart failure. *The Cochrane Database of Systematic Reviews* 4: CD003331. https://doi.org/10.1002/14651858.CD003331.pub4.

Taylor, R., Unal, B., Critchley, J., and Capewell, S. (2006). Mortality reductions in patients receiving exercise-based cardiac rehabilitation: how much can be attributed to cardiovascular risk factor improvements? *European Journal of Cardiovascular Prevention and Rehabilitation* 13 (3): 369–374.

Thorp, A., Owen, N., Neuhaus, M., and Dunstan, D. (2011). Sedentary behaviors and subsequent health outcomes in adults: a systematic review of longitudinal studies, 1996–2011. *American Journal of Preventive Medicine* 41 (2): 207–215.

Torbeyns, T., Bailey, S., Bos, I., and Meeusen, R. (2014). Active workstations to fight sedentary behaviour. *Sports Medicine (Auckland, N.Z.)* 44 (9): 1261–1273.

Townsend, N., Wickramasinghe, K., and Bhatnagar, P. (2012a). *Coronary Heart Disease Statistics: 2012*. United Kingdom: British Heart Foundation.

Troiano, R., Berrigan, D., Dodd, K. et al. (2008). Physical activity in the United States measured by accelerometer. *Medicine and Science in Sports and Exercise* 40 (1): 181–188.

Turk-Adawi, K., Sarrafzadegan, N., and Grace, S. (2014). Global availability of cardiac rehabilitation. *Nature Reviews. Cardiology* 11 (10): 586–596.

WHO (2012). Prevention and control of noncommunicable diseases: Formal meeting of Member States to conclude the work on the comprehensive global monitoring framework, including indicators, and a set of voluntary global targets for the prevention and control of noncommunicable diseases; Report by the Director–General of the World Health Organization. World Health Organization.

Wasfy, J.H., Rosenfield, K., Zelevinsky, K. et al. (2013). A prediction model to identify patients at high risk for 30-day readmission after percutaneous coronary intervention. *Circulation. Cardiovascular Quality and Outcomes* 6 (4): 429–435. https://doi.org/10.1161/CIRCOUTCOMES.111.000093.

Williams, M.A., Haskell, W.L., Ades, P.A. et al. (2007). Resistance exercise in individuals with and without cardiovascular disease: 2007 update. *Circulation* 116 (5): 572–584. https://doi.org/10.1161/CIRCULATIONAHA.107.185214.

Witte, K. and Clark, A. (2009). Chronotropic incompetence does not contribute to submaximal exercise limitation in patients with chronic heart failure. *International Journal of Cardiology* 134 (3): 342–344.

Yohannes, A., Doherty, P., Bundy, C., and Yalfani, A. (2010). The long-term benefits of cardiac rehabilitation on depression, anxiety, physical activity and quality of life. *Journal of Clinical Nursing* 19 (19–20): 2806–2813.

CHAPTER 6

Psychosocial Health

Linda Speck[1], Nick Brace[2], and Molly Byrne[3]

[1] Health Psychology Service, Cwm Taf Morgannwg University Health Board, Princess of Wales Hospital, Bridgend, and University of South Wales, UK
[2] Department of Health Psychology, Swansea Bay University Heath Board, Neath Port Talbot Hospital, Port Talbot, UK
[3] School of Psychology, National University of Ireland, Galway, Ireland

Abstract

This chapter will discuss psychosocial health and outline some of the evidence and issues relevant to cardiovascular prevention and rehabilitation settings. It examines why psychosocial health is important for preventive, restorative, and supportive rehabilitation. There is a focus on practical applications of the psychological evidence base in the assessment and treatment of those attending a cardiovascular prevention and rehabilitation programme (CPRP). Specific attention will be given to the role of social support, group processes, and the importance of incorporating psychological principles into goal-setting. Consideration will be given to the appropriateness of interventions in CPRP settings, dependent on professional competencies within the team.

Keywords: *psychological, psychosocial, cardiovascular prevention and rehabilitation, health*

Cardiovascular Prevention and Rehabilitation in Practice, Second Edition.
Edited by Jennifer Jones, John Buckley, Gill Furze, and Gail Sheppard.
© 2020 John Wiley & Sons Ltd. Published 2020 by John Wiley & Sons Ltd.

Key Points

- Recognition of the importance of psychological reactions in cardio-vascular disease.
- Assessment of psychological factors relevant to cardiovascular prevention and rehabilitation programmes (CPRPs).
- Evidence-based psychological interventions.
- Incorporating psychological principles into the structure of CPRPs.
- Understanding the role of social support in recovery.
- Recognising the limits of competency of CPRP teams to manage psychosocial issues and when to refer to specialist services.

6.1   RATIONALE AND AIMS

Psychosocial health is recognised by the BACPR Standards and Core Components (2017) as essential for successful cardiovascular prevention and rehabilitation. The aim of this chapter is to consider some of the principles for successful delivery of this component.

Psychological distress, in its many and varied expressions, is implicated in the development of cardiovascular disease, recovery following acute cardiac events, and adjustment to living with cardiovascular disease. CPRPs that address psychosocial issues and incorporate effective evidence-based psychological interventions may contribute to reductions in cardiovascular morbidity and mortality.

The aim of rehabilitation is not to get 'back to normal', but rather to help individuals and their families to accept the situation, and adopt healthful lifestyle change and adaptive emotional reactions. Cardiovascular prevention and rehabilitation enables transition from life without the knowledge of cardiovascular disease, through acute phases of the experience to develop resilience and restore or improve quality of life, within the limitations that the objective condition may set.

6.2   PSYCHOLOGICAL FACTORS RELATED TO HEART DISEASE

Wide-ranging effects of having experienced a heart condition impact upon the person, their partner, family, and other people within their wider social context. All parties may have potentially very different experiences of a shared situation. Each may require significant psychosocial support to make a transition to life post-cardiac event. Various anxieties may be present, frequently around physical activities, including day-to-day tasks, returning to work, resumption of sexual relationships, and altered awareness of physical sensations.

Cardiac events can be unexpected and frightening, causing considerable psychological distress. Distress reactions including anxiety, depression, fear, helplessness, guilt, and anger are common and variable, with severity of a myocardial infarction apparently unrelated to psychological response (Cay et al. 1972; Waltz et al. 1988). Unfortunately psychological problems persist for a significant number of people long after hospital discharge and, if not appropriately treated or managed, may lead to poor outcomes (Dickens et al. 2008; Shibeshi et al. 2007).

6.2.1   Anxiety

Anxiety is a normal immediate response to acute cardiac events, particularly myocardial infarction. It is usually short-lived (Doefler and Paraskos 2004) with normal levels regained by four months post event (Byrne 1990).

High levels of anxiety post-myocardial infarction and following coronary artery bypass grafting are associated with increased risk of future non-fatal myocardial infarction and mortality (Rosenbloom et al. 2009; Shibeshi et al. 2007). Furthermore, anxiety might well be an independent risk factor for coronary heart disease and cardiac mortality (Roest et al. 2010).

6.2.2   Psychological Stress

Stress reactions occur in response to acute events, or persistent difficulties. People do not experience uniform amounts of stress in relation to what may outwardly appear to be similar circumstances, reacting differently with the meaning one attributes to events and perceived availability of coping mechanisms.

Stress has long been cited as a cause of coronary heart disease, although evidence is mixed. Nevertheless, it is well established that acute psychological stress triggers various physiological reactions within the body implicated in coronary heart disease, such as increasing cortisol and catecholamines, activating platelets, thereby increasing cholesterol levels.

The large-scale INTERHEART Study (Rosengren et al. 2004) found psychosocial stress to be related to increased risk of acute myocardial infarction. Chronic work stress, especially for people of less than 50 years of age, has also been associated with coronary heart disease (Chandola et al. 2008).

6.2.3   Depression

Mood changes are often apparent following acute cardiac events with the severity and duration of symptoms experienced to varying degrees. Symptoms may include low mood, loss of interest, reduced concentration, feelings of hopelessness and helplessness, and possibly suicidal thoughts. Prevalence rates are estimated between 15 and 31% post-myocardial infarction, with 20% of these being diagnosed with major depression (Thombs et al. 2006).

Major depression and depressive symptoms have been found to be related to morbidity and mortality post-myocardial infarction (Grace et al. 2005) and post-coronary artery bypass grafting (Connerney et al. 2001). A first episode of depression occurring after myocardial infarction is a significant predictor of cardiac mortality (Dickens et al. 2008) equivalent in magnitude to having had a previous myocardial infarction, diabetes, or ventricular dysfunction (Lespérance et al. 2002).

The course of depressive symptoms is also a factor in recovery; post-myocardial infarction depression increasing in severity is associated with further cardiac events (Kaptein et al. 2006). Many patients are understandably found to experience some level of minor depression or low mood (72%) pre-cardiac surgery, which usually resolves over a six-month period following surgery. However, some experience significant depression, with 14% reporting worsening symptoms during the following six months (Murphy et al. 2008).

Although depression may be apparent following cardiac events, it has been found to pre-date events in as many as 50% of depressed individuals (Freedland et al. 1992). One might ask whether depression could be an independent or causal risk factor for heart disease for many people and not simply a reaction to the cardiac event itself.

Regardless of the cause of depression it is important to recognise that the quality of life of individuals with coronary heart disease and depression will be adversely affected. Being depressed after an acute cardiac event reduces the likelihood of making recommended health behaviour changes, as well as poor adherence to pharmaceutical treatment regimens (Denollet and Pederson 2009), and is a barrier to participation in a CPRP (Lane et al. 2000). In a large study of patients following myocardial infarction, attending a CPRP was found to significantly reduce the risk of mortality for those with a diagnosis of depression (Meurs et al. 2015). The researchers emphasised the importance of attendance at a CPRP for depressed individuals post-myocardial infarction.

Vigilance for symptoms and signs of depression is essential, from presentation at CPRP assessments and individual or group sessions, not relying solely on questionnaire data, routinely obtained during the course of a programme.

6.2.4   Denial

Some people may experience a period of denial following an acute cardiac event but is denial a bad thing? In the short term following an acute event it may actually be considered a helpful coping strategy, as research indicates that attempts to discuss traumatic events too soon after the event can be actively unhelpful (Rose et al. 2002). However, there is a point where denial can become unhelpful, where it persists in the longer term, resulting in reduced recognition of the benefits of lifestyle change to lessen future cardiac risk, presenting both a morbidity and mortality issue.

6.2.5 Post-traumatic Stress Disorder

Acute cardiac events are potentially life-threatening; they may occur suddenly and unexpectedly, without any apparent warning signs. A cardiac event may give rise to symptoms classifiable as a post-traumatic stress disorder (PTSD) (intense fear and 'flashbacks' related to the event, avoidance, and hypervigilance), with prevalence varying from 10 to 14.8% (Bennett et al. 2001; Whitehead et al. 2006). Unlike many other causes of PTSD, cardiac events pose an internal threat that is more difficult to avoid, with ongoing symptoms, taking regular medication, and participation in a CPRP being constant reminders. Although symptoms may be apparent soon after the event, it is important not to intervene too early, as many symptoms are self-remitting and premature intervention has been found to exacerbate, rather than alleviate, symptoms (Bennett et al. 2001).

6.2.6 Post-traumatic Growth

Despite observably distressing events, individual responses to traumatic events may not always be negative and can lead to positive consequences, such as re-evaluating priorities and taking more enjoyment from everyday life. Leung et al. (2010) identified a number of factors related to greater growth, including lower depressive symptoms and greater social support. Those who considered their coronary heart disease to be more acute believed that they could exert more control over their future health and illness. A recent qualitative study of survivors of myocardial infarction revealed that those who had been smokers experienced post-traumatic growth (PTG) in a similar way to that previously reported. It also indicated positive changes in growth, together with awareness of what is important and valued in life, wishing to get on with life, plus greater emotional sensitivity (Morgan et al. 2018). It can be important to acknowledge and foster the expression of PTG in cardiac rehabilitation settings.

6.2.7 Resilience

The concept of resilience is an important factor in the way that people respond and adapt to significant challenges, in order to make successful transitions beyond exposure to life-changing circumstances. Personal resilience creates potential for constructive change or development at such times. A low level of resilience has been found to be associated with depression in those with coronary heart disease (Toukhsati et al. 2016) and high levels of resilience have been found to be related to improvements in cardiovascular rehabilitation outcomes (Chan et al. 2006).

6.2.8   Optimism

One factor associated with psychological resilience is trait optimism. Optimism is a characteristic way of thinking comprising hopeful expectations of a positive future, regardless of past or current situations and challenges (Carver et al. 2010). It has been demonstrated to confer advantages in numerous areas of life, including cardiovascular-related health benefits. Reduced heart failure risk (Kim et al. 2014), and reduced cardiovascular mortality (Giltay et al. 2006; Tindle et al. 2009) have been demonstrated to be associated with optimism. In long-term prospective studies, improved psychological wellbeing, cardiovascular health status, and increased adherence to recommended cardioprotective health behaviours following acute coronary syndrome are also associated with initial optimism (Millstein et al. 2016; Ronaldson et al. 2015). Increased physical activity and lower rates of hospital readmission at six months in those with acute coronary syndrome (Huffman et al. 2016) have also been reported in the growing literature in this area.

6.2.9   Positive Affect

Similarly, Sin et al. (2015) considered positive affect, which is the subjective experience of positive moods, including enthusiasm, alertness, and excitement, and its relationship to several behaviours associated with cardiovascular health (namely, physical activity, sleep quality, adherence to prescribed medication, alcohol use, and smoking behaviour). They reported that, with the exception of alcohol use, positive affect was associated with healthful behaviour choices. They note that psychological wellbeing has been associated in the literature with increased self-efficacy for health behaviour change, motivation, and persever-ance in engagement with cardioprotective behaviours, and that those with better psychological wellbeing have been found to be more skilled at processing health risk-related information, and are better able to focus on healthful goals.

6.2.10   Psychosocial Impact on Partners

Partners are often as distressed as patients after a myocardial infarction (see e.g. Coyne and Smith 1991). The predominant partner reaction is anxiety. Spouses may be at increased risk of anxiety, depression, and suicide (Føsbol et al. 2013). It is understandable that partners may feel considerable psychological distress, not only because of their concerns for the wellbeing and future health of their spouse/partner, but also because of the uncertainties they may face, including practical considerations, changing roles and responsibilities, and additional burdens.

Spousal anxiety and depression have been found to be higher in some partners than patients, and so psychosocial adjustment of patients may suffer (Moser and Dracup 2004). Estimates of the prevalence of partner distress vary considerably. In a recent study over a third of partners were classified as being anxious and/or depressed twelve months after the cardiac event (Saltmarsh et al. 2016). These findings have implications for cardiovascular prevention and rehabilitation practice where the primary focus of care is understandably often patients, with only scant and passing attention to partners.

6.2.11   Sexuality and Cardiovascular Disease

Sexual problems are common with cardiovascular disease. Rates of erectile dysfunction amongst men with cardiovascular disease are twice as high as those in the general population, with similar rates of sexual dysfunction in females with cardiovascular disease (Kriston et al. 2010). These problems are important as they can negatively impact quality of life, psychological wellbeing, and relationship satisfaction (Traeen and Olsen 2007). They can also cause stress to patients' partners (O'Farrell et al. 2000). Reasons for the association between cardiovascular disease and sexual problems include: physical vascular causes, lack of knowledge about the sexual aspects of cardiovascular disease, fear of sexual activity provoking cardiac symptoms or a cardiac event, patient/partner relationship changes following a cardiac event, and associations with psychological problems such as depression (Schumann et al. 2010).

We know that sexual problems are rarely addressed during cardiac rehabilitation (Doherty et al. 2011), yet many people with cardiovascular disease wish to receive sexual education and counselling (D'Eath et al. 2013). Health professionals are frequently reluctant to address this personal aspect of patients' lives (Steinke and Swan 2004). Most cardiologists, nurses, and primary care physicians do not routinely ask cardiac patients about sexual problems, and patients are often reluctant or embarrassed to mention sex (Kloner et al. 2003). Even amongst clinicians who acknowledge the relevance of addressing sexual issues in their patients, there is a general lack of understanding of the optimal approach for sexual problem identification and recognition, and cardiac rehabilitation programmes typically fail to address the importance of sexual dysfunction concerns in their patients (Hatzichristou and Tsimtsiou 2005).

Research suggests that both male and female patients with coronary heart disease express regret that their primary care physician, cardiologist, or surgeon had not broached the subject of sexual function before or after an acute coronary illness episode (Renshaw and Karstaedt 1988).

Barriers to providing sexual counselling as identified by health professionals include: too little time, lack of knowledge or training, negative attitudes and beliefs about sexuality, a perception that it is someone else's job, patient's lack of readiness, sexuality not seen as a problem by health practitioners, patients perceived as too ill to address sexual issues, concerns about increasing patient anxiety, and discomfort in discussing the topic and views about the inappropriateness of sex in later life (Byrne et al. 2010; Doherty et al. 2011). There also appear to be a number of barriers that prevent patients from initiating discussions, including a perception that individual practitioners do not appear to be experienced or mature enough to understand the patient's problems or feelings of shyness and embarrassment. Also, age and gender issues may discourage the patient from expressing their concerns (Albarran and Bridger 1997; Byrne et al. 2013).

6.2.12   Personality-Related Factors

A Type A behaviour pattern has been linked to coronary heart disease. Originally identified by Friedman and Rosenman (1959), it is 'characterised by intense ambition, competitive "drive," constant preoccupation with "deadlines" and a sense of time urgency'. However, only hostility and anger within Type A have emerged as significantly related to coronary heart disease (Chida and Steptoe 2009).

More recently, a Type D (distressed) personality has been investigated. People described as Type D personalities are quite negative in their outlook, irritable, frequently worrying, socially withdrawn and inhibited, with a coping style of not expressing their emotions and holding back their thoughts and feelings. They are identified as being at increased risk of further cardiac events and having a poorer quality of life (Denollet and Conraads 2011).

6.3   DEVELOPING PSYCHOLOGICAL AWARENESS IN TEAMS

Psychosocial aspects of cardiac rehabilitation can be best addressed by a multidisciplinary team, adopting a biopsychosocial approach. Being psychologically aware and providing psychosocial support is the remit of all team members, who should receive training in communication and listening skills. Such training has been reported to be useful in other services such as cancer care, when delivered by skilled practitioners with comprehensive knowledge of its theoretical underpinnings (Fallowfield and Jenkins 1999).

6.3.1 Who Should Lead the Psychosocial Component?

According to Roth and Fonagy (2005), efficacy in psychological treatment settings depends at least in part on the knowledge and skills of the practitioners. In order to deliver effective and comprehensive psychological therapies within CPRPs, services require staff with appropriate specialist training that equips them with the knowledge and skills to be able to tailor complex psychological interventions, ideally drawing on a range of therapeutic models, as one approach will most certainly not fit all.

Highly skilled practitioners can also provide training to enhance the psychological awareness of non-psychology colleagues, further enhancing psychosocial support, thus reducing referrals of those with psychological issues outside of the CPRP. Yet, despite this, psychological practitioners remain largely absent from CPRP teams (British Heart Foundation National Audit of CR 2018).

So, whilst psychosocial 'support' is the domain of all CPRP staff, psychological 'intervention' requires specific high-level psychological knowledge and skills. Staff with this knowledge and skill should lead psychological aspects of cardiovascular prevention and rehabilitation.

6.4 ASSESSMENT ISSUES

The minimum factors considered necessary for suitable and comprehensive assessment in cardiovascular prevention and rehabilitation are listed below:

- Mood, distress, and emotional state.
- Quality of life.
- Understanding of, and beliefs about, the condition and its consequences.
- Impact of cardiac experience to date.
- Expectations and desires for attending rehabilitation.
- Perceptions of family relationships and social support.
- Adherence to prescribed medications.
- Historical adaptation to illness, health conditions, and significant life transitions.

An understanding of these issues for each individual will better inform the process of delivering and tailoring key messages of cardiovascular prevention and rehabilitation at both individual and group levels. In addition to discursive assessment of these issues, sound baseline measures of psychological state and quality of life should be sought.

6.4.1   Questionnaire Measures

When using questionnaire measures to inform assessment it is important to explain the way they should be completed, paying particular attention to the specific instructions relevant for each questionnaire in order to produce valid responses.

- *Anxiety and depression questionnaires.* Although no complete agreement exists regarding optimal measures for assessing psychological functioning amongst people attending CPRPs, guidance is available from the National Audit of Cardiac Rehabilitation (NACR). NACR advocates the use of the Hospital Anxiety and Depression Scale (HADS) (Zigmond and Snaith 1983), a 14-item questionnaire assessing symptoms of anxiety and depression. Scores on the questionnaire can be categorised clinically as normal range (0–7), borderline symptoms (8–10) and significant symptoms (11 or more) for both anxiety and depression.
- *Quality of life questionnaires.* NACR recommends the CO-OP Charts (Dartmouth Primary Care Cooperative [CO-OP] Information Project) (Nelson et al. 1987). The CO-OP consists of nine scales (physical endurance, emotional health, role function, social function, overall health, change in health, level of pain, overall quality of life, and social resources/support).

In addition, the authors have found further questionnaires to be clinically useful adjuncts to assessment. A number of generic quality of life measures are particularly useful when comparing different disease conditions. One such measure widely used in research is the Short-Form 36 (SF-36) (Ware and Sherbourne 1992), which measures quality of life along eight dimensions.

The MacNew Heart Disease Questionnaire (Oldridge et al. 1991; Valenti et al. 1996.) is heart-disease specific, designed to be sensitive to change in specific aspects of life for all cardiac patients across the domains of physical, social, and psychological functioning. It is highly sensitive to the changes and progress seen in CPRPs and can be particularly useful when reporting on patient progress.

6.4.2   Distress

The Distress Thermometer, recommended for use by the National Comprehensive Cancer Network (2003), with an associated problem list (Brennan et al. 2012), and the subsequent Emotion Thermometer, have been widely used to assess distress in cancer populations. The Emotion Thermometer tool has been further trialled in a British cardiovascular disease population by Mitchell et al. (2012) and on a heart failure population (Holly and Sharp 2012).

6.4.3   Illness Representations

Individual cardiac-related beliefs have been described as central to the under-standing of disability and quality of life issues in people following a diagnosis of coronary heart disease (Lewin 1999).

Illness representations comprise individual understanding of the condition, its causes, its consequences, expected duration, and how it can be best cured or managed. Formal assessment can be made using the Revised Illness Perceptions Questionnaire (Moss-Morris et al. 2002) or the Brief Illness Perceptions Questionnaire (Broadbent et al. 2006). However, for the purposes of assessment at a CPRP, it may be pragmatic to explore perceptions using simple open questions, as suggested below.

Open Questions to Elicit Illness Perceptions

Identity
Could you tell me in your own words what has happened to you?

Cause
What do you consider may have been the cause of your heart condition?
What do you see as the most likely causes of heart problems?

Time line
How predictable is your condition from day to day?
How do you think your condition will change in the future?
How long do you understand that you will have to take the medication for?

Consequences
How do you think that your condition will impact on your life in the future?
What would you say are the main consequences of having a heart condition?
How easy has it been to live with the condition so far?

Cure/control
What do you think you/we can do to help to manage your condition from now on?
What advice would you give to someone else if they were to be in your situation?
How effective do you think the treatment will be for your condition?

6.4.4   Self-Efficacy

Self-efficacy refers to an individual's perceived capability to undertake a specific task. This may not correspond with actual capability as it is a person's level of confidence to attempt a task that is worth exploring. A person's self-efficacy varies with circumstances and across situations; it is not an unchanging fixed characteristic of personality (see Chapter 4).

Bandura (1997) asserts that self-efficacy should be task specific. Likert-type scales and scaling questions, flexibly prepared to suit individual needs, are useful (see Figure 6.1 for an example of a scaling question). As self-efficacy is a measure of perceived capability, items should be devised asking 'can do' rather than 'will do' questions, as below. It is important not to fall into the trap of asking 'will do' questions, as it implies intention rather than perceived capability.

How confident are you that you can [insert specific stressor, e.g. manage your anxiety] (Mark on the line below).

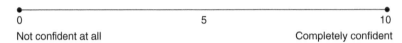

| 0 | 5 | 10 |
| Not confident at all | | Completely confident |

FIGURE 6.1 Example of a scaling question.

6.5 INTERVENTIONS

6.5.1 Aims of Psychosocial Interventions

The aims of psychosocial interventions in CPRPs might be summarised as follows.

- Assisting understanding of cardiovascular disease and its management.
- Addressing misconceptions.
- Supporting engagement in appropriate healthful behaviour choices.
- Increasing understanding of psychological factors influencing recovery.
- Enabling best possible adjustment to living with cardiovascular disease.
- Supporting development of realistic optimism, resilience and coping skills, facilitating reduction of psychological distress.
- Facilitating relevant goal-setting.
- Facilitating meaningful participation in all aspects of life.
- Encouraging independence from health services as people develop skills to manage their condition for themselves.

6.5.2 Education

Resist the urge to teach, even if this is what the group expects!

Teaching is only applicable where knowledge gaps are the most important factor. Discursive input helps to maximise personal salience of an intervention for participants. Experiential and skills-based learning, as in the case of initial relaxation skills practice, or physical activity sessions is also important. For further discussion, see Chapter 4 of this book.

6.5.3   Stressful Life Events and Coping

Coping is a dynamic interaction between life events that are appraised as stressful and a person's perceived ability to manage those events, as highlighted in the transactional model of stress and coping (Lazarus and Folkman 1984). Each potentially challenging situation is unique and perceived coping capacity likewise. Coping is the dynamic interaction between perceived challenges and burdens and the person's perceived skills to manage those challenges. Stress occurs when a person perceives life events as taxing or exceeding their coping resources (Lazarus and Folkman 1984, p. 19). Individual perceptions of stressful events and coping capacity are more important than the events themselves.

In CPRP settings it is useful to be aware that people use the term 'stress' in very different ways. For some it indicates the stress response itself, e.g. symptoms such as increased heart rate, whereas for others it relates to the cause of stress, e.g. work. A further distinction is that people may view stress as either chronic, perhaps related to a long-term illness, or acute, following a traumatic event. Understanding the varying usage of stress can be helpful, not only in explaining the concept but also the potential benefits from participating in the stress management input to programmes.

Coping skills and resilience are not meant to eliminate stress from life. They simply help to manage stressful aspects of life. Attendance at a CPRP helps with building coping skills and resilience by enabling people to recognise their progress and a sense of wellbeing, supporting their transition to a new life, developing optimism for a successful future, achieving meaningful goals, engaging in problem-solving, and encouraging healthful behaviours.

6.5.4   Stress and Emotions Management

Stress management may be facilitated in a number of ways, including cognitive-, behavioural-, systemic-, and acceptance-based approaches to living better with cardiovascular disease.

It is useful to highlight where emotional reactions can be unhelpful, in regard to recovery and transition to a new life with cardiovascular disease, and how they can influence self-efficacy and self-management. Discursive education regarding associations between stress and heart disease may be useful, especially in helping people to develop control of angina symptoms through understanding predisposing factors, and methods by which angina symptoms are better managed.

Participants can be encouraged to highlight stressors in their lives, and to work out which of these situations are modifiable. Where a situation can be modified, stress responses can be reduced, or even eliminated. Where stressors cannot be eliminated, modifications can still sometimes be made to influence the situation. Encouraging planned, graded, progressive steps to manage the situation can be helpful. Success in the initial stages in managing a problem develops confidence to progress to more challenging aspects. Of primary importance is that people are advised to become comfortable with each stage of the process, before making further progressions. Taking manageable steps facilitates learning that progress can be made, whilst pushing too far, too quickly can result in being overwhelmed and learning that one cannot manage a situation.

Assertiveness training, requesting appropriate help, and sharing emotional issues with suitable individuals can also be useful in managing some of the stressful situations encountered, especially regarding familial support offered. Shared responsibility should be encouraged, with supportive individuals asking, 'would it be helpful if...', rather than simply taking over tasks. Similarly, those looking for support might be advised to guide others as to what might be helpful, in order to increase the likelihood of receiving the kind of support they desire.

It is important to acknowledge that whilst those attending a CPRP should be encouraged and supported in the development of these skills many people are fully able to successfully manage busy lives and that such situations are not necessarily harmful to their cardiovascular health. On the contrary, it is likely that some people will be overly cautious in their approaches to rehabilitation, perhaps borne of misunderstandings about what is safe, or otherwise. This may result in avoidance of a number of things such as physical exercise, emotional situations, or sexual relationships (Perkins-Porras et al. 2015).

6.5.5   Relaxation Skills Training

Stress management usually involves basic information about the nature of stress and the practice of relaxation techniques. It is important to establish links between stress, distress, anxiety, and depression, and the cognitive and behavioural factors that trigger and maintain problems. Stress management is about skill acquisition. Relaxation is a set of internal individual skills that directly reduce physiological arousal and can be deployed in most situations. Where people are familiar with the use of relaxation CDs, but consider them to be ineffective in managing the stress of everyday life, or irrelevant in regard to cardiac symptoms, they will often be dismissed out of hand. This should be addressed and challenged.

6.5.6   Setting Up a Relaxation Session

It is a useful starting point to find out what participants consider relaxation to be and what experience they have had of using relaxation in the past. People often confuse inactive or enjoyable pastimes with relaxation. Relaxation should be taught as an active coping skill and integrated into the teaching of stress management. The process begins by teaching relaxation skills and moving on to incorporating thought management, employing some aspects of cognitive behaviour therapy.

Teaching Relaxation

- Explain that relaxation is a skill, and different from fun activities and inactivity.
- Practise once during clinical contact time, encouraging correct technique.
- Encourage regular (daily if possible) practice at home to improve skills.
- Use as part of a problem-solving package for managing anxiety, distress, and tension.
- Lifelong use of a CD is *not* what relaxation skills training is about.
- Resist the urge to repeatedly set up ideal conditions for practice (lying people down or sitting them in comfy chairs in a perfectly quiet and darkened room). The real world does not provide ideal conditions.
- Over time, help people to apply skills in situations in which they are tense or anxious.

Care needs to be taken in practising relaxation skills, especially with those who have abusive histories, who may find experiences of letting go and being guided by someone else extremely challenging.

It is advisable to encourage feedback about progress in practising at home, ensuring that relaxation is used as one of the skills of managing the cardiac condition.

6.5.7   Changing Thought Patterns

It is important to increase participants' awareness of the role of unhelpful or negative thought patterns, to enable them to develop helpful or realistically optimistic ways of thinking, and to focus their attention on modifiable internal aspects of coping, reducing attention given to uncontrollable external stressors.

However, CPRP professionals should be mindful of the potential oversimplification of messages surrounding positive thinking and positive mental attitude.

During group discussions, sensitively highlight instances of unhelpful thinking. Initially, people may find identifying and challenging unhelpful thoughts difficult. This can be aided by opening discussion to the group and sharing helpful alternatives to unhelpful thoughts, or presenting commonly held unhelpful thoughts to the group and generating alternatives to depersonalise the situation.

Unhelpful negative thoughts are characteristically quick to come to mind, easy to believe, often have no basis in truth, and are difficult to stop. They often act to perpetuate problem situations. Alternative thoughts have to be believable in order to have a desirable effect on mood. 'Positive' thoughts that appear less believable than their negative counterparts are likely to have minimal impact. Therefore, thoughts that are realistically optimistic should be encouraged, rather than simply advising positive thinking. When helpful optimistic alternatives are generated, it should not be expected that emotional changes will necessarily follow immediately. What is helpful is individual to each person, so practitioners are discouraged from identifying 'the right thought' for a participant.

When challenging unhelpful thoughts, it is useful to encourage participants to ask the following questions:

- How do I know this to be true?
- What is the evidence?
- What other ways could I think about this?
- What alternative ways can I manage this?

The following are some thought alternatives to managing unhelpful thoughts.

Unhelpful negative thought	Helpful alternative
I'm having a heart attack	I've had these symptoms before. My doctor says my heart is okay. I know I can manage this by...
I'll never be better	There is no reason why I can't get better. I can do this within my tolerances and gradually improve. If I look back to the day I left hospital, I'm already getting better.
I wish I could go back to normal	I cannot be the same as I was before, but by doing the right things I can be the best I can be. It's okay that this takes time. I'm going forwards, not backwards.
Other people judge me for my weakness	Having a heart condition does not make me weak. In any case, what others think matters little; it's what I do and my own sense of genuineness that matters.

Practice in identifying unhelpful negative thoughts when they happen and trying to think of a helpful (and believable) response is the key to making helpful thoughts more salient.

It may also be helpful to encourage participants to write coping self-statements when they are feeling okay, in order that they might use them when they feel low or anxious. Some coping statements are suggested here:

- Perfection is unachievable, but if I keep practising, my confidence will build.
- If I put relaxation into practice, I'll feel rather better.
- It's been like this before, and I was okay.
- I'm having a bad day; tomorrow will be better.
- Overall I am making good progress.

Some situations faced by those attending CPRPs are extremely challenging and potentially unpleasant. It is important that practitioners adopting this approach to thought challenges avoid the trap of invalidating the concerns of participants. Sometimes, an acknowledgement that life is difficult is important.

In this regard, it may be useful to adopt principles from Acceptance and Commitment Therapy (ACT), focusing on development of internal skills to effectively manage unpleasant and painful thoughts. This reduces the influence of such thoughts on emotions and helps to identify aspects of life that are important in order to become more motivated towards achieving truly fulfilling goals. Readers are directed towards *ACT Made Simple* (Harris 2009) for further introduction to this approach.

6.5.8 Goal-setting

Even when people set apparently physical goals, the physical activity required to achieve them is often psychologically underpinned. Goal-setting processes are discussed in Chapter 4 of this book. Sufficient time needs to be devoted to shaping ill-defined goals (such as 'I want to get back to normal') into mutually agreeable, achievable targets.

6.5.9 Improving Resilience through Optimism

Cognitive behavioural approaches to treatment, focusing on the use of optimistic mental imagery, have been shown to be effective in increasing optimism (Meevissen et al. 2011; Riskind et al. 1996), and an intervention comprising optimism, kindness, and gratitude has been shown to be effective in improving optimism in a population of heart failure and acute coronary syndrome patients (Huffman et al. 2011).

6.5.10   Problem-solving

People can become entrenched in a particular problem, making it difficult to view that problem objectively and take a problem-solving position. It may be helpful to take a generic problem and apply a group-based problem-solving approach. Problems may be related to other issues such as communication or assertiveness, and space should be dedicated to any such issues that arise within the group.

It is potentially useful to offer a reflective perspective in group discussion by asking what happened, what was helpful (and not helpful), and a future-based perspective regarding how things can be done differently. A solution-focused problem-solving approach (see Chapter 4) needs to be explicitly explained, in order that participants develop ownership of it, facilitating its future use as a self-help approach.

6.5.11   Sleep Interventions

Disruption of normal sleeping patterns is common post-cardiac event. For some, delayed onset of sleep, early morning wakening, or too much sleep can be a symptom of depression and careful assessment of the precipitating events and behaviours surrounding sleeplessness should be undertaken. Ascertaining how long the problem has existed, as many people have long-standing sleeping difficulties pre-dating their cardiac event, is also important.

Mooe et al. (2001) report that those with obstructive sleep apnoea are at significantly increased risk of cardiovascular ill-health and cardiac mortality. Hargens et al. (2015) reported that obstructive sleep apnoea is further associated with compromised cardiac function in CPRP attendees. Furthermore, research in shift-workers has demonstrated associations with cardiovascular ill-health in those with obstructive sleep apnoea, insomnia, and either excessive or foreshort-ened sleep time (Gallagher et al. 2015). Sleep difficulties are therefore something that should be considered in CPRPs.

Various interventional strategies have been researched and employed clini-cally with differing levels of effectiveness. They include physical considerations, and psychological strategies. More recent interventions have employed 'constructive worry', designed to reduce the likelihood of intrusive thoughts interfering with sleep onset, or returning to sleep after night-time waking (Jansson-Fröjmark et al. 2012).

It is essential to help people to create associations with bed and sleep. Equally it is important to break any associations of bed and sleeplessness or pat-terns of sleeping at undesirable times. It is also worth considering brief educa-tion about sleep structure and sleep needs, facilitating normalisation of variable sleep patterns, reduced sleep time, and self-perceived tiredness (in situations where there are few negative consequences for the amount of sleep obtained).

This can reduce the worry associated with changes in sleep habits, potentially improve sleep efficiency, or at least increase sleep satisfaction.

Gallagher et al. (2015) highlight that cognitive behaviour therapy for insomnia (CBT-I) has been demonstrated to be more effective in the longer term than pharmacological treatments (Morin et al. 2009), although access to appropriately trained practitioners to deliver CBT-I is lacking (Espie 2009).

6.6 SEXUAL ASSESSMENT AND COUNSELLING

A consensus document endorsed by the American Heart Association and the European Society of Cardiology recommends that all patients with cardiovascular disease should be assessed for sexual concerns and offered sexual counselling as part of cardiac rehabilitation (Steinke et al. 2013). Sexual counselling can be defined as an interaction between provider and patients where the provider provides information on sexual concerns and safe return to sexual activity, assessment, support, and specific advice related to psychological and sexual problems. Sexual counselling interventions can improve the frequency of sexual intimacy and the quality of sexual functioning for patients and should be offered regardless of age, gender, culture, or sexual orientation. Cognitive behavioural techniques, patient education, and therapeutic communication strategies have been used successfully in sexual counselling with cardiac patients. Sexual counselling should include a review of medications and any potential effects on sexual function, any risk related to sexual activity, the role of regular exercise in supporting intimacy, use of a comfortable familiar setting to minimise any stress with sexual activity, use of sexual activities that require less energy expenditure as a bridge to sexual intercourse, avoidance of anal sex, and the reporting of warning signs experienced with sexual activity. It can be beneficial to provide sexual counselling through several meetings and to offer the option of including partners or spouses.

6.7 RUNNING GROUPS

This focuses predominantly on the group stage of rehabilitation, although recognising that consistency of message and approach is important throughout. Effective use of groups to share concerns related to psychological adjustment with others similarly affected can have significant benefits. Group facilitators should sensitively manage patients' concerns so that others may be encouraged to do likewise.

Initially, people may be quite anxious about group participation. Early opportunity to speak, in a non-threatening way, in the form of a basic introduction is advantageous. This prevents 'build up' of difficulty in speaking publicly, and develops group cohesion.

Throughout a CPRP, attendees can be encouraged to actively participate in feedback discussions, airing experiences, increasing insight into difficulties and exploring possible solutions with the help of other group members and practitioners. This is an opportunity to share knowledge and skills, normalise commonly experienced distress, create mutual support, widen perspectives on problem-solving, and develop motivation to change. See Chapter 4 of this book for some suggestions for developing successful group support.

One of the challenges practitioners may experience when directing open discussions within a group is the anxiety associated with keeping people on track, or opening up something that is beyond the remit of the group, such as a major stressor or historical psychological trauma. Clear group guidelines, as discussed in Chapter 4, minimise the chances of such disclosures. The offer of discussion on an individual basis with a relevant team member can be made where there is significant emotional content present in what the participant is reporting.

6.8   THE INFLUENCE OF SOCIAL SUPPORT AND HOW WE CAN IMPROVE THIS

6.8.1   Social Support

Social support is a complex but important factor in cardiovascular rehabilitation, often involving other people. Considerable variation in the amount and quality of support received by each individual will exist. Some people are truly socially isolated and the lack of a supportive social network has been found to be related to increased morbidity, including clinical depression, and mortality after an acute myocardial infarction (Mookadam and Arthur 2004).

Cardiovascular prevention and rehabilitation teams should be alert to people who do not have significant social support, recognising that they may require additional input from services, especially during initial recovery. Those with limited support at 1 month post-event may have significantly poorer outcomes at 12 months (Leifheit-Limson et al. 2012).

Lack of social support may pre-date the cardiac event for some, doubling cardiovascular risk for both initial and recurrent cardiac events (Lett et al. 2005). Regardless of the amount of social support, satisfaction with the quality of support is particularly important (Sarason et al. 1983). Women often receive less social support than men, especially practically, up to 12 months post-myocardial infarction, with men being more likely to involve their partners in their recoveries (Kristofferzon et al. 2003).

CPRPs designed to maximise group support through sharing of concerns and progress with other group members can be very helpful for those with weaker social support networks. Continuing links with fellow group members may be established, as discussed earlier.

6.8.2   Partner Support

Inviting a partner, or someone else close to the cardiac patient, to CPRP sessions can be helpful in fostering appropriate social support, as well as to gain more understanding of the cardiac condition.

Positive support received from partners may be as important a factor in successful adaptation as an individual's own coping responses (Taylor et al. 1992). Social support from partners has been found to be protective against distress for men (Connell and Bennett 1997). Patients with heart failure who are married are more likely to have had an event-free survival when followed up for a period of four years (Chung et al. 2009). In reality some partners can be adversely affected by cardiac events, finding adjustment difficult, and consequently do not provide effective support for the patient (Moser and Dracup 2004).

Partners sometimes make well-meaning attempts to protect patients with unintentional detrimental long-term effects. Partner overprotectiveness is related to patients' increased anxiety and depression (Clarke et al. 1996) and decreased quality of life (Joekes et al. 2007b), even where overprotectiveness is not recognised by either partner (Joekes et al. 2007a).

Marriages and close relationships can be affected by illness and the extent of the disruption may be a function of the marital relationship pre-dating the onset of the health problem (Croog and Fitzgerald 1978). Emotionally close relationships are associated with positive support, whereas spouse conflict and interpersonal problems are associated with negative support (Waltz 1986). It is important to also consider the context in which partner distress may be experienced. The quality of the relationship prior to the cardiac event has been found to be predictive of partner distress 12 months later (Saltmarsh et al. 2016).

Appropriate partner support predicts improved psychological health, whereas spousal control is predictive of decreased patient health behaviour and mental health six months post-myocardial infarction or cardiac revascularisation (Franks et al. 2006).

CPRPs may be designed to provide support to partners, encouraging them to be appropriately supportive rather than overprotective or controlling. Inviting partners to attend group sessions should be routinely undertaken, to ensure that partners are cognizant of the pertinent issues related to recovery from cardiac events, thereby facilitating appropriate patient support. Staff facilitation of partner-only group sessions, with dedicated time to discuss concerns and issues, can also be helpful in providing partners the opportunity to air their worries with others in comparable situations who share similar difficulties. Skilful group facilitation is needed, avoiding blame for feelings and actions whilst encouraging sharing concerns and working through current relationship dilemmas.

6.9   PREPARING FOR THE END OF THE GROUP

Towards the end of a CPRP, participants may develop concerns about 'going it alone'. The loss of support can be challenging. Some express a need for more time to consolidate learning. It is useful to encourage them away from further help-seeking at this point, enabling them to put into practice cardiovascular rehabilitation skills in a lifelong self-managing way. Metaphors that normalise the CPRP experience as the foundation on which to build your own house, or the basis that allows you to pass a driving test, can be helpful, thereby reiterating a self-management message. That said, at the point of discharge from NHS CPRPs, many areas now offer extended exercise-only sessions. In addition, group members may wish to meet to maintain support. This can be effective, providing the focus remains on helpful aspects of their CPRP experience, continuing a solution focus, rather than a problem focus.

Prior to group conclusion, participants may benefit from preparation for separation; revising the management skills discussed, recognising successes, and acknowledging the normality of 'ups and downs' in the future.

6.10   VOCATIONAL INTERVENTIONS

Evidence suggests people's perceptions of illness duration and seriousness are related to speed of return to work (Petrie et al. 1996). Wherever the objective limitations of the condition allow, participants can be encouraged to return to work and can be supported to do so.

Given the recent events that participants will have experienced, they may be considering role changes, looking to retire, or to develop new interests. Whilst employment is recognised as healthful, alternative vocations can be equally fulfilling, provided they are adequately prepared for. Such alternatives might be encouraged as potential options where they are desired by participants.

6.11   WHEN TO REFER ON

Recovering from a cardiac event should, wherever possible, be framed in terms of the effects of dramatic change in peoples' context, rather than shortcomings in the person's psychological health or personality traits.

6.11.1 Significant Psychological Distress

Referral to mental health services for significant psychological distress should be considered alongside the potential stigma and discrimination that can be associated with mental health (NICE 2009). Integrating skilled psychological staff into CPRP teams serves to increase the skill mix within the team and normalises the psychological challenge of rehabilitation. Therefore, wherever possible, it is suggested that psychological wellbeing is best managed within the CPRP, and that staffing of services should reflect this, with employment of appropriate highly skilled staff to deliver psychologically underpinned interventions.

A common misconception regarding referral to psychological services seems to be around cut-off scores for screening questionnaires. Practitioners are advised against the use of widespread referral of individuals who score within clinical ranges on screening questionnaires without supportive evidence of the need for further professional help.

What and when to refer on can be only properly determined within the context of each service. We mentioned the variability of composition of CPRP multidisciplinary teams earlier. This is clearly something to keep in mind when considering external referrals of those with perceived psychological difficulties. Teams that report having a psychologist (or another highly skilled and professionally trained psychological practitioner) ought to be able to manage more complex psychological difficulties. Teams where there is no integral psychology service, and where those offering psychological support have been only briefly trained in psychological skills as an adjunct to their core professional skills, will need to refer out more frequently, as it will be beyond their competence, with the implications discussed above.

If psychological problems are long-standing, pre-dating the cardiac event, and significantly severe, this may warrant referral to mental health services, or liaison with primary care practitioners. If psychological problems have occurred secondary to the cardiac condition, consideration needs to be made regarding the stage of rehabilitation and degree of normality of the distress, given the person's circumstances.

6.11.2 Substance Misuse

Substance misuse in the form of both alcohol and drug misuse are significant health issues. Alcohol use is associated with an increased risk of cardiovascular disease by raising blood triglycerides, elevating blood pressure, and causing atrial fibrillation (World Health Organization 2014). Cardiomyopathy is reported to be associated with heavy alcohol consumption, although drinking patterns are also important to consider (Djoussé and Gaziano 2008). As greater economic wealth is associated with more alcohol consumption, people living in the western world are at increasing cardiovascular risk. A complicating factor is society's permissive attitude to moderate, or even greater alcohol use in some groups, especially as social events often centre around drinking. The World Health Organization estimates that 2% of coronary heart disease in developed countries is due to alcohol intake (World Health Report 2002).

Drug misuse is more common than many might expect with 35% of adults (16–59 years) having taken drugs at some point in their lifetime and 1 in 12 (8.4%) in the last year (Home Office 2016). Drug misuse can give rise to cardiovascular problems, such as abnormal heart rhythms and myocardial infarction. Although cannabis is the most widely used drug, cocaine is more prevalent in certain areas of the UK. The use of cocaine has significant cardiovascular risks leading to thickening of heart muscle, hypertension, and stiffening of arteries.

It is apparent from working in cardiovascular prevention and rehabilitation settings that increasing numbers of cardiac patients are reporting either having used drugs recently or at least in their past, and this is a challenge for CPRPs. Recognising the need for referral to specialist drug and alcohol services is extremely important, in order that each individual is offered the opportunity to engage with the most effective psychological and physical interventions to manage any dependence issues. The role of CPRP professionals is to help individuals understand the health issues related to drug and alcohol misuse, aiming to resolve ambivalence to change and supporting change whilst seeking out appropriate services to refer on to. Employing some of the principles already outlined, such as those underpinning motivational interviewing and solution-focused interventions, are paramount in this setting, but offering anything more specialist is not recommended. It is essential to seek out specialist services to refer on to, whilst simultaneously pursuing cardiovascular prevention and rehabilitation.

6.11.3 Geographical Variation in Referral

Referral options are subject to geographical variation. They may include short-term and longer-term psychological therapies, delivered in one-to-one or group settings, with services in some localities delivering cardiac-specific psychological interventions.

Increasing Access to Psychological Therapies (IAPT) in England has potentially made support for those with cardiac-related psychological difficulties more freely available. However, this does not appear to always be the case, and is certainly not so in regions where IAPT has not been implemented. Talking to mental health service providers in your area is the only real way to ensure appropriate referrals are made.

The obvious solution to this situation is to increase access to professional psychological management through employment of qualified psychological staff, as core members of the multidisciplinary CPRP team.

6.12 CONCLUSION

In this chapter we have discussed psychosocial health and outlined the basic principles that are needed to successfully support people through a CPRP. Psychological variables are related to the development of cardiovascular disease and are implicated in adjustment to, recovery from, and prevention of further cardiac events. Identification and management of psychological distress is essential to ensure optimal outcomes in cardiac health and improved quality of life. Assessment of psychological distress can be informed by the use of widely available validated questionnaire measures but these should not be used in isolation of professional clinical judgement.

This chapter has considered the delivery of evidence-based psychologically informed interventions to assist transition to successful self-management of living well with cardiovascular disease. Recognition is given not only to the individual with the condition but also to the social context in which people live. The potential for the co-existence of psychological distress for partners and the implications thereof should be acknowledged in cardiovascular prevention and rehabilitation settings. Consideration has been given to the remit of cardiovascular rehabilitation in the management of psychological distress. Whilst all CPRP staff should be psychologically informed, the boundaries of therapeutic interventions will be determined by the professional psychological skills within the composition of teams. From time to time there may be a need to refer to specialist services for those with severe and enduring mental health or drug misuse problems.

REFERENCES

Albarran, J.W. and Bridger, S. (1997). Problems with providing education on resuming sexual activity after myocardial infarction: developing written information for patients. *Intensive & Critical Care Nursing* 13 (1): 2–11.

Bandura, A. (1997). *Self-Efficacy: The Exercise of Control*, 2e. New York, NY: W.H.Freeman and Co.

Bennett, P., Conway, M., Clatworthy, J. et al. (2001). Predicting post-traumatic symptoms in cardiac patients. *Heart and Lung* 30 (6): 458–465.

Brennan, J., Gingell, P., Brant, H., and Hollingworth, W. (2012). Refinement of the distress management problem list as the basis for a holistic therapeutic conversation among UK patients with cancer. *Psycho-Oncology* 21 (12): 1346–1356.

British Association for Cardiovascular Prevention and Rehabilitation (2017). *The BACPR Standards and Core Components for Cardiovascular Disease Prevention and Rehabilitation (3rd Edition)*. London: BACPR. www.bacpr.com.

British Heart Foundation National Audit of Cardiac Rehabilitation (2018). *National Audit of Cardiac Rehabilitation Quality and Outcomes Report 2018*. London: British Heart Foundation. http://www.cardiacrehabilitation.org.uk/reports.htm.

Broadbent, E., Petrie, K.J., Main, J., and Weinman, J. (2006). The brief illness perception questionnaire (BIPQ). *Journal of Psychosomatic Research* 60: 631–637.

Byrne, D.G. (1990). Psychological aspects of outcomes and interventions following heart attack. In: *Anxiety and the Heart* (eds. D.G. Byrne and R.H. Rosenman), 369–396. New York: Hemisphere.

Byrne, M., Doherty, S., McGee, H.M., and Murphy, A.W. (2010). General practitioners' views about discussing sexual issues with patients with coronary heart disease: a national survey in Ireland. *BMC Family Practice* 11: 40.

Byrne, M., Doherty, S., Murphy, A.W. et al. (2013). The CHARMS study: cardiac patients' experiences of sexual problems following cardiac rehabilitation. *European Journal of Cardiovascular Nursing* 12 (6): 558–566.

Carver, C.S., Scheier, M.F., and Sergerstrom, S.C. (2010). Optimism. *Clinical Psychology Review* 30: 879–889.

Cay, E., Vetter, N., Philip, A., and Dugard, P. (1972). Psychological status during recovery from an acute heart attack. *Journal of Psychosomatic Research* 16 (6): 425–435.

Chan, I.W.S., Lai, J.C.L., and Wong, K.W.N. (2006). Resilience is associated with better recovery in Chinese people diagnosed with coronary heart disease. *Psychology and Health* 21 (3): 335–349.

Chandola, T., Britton, A., Brunner, E. et al. (2008). Work stress and coronary heart disease: what are the mechanisms? *European Heart Journal* 29 (5): 640–648.

Chida, Y. and Steptoe, A. (2009). The association of anger and hostility with future coronary heart disease. *Journal of the American College of Cardiology* 53: 936–946.

Chung, M.L., Lennie, T.A., Riegel, B. et al. (2009). Marital status as an independent predictor of event-free survival of patients with heart failure. *American Journal of Critical Care* 18 (6): 562–570.

Clarke, D.E., Walker, J.R., and Cuddy, T.E. (1996). The role of perceived overprotectiveness in recovery 3 months after myocardial infarction. *Journal of Cardiopulmonary Rehabilitation* 16 (6): 372–377.

Connell, H. and Bennett, P. (1997). Anticipating levels of anxiety and depression in couples where the husband has survived a myocardial infarction. *Coronary Health Care* 1 (1): 22–26.

Connerney, I., Shapiro, P., McLaughlin, J. et al. (2001). Relation between depression after coronary artery bypass surgery and 12-month outcome: a prospective study. *Lancet* 358 (9295): 766–1771.

Coyne, J.C. and Smith, D.A. (1991). Couples coping with a myocardial infarction: a contextual perspective on wives' distress. *Journal of Personality and Social Psychology* 61 (3): 404–412.

Croog, S. and Fitzgerald, E. (1978). Subjective stress and serious illness of a spouse: wives of heart patients. *Journal of Health and Social Behavior* 19 (2): 166–178.

D'Eath, M., Byrne, M., Doherty, S. et al. (2013). The CHARMS study: A qualitative enquiry of patient, general practitioner and cardiac rehabilitation staff views on sexual assessment and counselling for cardiac patients. *Journal of Cardiovascular Nursing* 28 (2): E1–E13. https://doi.org/10.1097/JCN.0b013e318281d0b3.

Denollet, J. and Conraads, V.M. (2011). Type D personality and vulnerability to adverse outcomes in heart disease. *Cleveland Clinic Journal of Medicine* 78 (Suppl. 1): S13–S19.

Denollet, J. and Pederson, S.S. (2009). Anger, depression, and anxiety in cardiac patients. *Journal of the American College of Cardiology* 53 (11): 947–949.

Dickens, C., McGowan, L., Percival, C. et al. (2008). New onset depression following myocardial infarction predicts cardiac mortality. *Psychosomatic Medicine* 70 (4): 450–455.

Djoussé, L. and Gaziano, M. (2008). Alcohol consumption and heart failure: a systematic review. *Current Atherosclerosis Reports* 10 (2): 117–120.

Doefler, L.A. and Paraskos, J.A. (2004). Anxiety, posttraumatic stress disorder and depression in patients with coronary heart disease: a practical review for cardiac rehabilitation professionals. *Journal of Cardiopulmonary Rehabilitation* 24 (6): 414–421.

Doherty, S., Byrne, M., Murphy, A.W., and McGee, H.M. (2011). Cardiac rehabilitation staff views about discussing sexual issues with coronary heart disease patients: a national survey in Ireland. *European Journal of Cardiovascular Nursing* 10 (2): 101–107.

Espie, C.A. (2009). 'Stepped care': a health technology solution for delivering cognitive behavioural therapy as a first line insomnia treatment. *Sleep* 32 (12): 1549–1558.

Fallowfield, L. and Jenkins, V. (1999). Effective communication skills are the key to good cancer care. *European Journal of Cancer* 35 (11): 1592–1597.

Føsbol, E.L., Peterson, E.D., Weeke, P. et al. (2013). Spousal depression, anxiety, and suicide after myocardial infarction. *European Heart Journal* 34 (9): 649–656.

Franks, M., Stephens, M., Rook, K. et al. (2006). Spouses' provision of health-related support and control to patients participating in cardiac rehabilitation. *Journal of Family Psychology* 20 (2): 311–318.

Freedland, K., Carney, R., Lustman, P. et al. (1992). Major depression in coronary artery disease patients with vs. without a prior history of depression. *Psychosomatic Medicine* 54 (4): 416–421.

Friedman, M. and Rosenman, R. (1959). Association of specific overt behavior pattern with blood and cardiovascular findings; blood cholesterol level, blood clotting time, incidence of arcus senilis, and clinical coronary artery disease. *Journal of the American Medical Association* 169 (12): 1286–1296.

Gallagher, J., Parenti, G., and Doyle, F. (2015). Psychological aspects of cardiac care and rehabilitation: time to wake up to sleep? *Current Cardiology Reports* 17 (12): 111.

Giltay, E.J., Kamphuis, M.H., Kalmijn, S. et al. (2006). Dispositional optimism and the risk of cardiovascular death: the Zutphen elderly study. *Archives of Internal Medicine* 166: 431–436.

Grace, S., Abbey, S., Kapral, M. et al. (2005). Effect of depression on five-year mortality after an acute coronary syndrome. *The American Journal of Cardiology* 96 (9): 1179–1185.

Hargens, T.A., Aron, A., Newsome, L.J. et al. (2015). Effects of obstructive sleep apnea on hemodynamic parameters in patients entering cardiac rehabilitation. *Journal of Cardiopulmonary Rehabilitation and Prevention* 35 (3): 181–185.

Harris, R. (2009). *ACT Made Simple*. Oakland, CA: New Harbinger.

Hatzichristou, D. and Tsimtsiou, Z. (2005). Prevention and management of cardiovascular disease and erectile dysfunction: toward a common patient-centered care model. *The American Journal of Cardiology* 96 (12, supplement 2): 80–84.

Holly, D. and Sharp, J. (2012). Distress thermometer validation: heart failure. *British Journal of Cardiac Nursing* 7 (12): 595–602.

Home Office (2016). *Drug Misuse: Findings from the 2015/16 Crime Survey for England and Wales*, Statistical Bulletin 07/16. London: Home Office.

Huffman, J.C., Beale, E.E., Celano, C.M. et al. (2016). Effects of optimism and gratitude on physical activity, biomarkers, and readmissions after acute coronary syndrome: the gratitude research in acute coronary events study. *Circulation. Cardiovascular Quality and Outcomes* 9 (1): 55–63.

Huffman, J.C., Mastromauro, C.A., Boehm, J.K. et al. (2011). Development of a positive psychology intervention for patients with acute cardiovascular disease. *Heart International* 6: 47–54.

Jansson-Fröjmark, M., Lind, M., and Sunnhed, R. (2012). Don't worry, be constructive: a randomised controlled feasibility study comparing behaviour therapy singly and combined with constructive worry for insomnia. *British Journal of Clinical Psychology* 51 (2): 142–157.

Joekes, K., Maes, S., and Warrens, M. (2007a). Predicting quality of life and self-management from dyadic support and overprotection after myocardial infarction. *British Journal of Health Psychology* 12 (4): 473–489.

Joekes, K., Van Elderen, T., and Schreurs, K. (2007b). Self-efficacy and overprotection are related to quality of life, psychological well-being and self-management in cardiac patients. *Journal of Health Psychology* 12 (1): 4–16.

Kaptein, K.I., de Jonge, P., van den Brink, R.H.S., and Korf, J. (2006). Course of depressive symptoms after myocardial infarction and cardiac prognosis: a latent class analysis. *Psychosomatic Medicine* 68 (5): 662–668.

Kim, E.S., Smith, J., and Kubzansky, L.D. (2014). Prospective study of the association between dispositional optimism and incident heart failure. *Circulation: Heart Failure* 7: 394–400.

Kloner, R.A., Mullin, S.H., Shook, T. et al. (2003). Erectile dysfunction in the cardiac patient: how common and should we treat? Part 2 of 2. *Journal of Urology* 170: S46–S50.

Kristofferzon, M., Lofmark, R., and Carlsson, M. (2003). Myocardial infarction: gender difference in coping and social support. *Journal of Advanced Nursing* 44 (4): 360–374.

Kriston, L., Gunzler, C., Agyemang, A. et al. (2010). Effect of sexual function on health-related quality of life mediated by depressive symptoms in cardiac rehabilitation: findings of the SPARK project in 493 patients. *The Journal of Sexual Medicine* 7 (6): 2044–2055.

Lane, D., Carroll, D., Ring, C. et al. (2000). Effects of depression and anxiety on mortality and quality-of-life 4 months after myocardial infarction. *Journal of Psychosomatic Research* 49 (4): 229–238.

Lazarus, R.S. and Folkman, S. (1984). *Stress, Appraisal and Coping*. New York: Springer.

Leifheit-Limson, E., Reid, K., Kasl, S. et al. (2012). Changes in social support within the early recovery period and outcomes after acute myocardial infarction. *Journal of Psychosomatic Research* 73 (1): 35–41.

Lespérance, F., Frasure-Smith, N., Talajic, M., and Bourassa, M. (2002). Five-year risk of cardiac mortality in relation to initial severity and one-year changes in depression symptoms after myocardial infarction. *Circulation* 105 (9): 1049–1053.

Lett, H., Blumenthal, J., Babyak, M. et al. (2005). Social support and coronary heart disease: epidemiologic evidence and implications for treatment. *Psychosomatic Medicine* 67 (6): 869–878.

Leung, Y.W., Gravely-Witte, S., MacPherson, A. et al. (2010). Post-traumatic growth among cardiac outpatients: degree comparison with other chronic illness samples and correlates. *Journal of Health Psychology* 15 (7): 1049–1063.

Lewin, R.J.P. (1999). Improving quality of life in patients with angina. *Heart* 82 (6): 654–655.

Meevissen, Y.M.C., Peters, M.L., and Alberts, H.J.E.M. (2011). Become more optimistic by imagining a best possible self: effects of a two week intervention. *Journal of Behavior Therapy and Experimental Psychiatry* 42: 371–378.

Meurs, M., Burger, H., van Riezen, J. et al. (2015). The association between cardiac rehabilitation and mortality risk for myocardial infarction with and without depressive symptoms. *Journal of Affective Disorders* 188: 278–283.

Millstein, R.A., Celano, C.M., Beale, E.E. et al. (2016). The effects of optimism and gratitude on adherence, functioning and mental health following acute coronary syndrome. *General Hospital Psychiatry* 43: 17–22.

Mitchell, A., Morgan, J., Petersen, D. et al. (2012). Validation of simple visual-analogue thermometer screen for mood complications of cardiovascular disease: the emotion thermometers. *Journal of Affective Disorders* 136 (3): 1257–1263.

Mooe, T., Franklin, K.A., Holstrom, K. et al. (2001). Sleep-disordered breathing and coronary artery disease: long-term prognosis. *American Journal of Respiratory and Critical Care Medicine* 10 (1): 1910–1913.

Mookadam, F. and Arthur, H. (2004). Social support and its relationship to morbidity and mortality after acute myocardial infarction: systematic overview. *Archives of Internal Medicine* 164 (14): 1514–1518.

Morgan, S., Moses, J., and Speck, L. (2018). 'Getting on with life': smokers' experiences of posttraumatic growth following a myocardial infarction. British Psychological Society.

Morin, C.M., Vallières, A., Guay, B. et al. (2009). Cognitive behavioural therapy, singly and combined with medication, for persistent insomnia: a randomized controlled trial. *JAMA* 301 (19): 2005–2015.

Moser, D.K. and Dracup, K. (2004). Role of spousal anxiety and depression in patients' psychosocial recovery after a cardiac event. *Psychosomatic Medicine* 66 (4): 527–532.

Moss-Morris, R., Weinman, J., Petrie, K.J. et al. (2002). The revised illness perception questionnaire (IPQ-R). *Psychology and Health* 17 (1): 1–16.

Murphy, B.M., Elliott, P.C., Higgins, R.O. et al. (2008). Anxiety and depression after coronary artery bypass graft surgery: most get better, some get worse. *European Journal of Cardiovascular Prevention and Rehabilitation* 15 (4): 210–215.

National Comprehensive Cancer Network (2003). Distress management. Clinical practice guidelines. *Journal of the National Comprehensive Cancer Network* 1 (3): 344–374.

National Institute for Health and Care Excellence (NICE) (2009). *Depression in Adults with a Chronic Physical Health Problem, Treatment and Management: National Clinical Practice Guideline 91*. London: NICE.

Nelson, E., Wasson, J., Kirk, J. et al. (1987). Assessment of function in routine clinical practice: description of the COOP chart method and preliminary findings. *Journal of Chronic Diseases* 40 (Suppl 1): 55S–63S.

O'Farrell, P., Murray, J., and Hotz, S.B. (2000). Psychologic distress among spouses of patients undergoing cardiac rehabilitation. *Heart & Lung* 29 (2): 97–104.

Oldridge, N., Guyatt, G., Jones, N. et al. (1991). Effects on quality of life with comprehensive rehabilitation after acute myocardial infarction. *The American Journal of Cardiology* 67 (13): 1084–1089.

Perkins-Porras, L., Joekes, K., Bhalla, N. et al. (2015). Reporting of posttraumatic stress disorder and cardiac misconceptions following cardiac rehabilitation. *Journal of Cardiopulmonary Rehabilitation and Prevention* 35 (4): 238–245.

Petrie, K.J., Weinman, J., Sharpe, N., and Buckley, J. (1996). Role of patients' view of their illness in predicting return to work and functioning after myocardial infarction: longitudinal study. *British Medical Journal* 312: 1191–1194.

Renshaw, D. and Karstaedt, A. (1988). Is there (sex) life after coronary bypass? *Comprehensive Therapy* 14 (4): 61–66.

Riskind, J., Sarampote, C.S., and Mercier, M.A. (1996). For every malady a sovereign cure: optimism training. *Journal of Cognitive Psychotherapy* 10: 105–117.

Roest, A.M., Martens, E.J., de Jonge, P., and Denollet, J. (2010). Anxiety and risk of incident coronary heart disease. *Journal of the American College of Cardiology* 56 (1): 38–46.

Ronaldson, A., Molloy, G.J., Wikman, A. et al. (2015). Optimism and recovery after acute coronary syndrome: a clinical cohort study. *Psychosomatic Medicine* 77: 311–318.

Rose, S., Bisson, J., Churchill, R., and Wessely, S. (2002). Psychological debriefing for preventing post traumatic stress disorder (PTSD) (review). *Cochrane Database of Systematic Reviews* (2): CD000560. https://doi.org/10.1002/14651858.CD000560.

Rosenbloom, J.I., Wellenius, G.A., Mukamal, K.J., and Mittleman, M.A. (2009). Self-reported anxiety and the risk of clinical events and atherosclerotic progression among patients with coronary artery bypass grafts (CABG). *American Heart Journal* 158 (5): 867–873.

Rosengren, A., Hawken, S., Ounpuu, S. et al. (2004). Association of psychosocial risk factors with risk of acute myocardial infarction in 11119 cases and 13648 controls from 52 countries (the INTERHEART study): case-control study. *Lancet* 364 (9438): 953–962.

Roth, A.D. and Fonagy, P. (2005). *What Works for Whom: A Critical Review of Psychotherapy Research*, 2e. New York: Guilford Press.

Saltmarsh, N., Murphy, B., Bennett, P. et al. (2016). Distress in partners of cardiac patients: relationship quality and social support. *British Journal of Cardiac Nursing* 11 (8): 397–405.

Sarason, I.G., Levine, H.M., Basham, R.B., and Sarason, B.R. (1983). Assessing social support: the social support questionnaire. *Journal of Personality and Social Psychology* 44 (1): 127–139.

Schumann, J., Zellweger, M.J., Di Valentino, M. et al. (2010). Sexual dysfunction before and after cardiac rehabilitation. *Rehabilitation Research and Practice*: 823060. https://doi.org/10.1155/2010/823060.

Shibeshi, W., Young-Xu, Y., and Blatt, C. (2007). Anxiety worsens prognosis in patients with coronary artery disease. *Journal of the American College of Cardiology* 49 (20): 2021–2027.

Sin, N.L., Moskowitz, J.T., and Whooley, M.A. (2015). Positive affect and health behaviours across 5 years in patients with coronary heart disease: the heart and soul study. *Psychosomatic Medicine* 77: 1058–1066.

Steinke, E. and Swan, J. (2004). Effectiveness of a videotape for sexual counseling after myocardial infarction. *Research in Nursing & Health* 27 (4): 269–280.

Steinke, E.E., Jaarsma, T., Barnason, S.A. et al. (2013). Sexual counseling for individuals with cardiovascular disease and their partners: A consensus document from the American Heart Association and the ESC Council on Cardiovascular Nursing and Allied Professions (CCNAP). *Circulation* 128. https://www.ahajournals.org/doi/10.1161/CIR.0b013e31829c2e53.

Taylor, C.B., Bandura, A., Ewart, C.K. et al. (1992). Exercise testing to enhance wives' confidence in their husbands' cardiac capability soon after clinically uncomplicated acute myocardial infarction. *American Journal of Cardiology* 55: 635–638.

Thombs, B.D., Bass, E.B., Ford, D.E. et al. (2006). Prevalence of depression in survivors of acute myocardial infarction. Review of evidence. *Journal of General Internal Medicine* 21 (1): 30–38.

Tindle, H.A., Chang, Y.-F., Kuller, L.H. et al. (2009). Optimism, cynical hostility, and incident coronary heart disease and mortality in the Women's Health Initiative. *Circulation* 120: 656–662.

Toukhsati, S.R., Jovanovich, A., Dehghani, S. et al. (2016). Low psychological resilience is associated with depression in patients with cardiovascular disease. *European Journal of Cardiovascular Nursing* 16 (1): 64–69.

Traeen, B. and Olsen, S. (2007). Sexual dysfunction and sexual well-being in people with heart disease. *Sexual and Relationship Therapy* 22 (2): 193–208.

Valenti, L., Lim, L., Heller, R.F., and Knapp, J. (1996). An improved questionnaire for assessing quality of life after myocardial infarction. *Quality of Life Research* 5 (1): 151–161.

Waltz, M. (1986). Marital context and post-infarction quality of life: is it social support or something more? *Social Science & Medicine* 22 (8): 791–805.

Waltz, M., Badura, B., Pfaff, H., and Schott, T. (1988). Marriage and the psychological consequences of a heart attack: a longitudinal study of adaptation to chronic illness after 3 years. *Social Science and Medicine* 27 (2): 149–158.

Ware, J.E. and Sherbourne, C.D. (1992). The MOS 36-item short-form health survey (SF-36) I. conceptual framework and item selection. *Medical Care* 30 (6): 473–483.

Whitehead, D.L., Perkins-Porras, L., Strike, P.C., and Steptoe, A. (2006). Post-traumatic stress disorder in patients with cardiac disease: predicting vulnerability from emotional responses during admission for acute coronary syndromes. *Heart* 92 (9): 1225–1229.

World Health Organization (WHO) (2002). *The World Health Report 2002: Reducing Risks, Promoting Healthy Life*. Geneva: WHO.

World Health Organization (WHO) (2014). *Global Status Report on Noncommunicable Diseases*. Geneva: WHO.

Zigmond, A.S. and Snaith, R.P. (1983). The hospital anxiety and depression scale. *Acta Psychiatrica Scandinavica* 67 (6): 361–370.

CHAPTER 7

Medical Risk Management

Joe Mills[1], Susan Connolly[2], Barbara Conway[3], Marie-Kristelle Ross[4], Samantha Breen[5], and Dorothy J. Frizelle[6]

[1] Liverpool Heart & Chest Hospital NHS Foundation Trust, Liverpool, UK
[2] Western Health and Social Care Trust, Enniskillen, Northern Ireland
[3] Department of Health Science, University of York, York, UK
[4] Hotel-Dieu de Lévis, Universite Laval Quebec City, Quebec, Canada
[5] Manchester Royal Infirmary and St Mary's Hospital, Manchester University NHS Foundation Trust, Manchester, UK
[6] The Mid Yorkshire Hospitals NHS Trust, Department of Clinical Health Psychology, Dewsbury District Hospital, Dewsbury, UK

Abstract

This chapter discusses the principles of medical risk management – how the measured values for systemic blood pressure, lipid fractions, and blood glucose are correlated with a continuum of risk for the development/progression of cardiovascular disease (CVD) and how interventions (pharmacological and complex device therapies) should be used to ameliorate vascular risk and improve prognosis. A number of therapies, which either result in the lowering of blood pressure, LDL-cholesterol, and average glucose levels, or are introduced in response to an acute CVD-related event, have been demonstrated to improve patient outcomes and reduce the rates of CVD-related morbidity and mortality. Therefore, the majority of individuals who are at moderate to high risk for the development of CVD and all of those with a confirmed CVD diagnosis will require structured assessment of their medical risk profile and the development of a detailed treatment plan.

Cardiovascular Prevention and Rehabilitation in Practice, Second Edition.
Edited by Jennifer Jones, John Buckley, Gill Furze, and Gail Sheppard.
© 2020 John Wiley & Sons Ltd. Published 2020 by John Wiley & Sons Ltd.

As with all of the individual core components, medical risk management overlaps significantly with a number of its counterparts. The control of blood pressure and blood sugar, and the initial prescribing of anti-platelet drugs, beta-blockers, renin-angiotensin system modulators, cholesterol-lowering therapies, etc., are all vitally important but only the first step towards CVD risk reduction. A cardiovascular prevention and rehabilitation programme (CPRP) and its dedicated teams of specialist staff are ideally placed to provide the necessary education, lifestyle advice, and behaviour change support to ensure optimal control of medical risk. Regularly monitoring the response to treatment, enquiring about side-effects, and supporting adherence are essential aspects to achieving sustained, maximised CVD risk reduction.

Keywords: *medical risk management, cardiovascular disease (CVD), risk reduction, drug therapies, education, behaviour change*

Key Points

- Medical risk management overlaps all of the core components and should be considered in the context of cardiovascular disease (CVD) in general.
- Blood pressure, lipid fractions, and blood glucose levels represent modifiable factors that contribute to an individual's risk of either developing CVD or exacerbating existing disease.
- All healthcare professionals delivering cardiac rehabilitation (CR) should have some understanding of the principles of medical risk management, including cardioprotective drugs and devices that a patient may need, and be able to reinforce the rationale for treatment.
- Ideally, a member of the CR team should be able to prescribe cardioprotective therapies, recognise side-effects, consider adherence, and adjust doses. This should be supported by a supervising physician if required. Close links with a patient's GP may be required.
- Use national, published guidelines to direct decisions regarding treatment targets and the optimum types/combinations of required interventions.
- Lifestyle recommendations, including advice on diet, alcohol intake, and exercise will have a significant impact on blood pressure, lipids, and blood sugar control.
- Most patients will have multiple risk factors and require numerous prescribed medications. Long-term adherence can be supported by the CPRP through active monitoring, education, and management of side-effects.

> ■ The presence of implanted cardiac devices (biventricular pace-makers or internal cardiac defibrillators) does not preclude patients from any of the key elements of CR, including the exercise components. However, specific issues pertaining to the device parameters may be important considerations for the CR team.

7.1 RATIONALE AND AIMS

CVD in general and coronary heart disease (CHD) in particular account for more deaths than any other cause in most developed countries. In the UK alone, there are more than a quarter of a million myocardial infarctions recorded each year – which works out as a heart attack approximately every two minutes – with 35 000 deaths from CHD and 30 000 deaths from stroke in 2009. However, death from CHD has been falling since the early 1980s in England and Wales, a trend that can now be demonstrated across the vast majority of European countries (Nichols et al. 2012). The reason for declining death rates is complex and cannot be attributed to any one particular factor, strategic decision, or government policy but key factors include access to modern treatments such as primary angioplasty and complex implantable cardiac devices, as well as effective CVD preventive measures, which include lifestyle modification, management of medical risk factors (blood pressure, lipids, glycaemia) and appropriate use of cardioprotective medication (Unal et al. 2004) (Figure 7.1). Cumulatively, these interventions have transformed the prognosis of CVD in the past few decades with many patients now able to live long and productive lives (British Cardiac Society 2005). CVD prevention programmes have a strong evidence base and should form an integral part of a modern effective comprehensive cardiovascular prevention and rehabilitation programme (CPRP) (Buckley et al. 2013; Clark et al. 2005). The aim of this chapter will be to highlight best-practice management of the principal, modi-fiable medical risk factors (blood pressure, lipids, and glycaemia) within the setting of the CPRP and to provide a review of currently recommended cardio-protective therapies with particular focus on the practical issues surrounding their introduction and subsequent surveillance. The wealth of scientific evi-dence that supports their integration into national/international guidelines will not be considered; rather, the rationale for each of these therapies will be highlighted in conjunction with specific considerations that are directly rele-vant to CR professionals and their patients such as side-effects, dose titration and monitoring, adherence, and patient education. For many reasons, the CPRP offers an ideal setting within which medical risk can be managed effectively. These include the duration of the programme and the therapeutic

Effect of Risk Factors and
Treatments on CHD Mortality

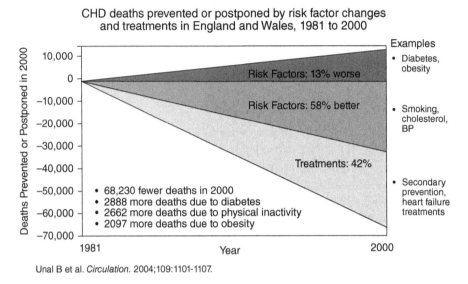

CHD deaths prevented or postponed by risk factor changes
and treatments in England and Wales, 1981 to 2000

Unal B et al. *Circulation.* 2004;109:1101-1107.

FIGURE 7.1   Contribution of various treatments and risk factors to CHD mortality.

relationship that typically develops between the CPRP healthcare professionals and patients over this period. The programme also provides frequent patient contact, allowing for repeated surveillance of the overall medical risk profile and adjustment of interventions (e.g. at the initial assessment and subsequently when attending the supervised exercise sessions). Medical risk management should be the responsibility of the cardiovascular specialist nurse or an independent prescriber (if there is one) working within the programme (which may or may not be a nurse). Liaison with the physician supporting the programme may also be appropriate as well as working collaboratively with the patient's primary care practitioner and other specialist services (e.g. diabetes) (Buckley et al. 2013).

7.2   BLOOD PRESSURE

7.2.1   Epidemiology/BP Targets

Clinic blood pressure (BP) bears an independent continuous relationship with the incidence of CVD (stroke, myocardial infarction, sudden death, heart failure, and peripheral artery disease) as well as of end-stage renal disease (ESRD) and

TABLE 7.1 Therapeutic targets for blood pressure, lipids, and glycaemia.

Target	NICE[a]	JBS3
Blood pressure	<140/90 mmHg <150/90 mmHg in those >80 years	<140/90 mmHg <130/80[b] mm Hg
Lipids (in CVD)	Aim for 40% reduction in non-HDL-cholesterol	LDL-c < 1.8 mmol/L Non-HDL-c < 2.5 mmol/L
Glycaemia	HbA1c personalised to patient. Not to be set <48 mmol/mol (6.5%)	HbA1c 48–58 mmol/mol (6.5–7.5%)

[a] NICE Hypertension CG127 2011, NICE Lipid Modification CG181 2014, NICE Type 2 Diabetes CG66 2008 (due update 2015).
[b] In those with cerebrovascular disease, chronic kidney disease with proteinuria and Type 1 DM.

this relationship holds true at all ages and in all ethnic groups. Blood pressure is normally distributed in the population and there is no natural cut-off point to define 'hypertension' (Mancia et al. 2013).

However, for pragmatic reasons, in clinical practice the threshold blood pressure determining the presence of hypertension is defined as the level of blood pressure above which treatment has been shown to reduce the development or progression of disease and this has also formed the basis of defining target BP. Previous UK guidance (JBS2) had defined a target of <130/80 mmHg (based on observational data) in those with CVD but evidence of benefit for this quite aggressive target has not been borne out by randomised controlled trials.

Therefore, a clinic target of <140/90 mmHg (<150/90 mmHg in those ≥80 years) is now recommended by NICE with a lower target of <135/85 mmHg for ambulatory and home blood pressure recordings (and <145/85 mmHg for these measures in the elderly) (Krause et al. 2011) – see Table 7.1 for a summary of targets.

A similar target of <140/90 mmHg is recommended in the recently published JBS3 Consensus Recommendations for the Prevention of Cardiovascular Disease (JBS3 Board 2014) with a lower target of <130/80 mmHg in certain groups (cerebrovascular disease, chronic kidney disease with significant proteinuria, and Type I diabetes mellitus).

7.2.2 Blood Pressure Measurement

An essential starting point in managing BP to target is accurate measurement of BP in a standardised fashion (O'Brien et al. 2003). BP can be highly variable, not just due to the inherent variability of BP, but also due to the influence of factors such as posture, room temperature, and discomfort/stress. Other contributing factors relate to the method used to measure BP and it is important that the correct cuff size and a validated automated monitor are used.

> **Key Message**
> In patients with atrial fibrillation (AF), use of an automated monitor is not appropriate and conventional clinic-based sphygmomanometry with auscultation is the only reliable method of measuring BP.

All healthcare staff working in and delivering a CPRP should be appropriately trained and competent in measurement of BP. BP levels should be measured at the initial assessment appointment in all patients and subsequently measured regularly (e.g. at the supervised exercise session) in those with elevated/low BP levels (e.g. systolic BP < 100 mmHg) at the initial assessment appointment, in those with symptoms (e.g. postural dizziness), or in those in whom cardioprotective drugs, e.g. ACE inhibitors are being up-titrated.

7.2.3   BP Management

Lifestyle measures remain very important including eating a cardioprotective diet rich in fruit and vegetables, avoidance of processed food (intrinsically high in salt), adhering to alcohol consumption recommendations, maintaining a healthy weight, and being regularly physically active (see Chapter 5). Lifestyle measures can achieve as much BP reduction as one drug and thus reduce the need for combination therapy as well as having an independent cardio-protective effect.

Nonetheless, it should be remembered that the majority of patients with truly elevated BP will also require drug therapy (especially in secondary prevention cases) and typically more than one therapeutic agent will be necessary to achieve control. It may be worth advising patients of this at the outset to avoid them feeling they are failing treatment when a second drug is indicated.

> **Key Message**
> Dual or even triple therapy are commonly required for good BP control in patients with hypertension.

7.2.4   Which Drug?

Meta-analyses have consistently shown that it is the BP reduction itself rather than the individual class of drugs that is responsible for reduction in cardiovascular risk. Nonetheless, in certain individuals one class of antihypertensive may be favoured over another and this decision should be based on several factors including patient characteristics (e.g. ethnicity, age, history of side effects) and also their medical history including diagnosis/treatment and renal function.

The NICE guidance provides an excellent evidence-based stepwise approach to BP management (see Figure 7.2) that is also very pragmatic and works well in clinical practice (Krause et al. 2011).

The following points are worth noting:

- Younger patients (<55 years) and Caucasians tend to have higher renin levels relative to older people or those of black African descent and so ACE inhibitors (or angiotensin receptor antagonists if ACE inhibitor intolerant) should be considered first line.
- In those with established CVD, however, ACE inhibitors (or angiotensin receptor antagonists if ACE inhibitor intolerant) should be used first line *irrespective of age and ethnicity* (particularly in those who are post-myocardial infarction) in view of their strong evidence base.
- Although beta-blockers have fallen out of favour in BP management (due to data suggesting they provide less protection against stroke) they remain very useful for treating hypertension in those with CVD, particularly in those post-myocardial infarction/heart failure where they have prognostic benefit.
- The combination of beta blockers and thiazide-like diuretics should be avoided due to the risk of precipitating diabetes mellitus in those at risk (e.g. those with impaired glucose tolerance, obesity, family history, etc.).

7.2.5 Know/Anticipate the Approximate Therapeutic Effects of What Is Being Prescribed

The following points are important to understand in managing BP to target (Law et al. 2003).

1. For the main groups of antihypertensives (e.g. ACE inhibitors, angiotensin receptor antagonists, thiazide-like diuretics, calcium channel blockers, alpha-blockers), each class at its standard dose (e.g. ramipril 10 mg) tends to provide approximately 9/5 mmHg BP lowering effect. There is, however, substantial variation from person to person and also the higher the initial BP, the larger the reduction seen.
2. Doubling an antihypertensive from its half standard dose to full dose tends to give only a further 20% BP reduction (e.g. ~2 mmHg reduction in systolic BP is gained on increasing amlodipine from 5 to 10 mg.

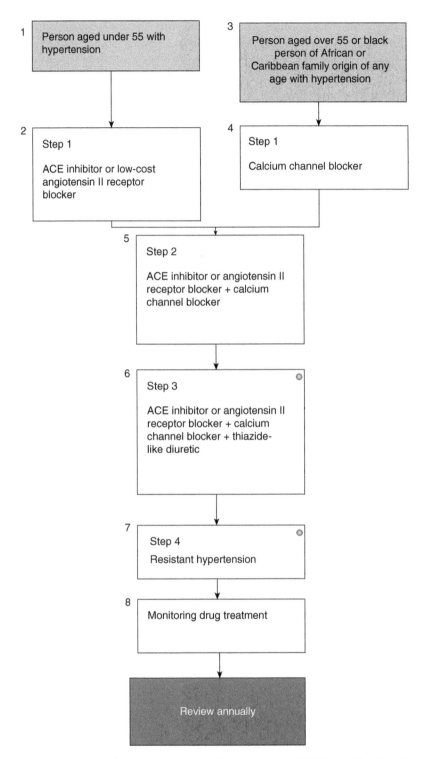

FIGURE 7.2   Choosing drugs for treatment of hypertension (NICE algorithm 2011).

3. Unlike ACE inhibitors and angiotensin receptor blockers, the risk of side-effects with calcium channel blockers, thiazide-like diuretics, and beta-blockers increases with increasing dose.

4. Therefore, it is often more effective to add in another drug rather than increasing the dose of the current drug (in the case of calcium channel blockers, beta-blockers, and diuretics) if a patient remains above target. For example, if a patient's BP is 152/101 mmHg and they are already on ramipril 10 mg and amlodipine 5 mg, the next step should preferentially be the addition of a third drug such as a thiazide-like diuretic rather than doubling the dose of the calcium channel blocker. The latter option will only result in a small incremental BP reduction and will likely cause side effects such as ankle swelling and result in subsequent cessation of the drug due to 'intolerance'.

5. For each antihypertensive added, one should expect the same BP lowering effect as if that drug was used in isolation, i.e. the effect of each drug is additive, but again the effect will vary from person to person.

7.2.6 Persistently Elevated Blood Pressure despite Treatment

Resistant hypertension is defined as a persistently elevated BP (>140/90 mmHg) despite the use of three antihypertensives (including a diuretic) at effective therapeutic doses (Krause et al. 2011). In these cases it is important to consider the following. 'Pseudoresistance' is more likely rather than true resistant hypertension. Pseudoresistance commonly occurs due to lack of adherence to therapy and it is estimated that up to 50% of patients discontinue taking their antihypertensives at one year. Reasons for this include:

- Cost
- Unclear instructions
- Lack of education
- Lack of involvement of patient in plan
- Side effects
- Complexity.

This is why an effective CPRP provides the ideal setting to overcome these barriers. Patient education and empowerment is key and the programme duration should allow sufficient time not only for patient education but also for potential side effects to emerge and be dealt with.

Other common causes of pseudoresistance include incorrect BP measurement (see start of section) and also dietary indiscretion (e.g. diet high in processed food, high alcohol consumption). That is why working in a team is so effective and liaison with the dietitian here is crucial. Concomitant drug use (e.g. non-steroidal anti-inflammatories, steroids, amphetamines, and erythro-poietin) can also raise BP and should always be asked about in the drug history.

Lastly, the white coat effect can also contribute to 'pseudoresistance' and a 24 hour ambulatory BP monitor can be very helpful to clarify habitual levels outside the clinical setting.

Genuine resistant hypertension represents a challenging clinical scenario and is particularly common in those with significant renal impairment and with increasing age. All such cases should be referred to a specialist clinic for further management.

> **Key Message**
> The effect of anti-hypertensive drugs is additive and most patients will require multiple therapeutic agents. However, inadequate BP control is common and this may be a consequence of poor adherence and/or adverse dietary factors.

7.3   LIPIDS

7.3.1   Epidemiology and Lipid Targets

Serum total cholesterol (TC) and LDL-cholesterol (LDL-c) levels also have a continuous relationship with the risk of CHD and, like BP, are normally distributed within the population with therapeutic targets based on levels below which benefit is seen in randomised controlled trials (Cooper and O'Flynn 2008).

In JBS2, the recommended target for all patients with established CVD was a TC < 4 mmol/L and an LDL-c of <2 mmol/L (or a 25% reduction in TC and a 30% reduction in cholesterol in LDL-c if that yielded a lower value). Similar targets were recommended by NICE in 2008 (Table 7.1).

However, the more recently published JBS3 guidelines have now lowered this target to an LDL-c of <1.8 mmol/L. It has also introduced the concept of using non-HDL cholesterol (total cholesterol – HDL-cholesterol [HDL-c]) both in risk estimation and as a therapeutic target (JSB3 Board 2014). Non-HDL-c is a sum of cholesterol contained in all atherogenic ApoB lipoproteins (LDL-c and VLDL-c). The rationale for this is that it obviates the need for fasting (see measurement of serum lipids) and provides a better prediction both of risk and treatment response than LDL-c (particularly in those with diabetes mellitus (DM)). Furthermore, a recent meta-analysis showed that non-HDL-c had the strongest association with cardiovascular events and that changes in non-HDL-c explained the largest proportion of the protective effect of statin intervention (Boekholdt et al. 2012).

A non-HDL-c target of <2.5 mmol/L is proposed by JBS3, which is equivalent to an LDL of <1.8 mmol/L (Table 7.1). Updated NICE guidance on lipid modification was published in July 2014 and this also recommends using non-HDL-c for risk estimation, using a blood sample that *does not* need to be taken in the fasting state. In addition, rather than titrating lipid-lowering agents according to the initial cholesterol profile, all patients with established CVD should be considered for high intensity statin therapy (i.e. atorvastatin 80 mg) unless there are potential drug interactions, high risk of adverse effects, or patient preference dictates otherwise. The NICE guideline also recommends repeat measurement of total cholesterol, HDL-c, and non-HDL-c at three months for all those individuals on high intensity statin. If non-HDL-c has not been reduced by greater than 40% then discussions regarding adherence to dose, timing, lifestyle, and diet should be undertaken (NICE 2014a).

7.3.2 Measurement of Serum Lipids

Measurement of serum lipids should be a standard part of the initial assessment in all patients attending the CPRP.

7.3.3 LDL-Cholesterol

Few laboratories measure LDL-c directly and it is usually calculated indirectly using the Friedewald formula (Friedewald et al. 1972).

Friedewald Formula

LDL-cholesterol = total cholesterol − HDL-cholesterol − (triglycerides/2.2)
Units mmol/L

The formula should *not* be used when triglycerides are >4 mmol/L and this is why traditionally a fasting state is recommended as post-prandial rises in triglyceride levels are common.

The following points are worth noting:

- High serum triglycerides in the fasting state suggests the possibility of obesity, poorly controlled diabetes mellitus, high alcohol consumption, hypothyroidism or, more rarely, some cases of genetic dyslipidaemias (e.g. familial combined hyperlipidaemia).
- In patients post-myocardial infarction and post-coronary artery bypass surgery, serum lipid levels tend to fall within the first 24 hours and do not return to habitual levels for at least eight weeks (Fyfe et al. 1971). Therefore, all such patients should have their lipid profile measured not

just at the initial assessment but also eight weeks from the time of their event.

- It is important to try and retrieve serum lipid levels at presentation before lipid-lowering therapy is initiated, i.e. within the first 24 hours of the hospital admission as this may be important in identifying those who may have genetic dyslipidaemias.
- A fasting total cholesterol >7.5 mmol/L and/or LDL-cholesterol >4.9 mmol/L (off lipid-lowering therapy), especially in conjunction with a family history of premature CVD, raises the possibility of familial heterozygous hyperlipidaemia and such patients should be referred to a specialist clinic for genetic screening, cascade testing of family members, and further management.
- Other laboratory tests should include assessment of renal function, liver and thyroid function tests, and creatine kinase (CK) levels.

Key Message
Non-HDL-c measurement can be performed in the non-fasting state and is used in preference to LDL-c for risk assessment. Lipid levels will vary by up to as much as 5–10% each time they are measured due to biological variation (Cooper and O'Flynn 2008).

7.3.4   Non-HDL Cholesterol

Non-HDL cholesterol represents the total cholesterol circulating in both LDL and apolipoprotein B-containing triglyceride-rich particles. It is easily calculated by subtracting HDL-c levels from total cholesterol. It does not need to be measured in the fasting state and a non-HDL-c of 2.5 mmol/L is equivalent to an LDL-c level of 1.8 mmol/L.

7.4   LIPID-LOWERING THERAPY

Lifestyle measures are important in helping to reduce serum lipid levels and dietary modification (e.g. reduction in saturated fat consumption and promotion of polyunsaturated fat consumption) should form part of the dietary intervention (see Chapter 5).

However, in established CVD, lifestyle measures alone are not sufficient to reduce cardiovascular risk and all patients with CVD should be offered 3-hydroxy-3-methylglutaryl coenzyme A (HMG CoA) reductase inhibitors, i.e.

statins, so that future risk of fatal and non-fatal CVD events can be significantly reduced and rapidly achieved (Cooper and O'Flynn 2008).

Statins reduce serum LDL-cholesterol by reducing endogenous hepatic cholesterol production, which results in increased LDL-receptor expression on hepatic cells increasing uptake of LDL particles by the liver and thus lowering serum LDL-cholesterol levels. Statins can also result in small increases in serum HDL-cholesterol levels (~5–10%) and reduce serum triglyceride levels by ~20–45%.

The four most commonly prescribed statins in the UK are atorvastatin, simvastatin, rosuvastatin, and pravastatin. As a general guide, high-intensity statin therapy refers to atorvastatin 40–80 mg and rosuvastatin 20–40 mg (approximately 45–55% LDL-c reduction), moderate intensity statins are atorvastatin 10–20 mg, rosuvastatin 5–10 mg, simvastatin 20–40 mg, and pravastatin 40–80 mg (30–40% LDL-c reduction), whilst simvastatin 10 mg and pravastatin 10–20 mg reflect low intensity therapy (20–25% LDL-c reduction).

7.4.1 Achieving Lipid Targets

A recent large updated meta-analysis estimated a 22% reduction in vascular event rate per 1 mmol/L reduction in LDL-c and also showed that statins typically reduce LDL-c by approximately 30% (Baigent et al. 2010). However, by using either higher doses of traditional statins or utilising newer, more potent, statins, LDL-c could be further reduced by up to 50%. These additional reductions in LDL-c (down to between 1 and 2 mmol/L) further reduce the incidence of vascular events and this is directly proportional to the absolute LDL-c reduction even when the starting level is already below 2 mmol/L (Cholesterol Treatment Trialists' (CTT) Collaboration et al. 2010). Furthermore, no significant adverse effects with this degree of LDL-c lowering were seen.

Whilst previously NICE recommended high intensity statins only for acute coronary syndromes (as opposed to stable coronary artery disease), this recent data, in combination with the fact that atorvastatin is now off patent (and so cost considerations no longer apply), strongly suggests that all patients with established atherosclerotic disease should be commenced on high intensity statins, e.g. atorvastatin 40–80 mg od (JSB3 Board 2014; NICE 2014a). Simvastatin 80 mg should be avoided as there is a significant risk of myopathy with this dose.

Key Message

It is important to remember the '6%' rule when prescribing statin therapy, i.e. doubling the dose of any statin only achieves an additional 6% LDL-c reduction. High intensity statin therapy may be the preferred option for most patients with established CVD.

7.4.2   Statin 'Intolerance' and Dealing with Side-effects

Statins have an excellent safety profile (even the high intensity statins) (Armitage 2007) yet statin 'intolerance' is reported in up to 1 in 5 patients in clinical practice. A large proportion of these patients, however, have 'perceived' intolerance and in fact if adverse effects are handled judiciously true statin intolerance (empirically defined as being intolerant of three different statins) is in fact extremely uncommon.

Adverse events associated with statins include headache, altered liver function, and gastrointestinal effects such as abdominal pain, diarrhoea, flatulence, nausea, and vomiting. The potential side effect that causes most concern to patients is muscle-related (see Table 7.2).

It is important to note that because of the cytochrome P450 enzymatic pathway (CYP3A4) through which atorvastatin and simvastatin are metabolised, the co-prescription of drugs or foods that inhibit CYP3A4 (see Table 7.3) will lead to an increased systemic exposure to statins and consequently a greater risk of adverse events such as myopathy.

7.4.3   Actions to Take if a Patient Develops Muscle Aches on Statin Therapy

1. Take a clear history. Muscle discomfort related to statins typically affects the large bulky muscles in the arms/legs, it is usually bilateral, and does not usually affect joints. It is important to distinguish symptoms from other causes of pain such as osteoarthritis or vitamin D deficiency. Also enquire about associated muscle weakness.
2. Measure a CK level.

TABLE 7.2   Summary of the principal muscle side-effects related to statins.

	Definition	Creatine kinase levels	Incidence
Myalgia	Muscle ache/ discomfort but no weakness	Typically normal	No higher than placebo in RCTs Up to 10% in clinical registries
Myopathy	Muscle discomfort also accompanied by weakness	Usually >10 times the upper limit normal	<0.01%
Rhabdomyolysis	Severe myopathy often with renal failure	Usually >40 times the upper limit normal	Less than 1/3 the incidence of myopathy

TABLE 7.3 MHRA[a] Update October 2012.

Interacting drug or food	Simvastatin prescribing advice	Atorvastatin prescribing advice
Grapefruit juice	Avoid grapefruit juice	Avoid grapefruit juice
Calcium antagonists (verapamil, diltiazem, amlodipine)	Do not exceed 20 mg	Use lowest necessary dose
Amiodarone	Do not exceed 20 mg	Use lowest necessary dose
Erythromycin/ clarithromycin, anti-fungals, HIV protease inhibitors	Contraindicated	Suspend until interacting drug discontinued and/or do not exceed 20 mg (clarithromycin), 40 mg (itraconazole)
Fibrates	Do not exceed 10 mg (higher doses can be used with fenofibrate)	Caution – increased risk of myopathy
Warfarin	INR surveillance at initiation and after dose changes	INR surveillance at initiation and after dose changes

[a] UK Medicines and Healthcare Products Regulatory Agency.

3. If the patient is not reporting weakness and the CK level is normal, the diagnosis is most likely statin myalgia. Ask the patient to take a statin break for a week or so. Generally, the symptoms will resolve quickly. If they don't other causes for the discomfort should be considered.

4. Challenge the patient with simvastatin 10 mg or atorvastatin 10 mg daily dose, choosing the statin that the patient has not previously taken. If tolerated, the dose can be gradually increased as required according to tolerance.

5. If not tolerated, prescribe low dose pravastatin at 10 mg daily dose or rosuvastatin at 5 mg daily dose. If necessary, rosuvastatin 5 mg can be pre-scribed every second day, or even once weekly) in accordance with patient preference and then titrated up, as required, if no side-effects occur.

6. If it is a statin myopathy, the statin must be stopped immediately and CK levels monitored until they return to normal. This does not mean statin therapy is now contraindicated and it may be retried at a lower dose at a later stage (see above) but ideally this should be done under specialist supervision.

7. Rhabdomyolysis requires hospital admission for administration of intra-venous fluid therapy and monitoring of renal function. Review of pos-sible precipitants is required and the risk/benefits of statin therapy in the future should be reviewed by a specialist.

7.4.4   CK Levels

It is worth measuring baseline CK levels. Some individuals may have a slightly elevated level at baseline, particularly if they are very physically active or involved in contact sports. CK levels, however, do not need to be measured rou-tinely thereafter and should only be checked if the patient develops symptoms. *Asymptomatic* moderate rises in CK levels do not require any action.

7.4.5   Hepatic Side Effects

It is estimated that ~7% of patients may have elevations in their transaminases at baseline. Common causes include non-alcoholic fatty liver disease, high alcohol consumption, or less commonly viral infections (e.g. hepatitis B) or other causes of chronic liver disease. Witholding statin therapy due to baseline liver dysfunction should be avoided where possible and only after consultation with a liver specialist. Non-alcoholic fatty liver is not a contraindication to statin therapy and may even be beneficial. Statins may be used in most cases of chronic liver disease although liaison with a hepatologist is advised alongside monitoring of liver function.

Less than 1% of patients will develop raised transaminases on statin therapy. This generally occurs in the first six months of initiating statin therapy and is usually asymptomatic.

Increases that are three times the upper limit of normal are considered significant but often resolve spontaneously even if statin therapy is continued. However, if they persist after one month it is generally an indication for stopping the statin. Liver abnormalities are more common with the higher intensity statins particularly atorvastatin 80 mg. Again, once transaminases return to normal the patient may be rechallenged with a lower dose statin with moni-toring of the liver function tests.

Key Message

Like blood pressure, the CPRP provides the ideal setting within which to achieve optimal lipid control. It therefore should be used as an opportunity to optimise statin therapy in conjunction with supporting adherence and assessing potential side-effects.

7.4.6 Other Lipid-lowering Drugs

Other lipid-lowering drugs should be considered in the following cases:

- Those with genuine statin intolerance or who cannot tolerate high dose statins
- Those who are not achieving target despite being on maximum tolerated statin
- Those with a mixed dyslipidaemia (e.g. high triglycerides) persisting despite lifestyle measures and statin therapy.

7.4.7 Ezetimibe

Ezetimibe inhibits cholesterol absorption in the gut and lowers LDL-c by about 15–20%. It is licensed for the treatment of hypercholesterolaemia (primary/familial). In addition, outcome data were published in 2015 demonstrating that combined simvastatin/ezetimibe therapy in patients with acute coronary syndromes resulted in fewer acute CVD events when compared with simvastatin alone (Cannon et al. 2015). As ezetimibe acts via a distinct pathway to that of statins, its side-effect profile is quite different and its LDL-c lowering effect is additive when used in combination with statin therapy.

7.4.8 Proprotein Convertase Subtilisin/Kexin Type 9 (PCSK9) Monoclonal Antibodies: Evolocumab/Alirocumab

This novel class of LDL-c lowering therapies, generally administered via fortnightly subcutaneous injection, have amassed a considerable wealth of persuasive biochemical and clinical data confirming efficacy and safety. Both evolocumab and alirocumab lower LDL-cholesterol by ~50–60% as either monotherapy or when added to statin therapy. Both drugs have been approved by NICE for use in certain patient groups with persistently high levels of LDL-c despite maximum tolerated lipid-lowering therapy. The details of the approved indications for use are detailed within their respective technology appraisal documents (NICE TA 393 2016; NICE TA 394 2016). More recently a CVD outcome study has shown further reduction in cardiovascular events when added to statin therapy in a high risk CVD population. The average LDL-c levels achieved in this trial were under 1 mmol/L, heralding a new era in lipid-lowering therapy and confirming that 'lower is better' (Sabatine et al. 2017). However, these drugs are expensive and thus should only be used in the highest risk groups (e.g. familial heterozygous hyperlipidaemia not at target, recurrent/ aggressive CVD, or in those with CVD who are genuinely statin intolerant), and under specialist supervision only.

7.4.9   Colesevelam

Colesevelam is a recently developed bile-acid binding resin that is better tolerated than previous such agents although gastrointestinal side-effects remain an issue. It may lower LDL-c by ~15–20% but should be avoided in hypertriglyceridaemia. For the truly statin intolerant, ezetimibe and colesevelam may be used in combination with an LDL-c lowering effect of up to 30% but this should only be done under specialist advice.

7.4.10   Fibrates

Fibrates increase HDL-c by about 10% and lower triglycerides by about 30% and thus may be indicated in those patients with persisting abnormalities in these parameters despite statin therapy (e.g. in some genetic dyslipidaemias). However, the evidence for fibrates in improving cardiovascular outcomes is weak (Jun et al. 2010) and therefore they should not be used as substitutes for statin therapy (Saha et al. 2007).

7.4.11   Nicotinic Acid/Niacin

This B vitamin was previously used in those with low HDL-c levels/ hypertriglyceridaemia but is no longer available in the UK after recent trials showed a lack of cardiovascular benefit and increased risk of side effects (Niacin in patients 2011; HPS2-THRIVE randomised 2013).

7.4.12   Fish Oils

High dose fish oils may be used as add on therapy in the treatment of hypertriglyceridaemia – again this should be under supervision of specialist clinic.

Key Message

Lifestyle/dietary intervention plus statin therapy is the most effective and evidence-based mechanism for reducing LDL-c and improving CVD risk profile. Side-effects can be managed by appropriate monitoring and changes to dose/preparation. True statin intolerance is rare.

7.5 DYSGLYCAEMIA

In those without diagnosed diabetes mellitus, blood glucose has a continuous relationship with CVD similar to that of blood pressure and cholesterol (British Cardiac Society 2005).

In those with diabetes, CVD risk differs according to the type of diabetes. In Type 1 diabetes, which is characterised by loss of pancreatic beta cell function and endogenous insulin production, there is a two- to threefold increase in the relative risk of developing CVD (Livingstone et al. 2012), with this risk being notably increased in those with diabetic nephropathy.

In Type 2 diabetes, which is much more common (90% of cases) and characterised by insulin resistance and eventual beta cell failure, cardiovascular risk is approximately double that of non-diabetic individuals (Emerging Risk Factors Collaboration et al. 2010) and this risk correlates with duration of diabetes and/or the presence of proteinuria.

Dysglycaemia is therefore common in patients presenting with CVD (both acute and stable) with approximately one third having a previous diagnosis of diabetes mellitus whilst a further 4 in 10 have hitherto undiagnosed abnormalities in their glucose metabolism (Bartnik et al. 2004).

7.5.1 Diagnosing Dysglycaemia/Diabetes Mellitus

All patients attending a CPRP should therefore have their glycaemic status assessed.

The gold standard diagnosis until recently has been the oral glucose tolerance test (OGTT), which typically consists of the oral administration of a 75 g glucose load with measurement of plasma glucose two hours later. Dysglycaemia may be classified into the following three categories (Table 7.4):

1. Impaired fasting glycaemia (IFG)
2. Impaired glucose tolerance (IGT)
3. Diabetes mellitus.

An OGTT has been the gold standard for the following reasons:

- Fasting plasma glucose alone fails to diagnose ~30% of cases of diabetes
- It is the only way of diagnosing impaired glucose tolerance, which itself is associated with an increased cardiovascular risk of ~1.5.

However, since 2011, the World Health Organization has also recognised glycated haemoglobin (HbA1c) as being a diagnostic test for DM (World Health

TABLE 7.4   World Health Organization Diagnostic Criteria for Dysglycaemia based on the oral glucose tolerance test (OGTT).

Diabetes	Fasting plasma glucose ≥ 7.0 μmol/L **or** 2–h plasma glucose[a] ≥11.1 μmol/L
Impaired glucose tolerance (IGT)	Fasting plasma glucose <7.0 μmol/L and 2 h plasma glucose[a] ≥7.8 and < 11.1 μmol/L
Impaired fasting glucose (IFG)	Fasting plasma glucose 6.1 to 6.9 μmol/L and (if measured)[b] 2 h plasma glucose[a] <7.8 μmol/L

[a] Venous plasma glucose two hours after ingestion of 75 g oral glucose load.
[b] If two hour plasma glucose is not measured, status is uncertain as diabetes or IGT cannot be excluded.

Organization 2011). HbA1c is formed via a non-enzymatic glycation pathway following exposure to blood glucose. Due to the half-life of haemoglobin, HbA1c will reflect the average plasma glucose over the previous two to three months and so can be used to assess glycaemic control in patients with DM.

A diagnosis of diabetes is made if the HbA1c is above 48 mmol/mol (6.5%) and in the absence of symptoms of diabetes (common) this should be measured on two separate occasions.

Note a value of less than 48 mmol/mol does not exclude DM already diagnosed using other glucose tests.

A HbA1c of 42–47 mmol/l indicates a high risk of developing DM and these patients should receive tailored intensive lifestyle advice and their primary care practitioner should be advised to monitor their HbA1c on an annual basis.

> **Key Message**
> The use of blood HbA1c levels to diagnose and monitor diabetes is advantageous since the patient does not need to be fasting and HbA1c does not have the variability of day-to-day glucose monitoring.

7.5.2   Is Glycaemic Control Important?

Whilst tight glycaemic control without doubt reduces the risk of microvascular disease (e.g. nephropathy, retinopathy) in both Type 1 (The Diabetes Control and Complications Trial Research Group 1993) and Type 2 DM (UK Prospective Diabetes Study Group 1998), the evidence for protection against macrovascular events is less clear cut (Nathan et al. 2005; Turnbull et al. 2009). A post-interventional study from UKPDS did find a benefit in cardiovascular outcomes in patients recently diagnosed with Type 2 DM (Holman et al. 2008), but contemporary studies that have used intensive treatment have failed to show similar benefit, with one trial even showing an increase in mortality, possibly due to severe hypoglycaemia episodes, which were more frequent in the intensive treatment arm (Ray et al. 2009). Two subsequent meta-analyses have been carried out (Ray et al. 2009; Turnbull et al. 2009) with one indicating that whilst cardiovascular outcomes were indeed reduced by intensive glucose control (Turnbull et al. 2009) this was principally in those with no previous history of CVD and neither meta-analyses showed an effect on all-cause mortality.

7.5.3 Glycaemia, HbA1c, and Targets

Given the lack of consistent, persuasive data, it is now recommended that the targets of glycaemia and HbA1c should be discussed and individualised for each patient. Whilst previously a target HbA1c of <6.5% (48 mmol/mol) (British Cardiac Society 2005; Home et al. 2008) was advised, it is now accepted that most patients should aim for an HbA1c between 6.5 and 7.5% (48–58 mmol/mol). Stricter control is not recommended and it is even sometimes adequate to aim for slightly less intensive control in specific populations, such as elderly patients or in those with established CVD (JSB3 Board 2014).

What has also becoming increasingly evident, however, is that there should be strong emphasis placed on control of other cardiovascular risk factors (e.g. blood pressure and lipids) in patients with DM as improvements in these parameters may have a more substantial impact upon CVD risk compared to that achieved by too rigid a focus on glucose control.

7.5.4 Management of Diabetes Mellitus in the CPRP

The responsibilities of the cardiovascular prevention and rehabilitation team should include assessment of glycaemic status in all patients attending the programme and in addition assessment of glycaemic control in those with DM. Blood pressure and lipids should be actively managed in these patients within the setting of the programme as discussed in previous sections.

However, alterations in oral hypoglycaemic therapy/insulin will usually fall outside the remit/skill of the multidisciplinary team and liaison with diabetes specialist nurse/specialist/primary care practitioner is therefore advised.

Physical activity is generally safe for patients with DM, but for specific recommendations on blood glucose management during exercise please refer to the Joint scientific statement of the BACPR, Diabetes UK, and the British Association of Sport and Exercise Sciences on 'Practical exercise considerations for the CR participant with diabetes' (JSB3 2014).

> **Key Message**
> Assessment of glycaemic status and optimisation of glucose control should be key aspects of the CPRP, which are performed in combination with other modifiable risk factor interventions. A rigid focus on achieving tight blood sugar levels is not recommended.

7.6   MEDICAL RISK FACTORS AND OTHER LONG-TERM CONDITIONS

With an ageing population that is increasingly overweight/obese and sedentary, the already high prevalence of hypertension, DM, and dyslipidaemia will continue to rise. It is therefore likely that most patients with long-term conditions such as CVD, chronic pulmonary disease, and degenerative/inflammatory arthritis will have accrued at least one modifiable, medical CVD risk factor. The basic principles of CVD risk assessment should be applied to all patients and this should include appropriate dietary and lifestyle recommendations. The need for pharmacological interventions should be considered in the context of each individual's co-morbidity and other prescribed therapies, but a general commitment to optimising CVD risk reduction should be pursued. Of course, overall prognosis, personal circumstances, and quality of life issues may impact on the nature and merits of any CVD risk reduction strategy.

7.7   CARDIOPROTECTIVE DRUG AND DEVICE THERAPIES

7.7.1   Dual Anti-platelet Therapy

7.7.1.1   Aspirin

The data supporting the benefits of aspirin pre-date contemporary interventional practice but the drug is inexpensive, well tolerated, and still recommended within national guidelines (NICE 2010b; NICE 2013). Genuine intolerance of aspirin is rare but anaphylaxis, acute bronchoconstriction, and pruritic rashes can occur and under such circumstances patients will be discharged on a different, single anti-platelet agent. A past history of upper gastrointestinal (GI) pathology is quite common and this may or may not be related to previous aspirin use. In general, most such patients should receive aspirin with an adjunctive proton pump inhibitor but if symptoms of upper GI pathology occur, e.g. indigestion, acid reflux, abdominal pain, or suspicion of blood in the faeces, then an urgent check of the full blood count and referral to a GI specialist would be reasonable (NICE 2004; NICE 2012). Low dose aspirin should be recommended as life-long therapy for patients who have experienced any symptomatic manifestation of CVD and rarely should it be discontinued (unless advised to do so by a specialist or in the setting of life-threatening bleeding).

7.7.1.2 Clopidogrel/Prasugrel

Clopidogrel and prasugrel are thienopyridines that bind irreversibly to the P2Y12 platelet receptor and thereby inhibit platelet aggregation. Clopidogrel has been the most widely used second anti-platelet drug (in combination with aspirin) for patients who have experienced acute coronary syndrome (ACS) or who have undergone revascularisation (PCI or CABG) for symptoms of stable angina (Cuisset et al. 2008; NICE 2010b). It may be associated with a pruritic rash and/or haemorrhagic complications with the latter affecting many patients in the form of easily bruised skin, whereby reassurance is all that is generally required. However, all combinations of dual anti-platelet therapy (DAPT) will significantly increase a patient's risk of more sinister forms of bleeding and healthcare professionals should have a low threshold for ordering blood tests and referring on for specialist advice. In general, clopidogrel therapy should be recommended for no more than 12 months, however, if consideration is being given to stopping clopidogrel early (or indeed any second anti-platelet drug) then advice from the patient's supervising cardiologist should always be sought. In general, anti-platelet drugs are prescribed to reduce the future risk of acute cardiovascular events – namely MI and stroke – but DAPT regimens are also crucial for reducing the risk of stent thrombosis and thus the importance of involving the cardiology team if any changes to these drugs are contemplated.

Prasugrel has been demonstrated in clinical trials to be superior to clopidogrel in patients receiving coronary stents for the acute treatment of ST-segment elevation myocardial infarction (STEMI) and, for patients with diabetes mellitus, non-ST-segment elevation myocardial infarction (NSTEMI) and unstable angina (Wiviott et al. 2007). The active metabolite of prasugrel is identical to that of clopidogrel but is achieved through a far less complex process of metabolism and thus less susceptibility to genetic factors that might impact on the metabolic pathway and reduce the bioavailability of the active drug (Lazar and Lincoff 2009).

7.7.1.3 Ticagrelor

Ticagrelor also acts upon the platelet P2Y12 receptor but binds reversibly and does not appear susceptible to genetic variation in efficacy. Data from the PLATO trial (Wallentin et al. 2009) and a NICE technology appraisal support the use of ticagrelor in the setting of STEMI, NSTEMI, and unstable angina, irrespective of treatment strategy (NICE 2011). In addition to the increased risk of haemorrhagic complications (as described above) a commonly reported side-effect of this drug is that of transient breathlessness. Patients may describe brief episodes of gasping for breath or needing to take deep, sighing breaths, often at entirely unpredictable times. The mechanism for this side-effect is not precisely understood but generally subsides within four weeks of drug initiation and does not exacerbate symptoms of asthma or chronic obstructive pulmonary disease (Storey et al. 2011). Patients should be reassured accordingly but if intolerable side-effects persist it may become necessary to contact the patient's cardiologist to discuss alternative anti-platelet therapy.

> **Key Message**
> Anti-platelet therapies reduce the risk of stent thrombosis and acute athero-thrombotic vascular events. Bleeding risk, especially upper GI bleeding, increases when agents are combined. A cardiologist should always be involved in any decision to alter or discontinue DAPT.

7.7.2　Beta-blocker Therapy

Beta-blockers are recommended for all patients with ACS and/or left ventricular systolic dysfunction (LVSD), including patients with peripheral vascular disease, erectile dysfunction, DM, and pulmonary disease (NICE 2010a; NICE 2013). A confirmed medical history of COPD should not preclude the use of cardioselective beta-blockers, in fact, data exists to suggest that such patients may even derive greater benefit from their inhaler therapies once established on beta-blocker drugs (Short et al. 2011). Beta-blockers should be continued for a minimum of 12 months and ideally life-long in the presence of persistent LVSD. Although it is important to up-titrate beta-blocker dose to the maximum tolerated/evidence-based level (Fiuzat et al. 2012; Goldberger et al. 2010), attempts to achieve this are often undermined by intolerable haemodynamic consequences (dizziness/syncope) or other unwanted side-effects such as fatigue/lethargy, cold/painful peripheries, erectile dysfunction, and wheeze/breathlessness.

　　For patients who have tolerated beta-blocker initiation then an assessment of their prescribed dose should be undertaken at approximately fortnightly intervals. As a rough guide, if the resting heart rate is above 60 beats per minute, and the systolic blood pressure above 100 mmHg, then a dose increment should be considered, particularly if the patient is free from beta-blocker associated side-effects. Asymptomatic patients do not require dose reductions irrespective of their haemodynamic parameters. Patients should be aware that beta-blockers may prolong their life and reduce the likelihood of acute CVD events occurring but that certain side-effects may arise. The CR professional is ideally placed to consider dose reductions or alternative agents in the setting of beta-blocker associated symptoms that may prevent continued adherence. On occasion, patients will not be able to tolerate even the smallest doses of cardioselective beta-blockers such as bisoprolol or nebivolol, and in the setting of ACS (though not with heart failure) there may be some cardioprotective benefit derived from the use of alternative heart rate slowing drugs such as verapamil or diltiazem (NICE 2013).

> **Key Message**
>
> Beta-blocker dose should be up-titrated, according to heart rate and blood pressure response, to the maximum tolerated level. Mild side-effects such as fatigue and cold peripheries may occur. Pulmonary disease, especially COPD, is not a contra-indication to the use of beta-blockers.

7.8   ACE INHIBITORS/ANGIOTENSIN II RECEPTOR BLOCKERS

ACE inhibitors have been shown to reduce cardiovascular mortality in patients with LVSD and/or acute myocardial infarction (with or without heart failure) (AIRE 1993; Flather et al. 2000; Yusuf et al. 2000). Angiotensin II receptor blockers (ARBs) should be reserved for those patients who are unable to tolerate ACE inhibitor therapy (NICE 2010a, 2013). The most frequently reported adverse effect of ACE inhibitors is that of dry cough and may affect up to 35% of patients (Dicpinigaitis 2006), with angio-oedema and rash occurring far less frequently. Both ACE inhibitors and ARBs will have an impact on glomerular filtration rate and this will lead to a rise in serum creatinine and potassium so it is essential that urea, creatinine, and electrolytes are checked prior to initiation and within two weeks of a dose adjustment.

The CR team is ideally placed to assess the ACE inhibitor dose and adjust in line with haemodynamic parameters whilst monitoring renal function and adverse symptoms. The ACE inhibitor or ARB dose should be up-titrated to evidence-based or maximally tolerated levels within four to six weeks of the acute CVD event (AIRE 1993; Yusuf et al. 2000) with dose adjustments dependent upon renal function and systolic blood pressure response. As a guide, a systolic blood pressure of greater than 100 mmHg and a serum creatinine that has not increased above 50% of that of baseline (or an absolute value of more than 266 μmol/L) should allow a dose up-titration. If potassium rises above 5.5 mmol/L or creatinine more than 100% of the baseline value (or more than an absolute value of 310 μmol/L) then the ACE inhibitor (or ARB) therapy should be discontinued and specialist advice obtained (SIGN 2007). A guide to the starting and target doses of ACE inhibitors and ARBs is shown in Table 7.5. In addition, symptomatic hypotension may also limit the degree to which ACE inhibitors or ARBs can be up-titrated.

TABLE 7.5   ACE inhibitor/ARB therapy starting and target doses.

ACE inhibitor	Starting dose	Target dose
Captopril	6.25 mg three times daily	50 mg three times daily
Enalapril	2.5 mg twice daily	10–20 mg twice daily
Lisinopril	2.5–5 mg once daily	20 mg once daily
Ramipril	2.5 mg twice daily	5 mg twice daily or 10 mg once daily
Perindopril	2 mg once daily	8 mg once daily
Trandolapril	0.5 mg once daily	4 mg once daily
ARB		
Candesartan	4 or 8 mg once daily	32 mg once daily
Valsartan	40 mg twice daily	160 mg twice daily

Most patients will tolerate a resting systolic blood pressure of 90–100 mmHg but postural hypotension can occur regardless of resting blood pressure, and if severe enough to result in collapse/syncope then a reduction in dose may have to be considered. It is important to review other medications and in particular to avoid other unnecessary drugs that may interfere with renal function (such as non-steroidal anti-inflammatory drugs) or exacerbate hypotension (such as α-blockers). Patients should be encouraged to report side-effects such as cough, rash, or dizziness so that appropriate interventions can be considered, which may, in turn, result in longer-term adherence. For example, patients with a pre-sumed ACE inhibitor-induced dry cough should be considered for ARBs, and symptoms of dizziness may be more tolerable if dosing is switched to a once daily preparation that can be taken at night.

Key Message
ACE inhibitor/ARB dose should be up-titrated, according to renal function and blood pressure response, to the maximum tolerated. ACE inhibitor-induced dry cough is a common side-effect that does not occur with ARB therapy.

7.9   MINERALOCORTICOID RECEPTOR ANTAGONIST

Two clinical trials, the Randomized Aldosterone Evaluation Study (RALES) (Pitt et al. 1999) and the Eplerenone Heart failure and Survival Study (EPHESUS) (Pitt et al. 2003), have convincingly indicated that mineralocorticoid receptor

TABLE 7.6 Serum potassium and MRA dose adjustment.

Serum potassium (mmol/L)	Action	Dose adjustment
<5.0	Increase	25 mg every other day to 25 mg once daily 25 mg once daily to 50 mg once daily
5.0–5.4	Maintain	No adjustment
5.5–5.9	Decrease	50 mg once daily to 25 mg once daily 25 mg once daily to 25 mg every other day 25 mg every other day to withhold
≥6.0	Withhold	Restart at 25 mg every other day when potassium levels fall to < 5.5 mmol/L

antagonists (MRAs) reduce mortality in patients with symptomatic heart failure (irrespective of aetiology) and systolic left ventricular dysfunction post-myocardial infarction on top of ACE inhibition. In particular, a reduction in the rate of sudden death was observed in both trials. Spironolactone is an MRA that also has anti-androgen properties and may lead to unwanted side-effects such as gynaecomastia, impotence, and loss of libido.

Eplerenone, also an MRA, is associated with a lower incidence of such side-effects but is currently more expensive and there appears little difference between the two drugs in terms of their cardioprotective properties (Chatterjee et al. 2012). It is recommended that in the ACS setting, MRAs are initiated 3–14 days after the index event and 25 mg daily is the usual starting dose, although if the baseline potassium level is in the high normal range and/or ACE inhibitor doses are still to be increased, then 25 mg alternate days should be considered. The main biochemical effect of MRAs result in a change in serum creatinine and serum potassium, both of which will increase, particularly if underlying renal function is abnormal. Serum biochemistry should be taken at baseline and then again within the first seven days of MRA initiation or dose adjustment. Once dosing is stable, then a further check at one month should be performed (Table 7.6).

7.10 LOOP DIURETICS

Furosemide and bumetanide are the most commonly prescribed loop diuretics and are generally used to treat hypertension or ameliorate oedema in patients with symptomatic heart failure. There is no convincing evidence that these drugs are directly cardioprotective but may, through careful dose adjustment in response to warning signs of decompensation (such as weight gain), prevent an unplanned hospital admission. Even for those patients without evidence of fluid overload a maintenance dose of loop diuretic may lead to a vastly improved quality of life by reducing or even eliminating exertional breathlessness. Serum urea and electrolytes should be monitored closely at the time of diuretic initiation and then within five to seven days after subsequent dose adjustments. Sodium and potassium levels will tend to fall and serum creatinine will rise (in response to the reduced renal blood flow) and specialist (cardiologist/nephrologist) input may be required if these changes continue without any obvious improvement in the patient's clinical condition. Ultimately, many patients with chronic heart failure may require a more palliative treatment strategy and it has recently been shown that furosemide can be given safely and effectively via a subcutaneous route in a community setting (Farless et al. 2012). Again, this may lead to rapid resolution of distressing symptoms and prevent acute hospital admission.

> **Key Message**
>
> MRAs may improve survival in patients with symptoms of heart failure and significant impairment of left ventricular systolic function. Eplerenone may be better tolerated than spironolactone and renal function should be monitored as potassium levels impact on dose adjustment. Loop diuretics alleviate symptoms of heart failure and, if used prophylactically, may prevent decompensation.

7.11 STATIN THERAPY

The rationale for high intensity statin therapy is covered in detail in Section 7.4 of this chapter.

7.12 ANTI-COAGULANT THERAPIES

For patients with atherothrombotic vascular disease, the presence of AF significantly complicates the issue of anti-platelet and anti-coagulant therapies. AF-related embolic events account for 15–20% of all strokes and there is good evidence that appropriate anti-coagulation with vitamin K antagonists (such as warfarin) or new oral anti-coagulants (NOACs) such as dabigatran, rivaroxaban, apixaban, and edoxaban can prevent more than 70% of these catastrophic events (Camm et al. 2012; Giugliano et al. 2013). However, in the ACS setting, particularly when intra-coronary stents have been implanted and a period of DAPT warranted, the timing of anti-coagulant initiation and the risk of haemorrhagic adverse events are important considerations.

A significant proportion of patients experiencing ACS will be admitted on anti-coagulant therapy or will develop a clinical need for anti-coagulation during the acute clinical phase (evidence of left ventricular thrombus or venous thrombo-embolism). Under these circumstances a combination of warfarin and clopidogrel should be considered even if intra-coronary stents have been implanted (NICE 2013). Patients should be aware of the increased risk of bleeding when anti-platelet and anti-coagulant agents are combined and that skin bruising and bleeding from the gums during tooth brushing are commonly reported adverse effects. Ensure that patients receiving warfarin are adequately monitored and review their international normalised ratio (INR) values with them. Once beyond the two to three months initiation phase, INR values below 1.7 or above 5 suggest poor INR control and issues around adherence should be discussed and specialist clinical advice should be obtained.

> **Key Message**
> Warfarin plus clopidogrel is currently recommended for patients who would otherwise require DAPT but who also have a clinical indication for concomitant anti-coagulant therapy. A NOAC may be a suitable alternative to warfarin for those patients who refuse warfarin therapy or have significant fluctuations in INR that are either unexplained or unavoidable.

7.13 IMPLANTABLE DEVICES

Cardiac resynchronisation therapy (CRT) is a proven treatment for heart failure-induced conduction disturbances and ventricular dyssynchrony, which ameliorates symptoms and improve cardiac function by restoring coordinated contraction between the ventricles. Implantable cardioverter defibrillators (ICDs) are recommended for patients who have either already experienced life-threatening ventricular arrhythmias or are at high risk of developing them. NICE (2014b) recommend CRT with a pacing device (CRT-P) or a defibrillator device (CRT-D) as a treatment option for people with heart failure and LVEF $\leq$ 35% according to the following ECG criteria and NYHA symptom class:

- QRS duration of $\geq$ 120 ms, with or without left bundle branch block (LBBB), NYHA class IV (CRT-P).
- QRS duration of 120–149 ms, with LBBB, NYHA II (CRT-D), or NYHA III (CRT-P/D).
- QRS duration of $\geq$ 150 ms, with or without LBBB, NYHA I or II (CRT-D); NYHA III (CRT-P/D).

NICE (2014b) recommend ICDs as options for treating people with previous serious ventricular arrhythmias, in the absence of a treatable cause, who fulfil any of the following criteria:

- Survived a cardiac arrest due to ventricular tachycardia (VT) or ventricular fibrillation (VF), or
- Spontaneous sustained VT with syncope/haemodynamic compromise, or
- Sustained VT with a left ventricular ejection fraction (LVEF) of $\leq 35\%$ and NYHA I, II, or III.

An ICD may also be implanted for prophylaxis in any of the following circumstances (NICE 2014b):

- Familial conditions with high risk of sudden death such as long QT syndrome, hypertrophic cardiomyopathy, Brugada syndrome, arrhythmogenic right ventricular dysplasia, or
- Successful surgical repair of congenital heart disease, or
- NYHA class I, II, or III symptoms with LVEF of $\leq 35\%$, irrespective of QRS duration.

Specialist assessment should be undertaken in order to make an evidence-based decision with regards device implantation and the CR team should consider referral to a cardiologist for repeat assessment in the event of a deterioration in clinical condition or a broadening of QRS complex on the ECG (with or without the development of [LBBB]).

7.14   SPECIFIC ISSUES FOR PATIENTS WITH DEVICES

7.14.1   Psychological

The incidence of psychological disorders for cardiac device patients is similar to that found in general cardiac populations and, as such, the usual approaches and interventions to manage adjustment, low mood, issues of loss, and strategies to help with coping are all applicable and relevant for device patients. However, ICD patients have been shown to also have specific ICD-related concerns such as fear of shock (and associated avoidance of activities believed to precipitate shock), fear of device malfunction and death. Various theoretical perspectives have been posited to help explain the occurrence of psychological symptoms post-implantation but easily the main focus for CR teams should be the presence of anxiety. ICD patients have been shown to be at increased risk of anxiety disorders (Pedersen et al. 2005) and, in turn, anxiety has been identified as a precipitant of ventricular arrhythmias. Anxiety may be related to concerns about the ICD firing, undertaking activity or exercise with an ICD, or any other aspect of living with an implanted cardiac device. Patients' concerns should be explored by the CR team and screening tools such as the ICD Patient Concerns Questionnaire may identify patients at risk for psychological morbidity.

7.14.2 Activity/Exercise

ICD shocks to terminate the arrhythmia are associated with reduced quality of life and increased mortality (Isaksen et al. 2012). Over half the recipients of a shock have reported an impact on subsequent avoidance behaviour, most commonly avoidance of exercise/physical activity (37%), but also included avoidance of specific objects (27%) and places (17%), which were least avoided. Such avoidance behaviour can have a devastating effect on quality of life as well as the physical health of some patients. A brief educational intervention or regular participation in ICD support groups is recommended to help dispel misinformation amongst patients and discourage inappropriate avoidance (Lemon et al. 2004). The important point, in terms of CR, is that prescribed exercise in most patients is well below the intensities associated with exercise-induced arrhythmias. Manchester Heart Centre exercise testing data (Doherty and Breen 2009) showed the average METs associated with exercise-induced arrhythmias was 9.4, which is higher than most prescribed intensity levels in CR programmes. Furthermore, evidence is emerging to demonstrate that patients with systolic heart failure are at no greater risk of shocks when exercise training (Davies et al. 2010). Both of these factors should increase practitioners' confidence in exercising this population group. In addition to the usual CR assessment process the following points should also be considered prior to prescribing exercise:

- Evaluation of current cardiac status which may vary from structural disease with a poor LVEF to patients with electrical cardiac disease who may have normal cardiac function.
- Knowledge of the ICD parameters:
  - ICD detection threshold setting in bpm
  - Whether the device is set for ventricular tachycardia (VT) or ventricular fibrillation (VF)
  - Rapid onset setting
  - Sustained ventricular tachycardia settings
  - ICD therapy, e.g. anti-tachycardia pacing or shocks.

- Knowledge of electrophysiology referral team contact details and communication links for the follow-up of missing referral information and to discuss any concerns.
- Knowledge of prior shock history.
- Knowledge of the relationship between the ICD and exercise training thresholds. To establish this, a submaximal functional capacity test is an essential element of the assessment process.

90% of patients will have assigned a cause to a shock (Sears et al. 2001) leading to avoidance behaviour. If a shock has been previously experienced on physical exertion this may be a barrier to exercise (Isaksen et al. 2012).

To reduce the risk of inappropriate therapy or the provocation of an arrhythmia, the exercise prescription should follow the recommended Association of Chartered Physiotherapists in Cardiac Rehabilitation (ACPICR) standards (ACPICR 2009) for structured exercise training in conjunction with a number of other considerations, including:

- Keep the exercise HR 10 bpm below ICD detection threshold using HR monitoring initially until effective use of RPE has been established.
- Keep horizontal and seated arm exercises to a minimum. Seated arm exercise is associated with reduced venous return, reduced end-diastolic volume, a concomitant decrease in cardiac output and increased likelihood of arrhythmia. If performed, the intensity should be lowered with emphasis on muscular endurance. Mild leg exercise, for example alternate heel raises, should be combined with arm exercise to reduce the haemodynamic response.
- Avoid breath hold and sustained isometric work which are associated with reduced venous return, reduced end-diastolic volume, a concomitant decrease in cardiac output and increased likelihood of arrhythmia. Isometric work, particularly of the abdominal region, should be avoided especially during arm exercise in patients with low functional capacity.
- Use Karvonen formula to set the target exercise intensity and reduce the exercise intensity initially to the lower end of moderate. The use of 75% MHR, in patients with slow ventricular tachycardia, will often mean that the target exercise HR is above the detection threshold of the ICD.
- Begin exercise training a minimum of six weeks post-device implantation to ensure lead integrity.
- Avoid extreme ipsilateral arm movements and/or highly repetitive vigorous shoulder movements which could cause lead rupture or dislocation.

7.14.3   What to Do in the Event of a Shock

It is important to have a protocol so that staff are aware of procedures to follow should a patient experience a shock during an exercise session:

1. Sit or lie the patient down.
2. If the patient recovers quickly and feels well after a shock they can continue to exercise, however, the patient should inform the follow-up centre as the device will need to be interrogated to check the appropriateness of the shock, following which medication and/or device settings may be altered.
3. If the patient is feeling unwell after a shock or more than one shock is delivered, an ambulance (999) should be called.
4. Exercise should be started again swiftly after the device has been interrogated to avoid the ICD discharge becoming a psychological block on future activity (Isaksen et al. 2012; Sears et al. 2001).

Appropriate regular physical activity should be encouraged in patients with an ICD, as this improves parasympathetic tone and HR variability, thereby reducing arrhythmia risk (Belardinelli 2003; Pigozzi et al. 2004). Some patients may wish to undertake certain, specific sporting endeavours and whilst in general this should be encouraged, there a number of factors worthy of consideration when formulating specific advice. Finally, it should be remembered that the ICD is designed to provide immediate emergency treatment rather than constricting activity due to fear of activity provoking an arrhythmia.

> **Key Message**
> Implantable device therapies may improve survival and improve symptoms in appropriately selected patients. Patient anxiety and avoidance behaviour, particularly of physical activity, may impair quality of life and must be assessed by the CR team and appropriate interventions offered. Structured exercise programmes are of benefit and ACPICR standards should be followed.

7.15   CARDIOPROTECTIVE THERAPIES AND OTHER LONG-TERM CONDITIONS

The national CVD outcomes strategy recommends a structured, integrated approach to the management of CVD, which should incorporate diabetes mellitus, chronic renal disease, and stroke. In addition, patients with established hypertension, hypercholesterolaemia, and impaired glucose tolerance may also be at increased risk for developing non-fatal and fatal CVD events. Therefore, all patients with these long-term conditions should be considered for cardio-protective therapies in line with national and international guidelines, bearing in mind that many patients will have a number of overlapping CVD conditions and potentially modifiable risk factors. The complex nature of such multi-morbidity invariably results in a lengthy list of prescribed drugs thus impacting on the challenge of long-term adherence. Patients must be centrally involved in the decision-making process and be fully informed of the rationale to introduce any new cardioprotective agent. They should be provided with sufficient opportunity to discuss side-effects, consider adjustments to dose or prescribed preparation, and report concerns about any aspect of their medical therapy. It is likely that, over time, effective CR programmes will become increasingly involved in the management of most patients with either established vascular disease or clusters of modifiable risk factors.

7.16   MEDICAL MANAGEMENT IN ERECTILE DYSFUNCTION

As discussed in Chapter 6, erectile dysfunction (ED) is a common issue in patients with CVD due to a commonality of risk factors (age, dyslipidaemia, hypertension, smoking, obesity, diabetes, and depression). Whilst the most common form of ED in CVD is physical ED, psychogenic ED can also contribute (the psychological 'hit' from a cardiovascular event resulting in anxiety, depression, or fear of sexual intercourse) and there can be substantial overlap. Figure 7.3 illustrates how to distinguish between physical and psychogenic ED and their common causes. The medications used to treat CVD can also impact. Therefore the management of ED in the cardiovascular patient can be challenging and is probably best done through a collaborative approach including involvement of the primary care physician, urologist, psychologist, etc.

7.16.1   Assessment of ED in the CVD Patient

Much of the assessment for ED overlaps with the assessment of the CVD patient in the CR setting, making it the ideal place to try and coordinate its management. The ED assessment should include smoking history, alcohol consumption,

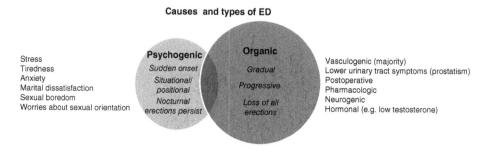

FIGURE 7.3   Causes and types of erectile dysfunction.

measurement of anthropometrics (e.g. central obesity), screening for diabetes, review of medications, and assessment of psychological health. Measurement of serum testosterone is also recommended and could be done through the primary care practitioner. Similarly, if the patient has significant lower urinary tracts symptoms (prostatism) the primary care physician can be alerted. It is helpful to use a validated questionnaire such as the 5-item Sexual Health Inventory for Men/International Index Erectile Function-5 (Table 7.7). Responses to the five questions range from 1 (worst) to 5 (best). Questions 2 to 4 may be graded 0 (if there is no sexual activity, or no sexual intercourse attempt) and the final score ranges from 1 to 25 points; a descending score indicates worsening of erectile function, with values ≤ 21 being diagnostic of ED (Vlachopoulos et al. 2013).

7.16.2 Cardiovascular Medications and ED

There is a lot of disinformation (e.g. social media, internet) regarding the impact of cardiovascular medications on erectile function, which in turn can affect adherence. The ASCOT data clearly demonstrated that if anything statins improve erectile function, which is not surprising as statins improve endothelial function, which is crucial for erectile health. The only cardiovascular medications clearly implicated are the thiazide and thiazide-like diuretics, and also spironolactone. Some of the older beta-blockers may also have a negative effect but the vasodilating nebivolol can actually improve erectile function. ACE-inhibitors, angiotensin-receptor blockers, and calcium channel blockers are reported to have neutral or even a positive effect on erectile function.

7.16.3 Sexual Activity and Cardiovascular Risk

After a cardiovascular event patients often have concern about resumption of sexual activity and counselling in this regard is an essential part of CR. Patients should be reassured that conventional sexual activity is typically regarded as mild-to-moderate physical activity in the range of three to four metabolic equivalents (METs). This is equivalent to walking 1 mile on the flat in 20 minutes or briskly climbing two flights of stairs.

7.16.4 Pharmacotherapies in the Management of Erectile Dysfunction

Lifestyle changes can help improve erectile function – namely weight loss, increasing physical activity, smoking cessation, and reduction in alcohol consumption (if the baseline consumption levels are above the recommended level) (Gupta et al. 2011). These should always be recommended as first line.

With regards to medical therapy, phosphodiesterase-5 (PDE5) inhibitors have transformed the management of erectile dysfunction and are the mainstay

TABLE 7.7 The sexual health inventory for men (SHIM) or IIEF-5 over the past six months.

1. How did you rate your confidence that you could get and keep an erection?		Very low 1	Low 2	Moderate 3	High 4	Very high 5
2. When you had erections with sexual stimulation, how often were your erections hard enough for penetration?	No sexual activity 0	Almost never or never 1	A few times 2	Sometimes 3	Most times 4	Almost always or always 5
3. During sexual intercourse, how often were you able to maintain your erection after you have penetrated your partner?	Did not attempt intercourse 0	Almost never or never 1	A few times 2	Sometimes 3	Most times 4	Almost always or always 5
4. During sexual intercourse, how difficult was it to maintain your erection to completion of intercourse?	Did not attempt intercourse 0	Extremely difficult 1	Very difficult 2	Difficult 3	Slightly difficult 4	Not difficult 5
5. When you attempted sexual intercourse, how often was it satisfactory to you?	Did not attempt intercourse 0	Almost never or never 1	A few times 2	Sometimes 3	Most times 4	Almost always or always 5

The IIEF-5 is administered as a screening instrument for the presence and severity of ED in conjunction with clinical assessment. The score is the sum of the response to the five items, so that the overall score may range from 1 to 25: no ED (total score, 22–25), mild (17–21), mild to moderate (12–16), moderate (8–11), and severe ED (1–7).

TABLE 7.8   The four commonly used PDE-5 inhibitors.

	Dose (initial and maximum)	Peak absorption post ingestion	Half-life	Take on empty stomach
Sildenafil	50–100 mg	1–2 h	3–5 h	Yes
Vardenafil	10–20 mg	1–2 h	3–5 h	Yes
Tadalafil	10–20 mg	2–4 h	12 h	No
Avanafil	50–200 mg	0.5 h	6 h	No

of treatment. Mechanistically, these drugs competitively inhibit PDE5, leading to a build-up of cyclic GMP (cGMP) upon nitric oxide (NO) release, initiating a cascade of events that lead to smooth muscle relaxation and promotion of an erection. There are four principal PDE5 inhibitors that have varying pharmaco-kinetics, which is important to be aware of (Table 7.8).

The medications must be ingested with adequate time to allow peak absorption of the drug before sexual intercourse. Sildenafil and vardenafil should be taken on an empty stomach because lipids in foods can decrease and delay absorption. Tadalafil and avanafil are not as strongly affected by food. It is generally recommended starting with the initiating dose and uptitrating to maximum dose. If one PDE5 inhibitor is not effective it is worth trialling the others. Tadalafil has an extremely long half-life and it is also an option to take this as a once daily dose (2.5–5 mg), much like the patient would take their statin. This removes the need for planning sexual activity and many couples prefer this approach as it allows more spontaneity. Success rates with PDE5 inhibitors are in the range 60–65% although this will be lower in certain populations (particularly if neurogenic in origin). Of note is if a patient is deficient in testosterone the efficacy of PDE5 inhibitors is improved with simultaneous testosterone hormone replacement.

Patients do need to be counselled regarding side-effects, which may include headache, dyspepsia, facial flushing, nasal congestion, and visual disturbances. Myalgia (muscle pain) is more common with tadalafil than the other PDE5 inhibitors.

Also, PDE5 inhibitors and α-adrenergic receptor blockers, often used for treatment of BPH, need to be taken at least four hours apart. It does appear, however, that combined use of PDE5 inhibitors and alpha-blockers results in additive favourable effects in men with erectile dysfunction and lower urinary tract symptoms suggestive of benign prostatic hyperplasia compared with PDE5 inhibitor monotherapy.

Sexual stimulation, both physical and mental, is still necessary to create arousal and initially raise the available levels of NO in an effort to generate cGMP production. Priapism (erection lasting >4 hours) is rare and occurs in less than 0.1% of users.

The use of PDE5 inhibitors in patients with CVD can often be of concern to primary care physicians but their safety in this population has been well demonstrated. There is no evidence of an increased risk of a cardiovascular event and they do not result in hypotension unless used with nitrate-containing medications, which include oral nitrates, GTN patches, GTN spray, or amyl nitrate (or 'poppers', which may be used in homosexual activity). Thus use of nitrates with PDE5 inhibitors is absolutely contraindicated in this regard.

Second-line therapies consist of an intra-urethral suppository (IUS) of prostaglandin E1 (alprostadil) and intracavernosal injection (ICI) with vasoactive substances. These therapies should be delivered under the remit of a specialist ED team (typically urology) and referral should be considered if PDE5 inhibitors are not effective. Surgical intervention is reserved as the final option after conservative options have been discussed or attempted (Yafi et al. 2016).

7.17 CONCLUSION

Medical risk management, which includes medical risk factor assessment/treatment and the introduction/adjustment of cardioprotective therapies, is very important for reducing the likelihood of future cardiovascular events as well as improving quality and (for certain patients and therapies) quantity of life. Therefore, the management of blood pressure, lipids, glycaemia, cardio-protective drugs, and complex devices forms an integral component of all modern, effective, evidence-based CPRP. The programme provides the ideal setting within which medical risk can be actively managed to achieve an optimum risk profile for each individual. This should be the responsibility of the CPRP nurse/independent prescriber but working in collaboration not just with the MDT but also the cardiologist, the patient's primary care practitioner, and other specialist services. The classes of medication that should be considered, the desired levels of dosing (to achieve either target values or to achieve maximum prognostic benefit), and the indications for implantable devices are all embedded within comprehensive local, national, and international guidelines, and are supported by a huge body of published clinical data. Despite this, however, patients with CVD are frequently exposed to excessive risk of future adverse cardiovascular events as a direct result of deficiencies in prescribed medication and/or a lack of specialist assessment. Cardiovascular rehabilitation programmes, delivered by a dedicated mix of healthcare professionals, are the perfect structures through which to ensure that patients with CVD are optimally managed. By virtue of this continuity of care and thus the close relationship that often develops between CR personnel and their patients, CR is uniquely placed to support patients with their sustained adherence to any of the recommended interventions to facilitate medical risk management.

REFERENCES

ACPICR (2009). ACPICR standards for physical activity and exercise in the cardiac population. Association of Chartered Physiotherapists in Cardiac Rehabilitation.

AIRE (1993). Effect of ramipril on mortality and morbidity of survivors of acute myocardial infarction with clinical evidence of heart failure. The Acute Infarction Ramipril Efficacy (AIRE) Study Investigators. *Lancet* 342: 821–828.

Armitage, J. (2007). The safety of statins in clinical practice. *Lancet* 370 (9601): 1781–1790.

Bartnik, M., Ryden, L., Ferrari, R. et al. (2004). The prevalence of abnormal glucose regulation in patients with coronary artery disease across Europe. The European heart survey on diabetes and the heart. *European Heart Journal* 25 (21): 1880–1890.

Belardinelli, R. (2003). Arrhythmias during acute and chronic exercise in chronic heart failure. *International Journal of Cardiology* 90 (2–3): 213–218.

Boekholdt, S.M., Arsenault, B.J., Mora, S. et al. (2012). Association of LDL cholesterol, non-HDL cholesterol, and apolipoprotein B levels with risk of cardiovascular events among patients treated with statins: a meta-analysis. *Journal of the American Medical Association* 307 (12): 1302–1309.

British Cardiac Society BHS/DU/HU/PCCST/SA (2005). 'JBS 2: joint British Societies' guidelines on prevention of cardiovascular disease in clinical practice. *Heart* 91 (suppl 5): v1–v52.

Buckley, J.P., Furze, G., Doherty, P. et al. (2013). BACPR scientific statement: British standards and core components for cardiovascular disease prevention and rehabilitation. *Heart* 99 (15): 1069–1071.

Camm, A.J., Lip, G.Y., De Caterina, R. et al. (2012). 2012 focused update of the ESC Guidelines for the management of atrial fibrillation: an update of the 2010 ESC Guidelines for the management of atrial fibrillation. Developed with the special contribution of the European Heart Rhythm Association. *European Heart Journal* 33 (21): 2719–2747.

Cannon, C.P., Blazing, M.A., Giugliano, R.P. et al. (2015). Ezetimibe added to statin therapy after acute coronary syndromes. *The New England Journal of Medicine* 372: 2387–2397.

Cannon, C.P., Giugliano, R.P., Blazing, M.A. et al. (2008). Rationale and design of IMPROVE-IT (IMProved Reduction of Outcomes: Vytorin Efficacy International Trial): comparison of ezetimibe/simvastatin versus simvastatin monotherapy on cardiovascular outcomes in patients with acute coronary syndromes. *American Heart Journal* 156 (5): 826–832.

Chatterjee, S., Moeller, C., Shah, N. et al. (2012). Eplerenone is not superior to older and less expensive aldosterone antagonists. *The American Journal of Medicine* 125 (8): 817–825.

Cholesterol Treatment Trialists' (CTT) Collaboration, Baigent, C., Blackwell, L. et al. (2010). Efficacy and safety of more intensive lowering of LDL cholesterol: a meta-analysis of data from 170,000 participants in 26 randomised trials. *Lancet* 376 (9753): 1670–1681.

Clark, A.M., Hartling, L., Vandermeer, B., and McAlister, F.A. (2005). Meta-analysis: secondary prevention programs for patients with coronary artery disease. *Annals of Internal Medicine* 143 (9): 659–672.

Cooper, A. and O'Flynn, N. (2008). Risk assessment and lipid modification for primary and secondary prevention of cardiovascular disease: summary of NICE guidance. *British Medical Journal* 336 (7655): 1246–1248.

Cuisset, T., Mudra, H., Muller, O. et al. (2008). Rationale and use of antiplatelet and antithrombotic drugs during cardiovascular interventions. *EuroIntervention* 4 (2): 183–186.

Davies, E.J., Moxham, T., Rees, K. et al. (2010). Exercise training for systolic heart failure: Cochrane systematic review and meta-analysis. *European Heart Journal* 12 (7): 706–715.

Dicpinigaitis, P.V. (2006). Angiotensin-converting enzyme inhibitor-induced cough: ACCP evidence-based clinical practice guidelines. *Chest* 129 (1 Suppl): 169S–173S.

Doherty, P.J. and Breen, S. (2009). Arrhythmia and Implanted Cardioverter Defibrillators. In: *Cardiac rehabilitation: exercise leadership for high risk groups*. Chichester: Wiley & Sons.

Emerging Risk Factors Collaboration, Sarwar, N., Gao, P. et al. (2010). Diabetes mellitus, fasting blood glucose concentration, and risk of vascular disease: a collaborative meta-analysis of 102 prospective studies. *Lancet* 375 (9733): 2215–2222.

Farless, L.B., Steil, N., Williams, B.R., and Bailey, F.A. (2012). Intermittent subcutaneous furosemide: parenteral diuretic rescue for hospice patients with congestive heart failure resistant to oral diuretic. *American Journal of Hospice & Palliative Medicine* 30 (8): 791–792.

Fiuzat, M., Wojdyla, D., Kitzman, D. et al. (2012). Relationship of beta-blocker dose with outcomes in ambulatory heart failure patients with systolic dysfunction: results from the HF-ACTION (Heart Failure: A Controlled Trial Investigating Outcomes of Exercise Training) trial. *Journal of the American College of Cardiology* 60 (3): 208–215.

Flather, M.D., Yusuf, S., Køber, L. et al. (2000). Long-term ACE-inhibitor therapy in patients with heart failure or left-ventricular dysfunction: a systematic overview of data from individual patients. ACE-Inhibitor Myocardial Infarction Collaborative Group. *Lancet* 355 (9215): 1575–1581.

Friedewald, W.T., Levy, R.I., and Fredrickson, D.S. (1972). Estimation of the concentration of low-density lipoprotein cholesterol in plasma, without use of the preparative ultracentrifuge. *Clinical Chemistry* 18 (6): 499–502.

Fyfe, T., Baxter, R.H., Cochran, K.M., and Booth, E.M. (1971). Plasma-lipid changes after myocardial infarction. *Lancet* 2 (7732): 997–1001.

Giugliano, R.P., Ruff, C.T., Braunwald, E. et al. (2013). Edoxaban versus warfarin in patients with atrial fibrillation. *The New England Journal of Medicine* 369 (22): 2093–2104.

Goldberger, J.J., Bonow, R.O., Cuffe, M. et al. (2010). Beta-blocker use following myocardial infarction: low prevalence of evidence-based dosing. *American Heart Journal* 160 (3): 435–442. e1.

Gupta, B.P., Murad, M.H., Clifton, M.M. et al. (2011). The effect of lifestyle modification and cardiovascular risk factor reduction on erectile dysfunction: a systematic review and meta-analysis. In: Database of Abstracts of Reviews of Effects (DARE): Quality-assessed Reviews [Internet]. York (UK): Centre for Reviews and Dissemination (UK). NCBI. https://www.ncbi.nlm.nih.gov/books/NBK81474.

Haynes, R., Jiang, L., Hopewell, J.C. et al. (2013). HPS2-THRIVE randomized placebo-controlled trial in 25 673 high-risk patients of ER niacin/laropiprant: trial design, pre-specified muscle and liver outcomes, and reasons for stopping study treatment. *European Heart Journal* 34 (17): 1279–1291.

Holman, R.R., Paul, S.K., Bethel, M.A. et al. (2008). 10-year follow-up of intensive glucose control in type 2 diabetes. *New England Journal of Medicine* 359 (15): 1577–1589.

Home, P., Mant, J., Diaz, J., and Turner, C. (2008). Management of type 2 diabetes: summary of updated NICE guidance. *British Medical Journal* 336 (7656): 1306–1308.

Isaksen, K., Morken, I.M., Munk, P.S., and Larsen, A.I. (2012). Exercise training and cardiac rehabilitation in patients with implantable cardioverter defibrillators: a review of current literature focusing on safety, effects of exercise training, and the psychological impact of programme participation. *European Journal of Preventive Cardiology* 19: 804–812.

JBS3 Board (2014). Joint British Societies' consensus recommendations for the prevention of cardiovascular disease (JBS3). *Heart* 100: ii1–ii1167. https://doi.org/10.1136/heartjnl-2014-305693.

Jun, M., Foote, C., Lv, J. et al. (2010). Effects of fibrates on cardiovascular outcomes: a systematic review and meta-analysis. *Lancet* 375 (9729): 1875–1884.

Krause, T., Lovibond, K., Caulfield, M. et al. (2011). Management of hypertension: summary of NICE guidance. *British Medical Journal* 343: d4891.

Law, M.R., Wald, N.J., Morris, J.K., and Jordan, R.E. (2003). Value of low dose combination treatment with blood pressure lowering drugs: analysis of 354 randomised trials. *British Medical Journal* 326 (7404): 1427.

Lazar, L.D. and Lincoff, A.M. (2009). Prasugrel for acute coronary syndromes: faster, more potent, but higher bleeding risk. *Cleveland Clinic Journal of Medicine* 76 (12): 707–714.

Lemon, J., Edelman, S., and Kirkness, A. (2004). Avoidance behaviors in patients with implantable cardioverter defibrillators. *Heart & Lung* 33 (3): 176–182.

Livingstone, S.J., Looker, H.C., Hothersall, E.J. et al. (2012). Risk of cardiovascular disease and total mortality in adults with type 1 diabetes: Scottish registry linkage study. *Public Library of Science - Medicine* 9 (10): e1001321. doi: 10.1371/journal.pmed.1001321.

Mancia, G., Fagard, R., Narkiewicz, K. et al. (2013). 2013 ESH/ESC guidelines for the management of arterial hypertension: the task force for the Management of Arterial Hypertension of the European Society of Hypertension (ESH) and of the European Society of Cardiology (ESC). *European Heart Journal* 34 (28): 2159–2219.

Nathan, D.M., Cleary, P.A., Backlund, J.Y. et al. (2005). Intensive diabetes treatment and cardiovascular disease in patients with type 1 diabetes. *New England Journal of Medicine* 353 (25): 2643–2653.

NICE (2004). Dyspepsia - management of dyspepsia in adults in primary care. NICE Clinical Guideline 17. National Institute for Health and Care Excellence.

NICE (2010a). Chronic heart failure: Management of chronic heart failure in adults in primary and secondary care. NICE Clinical Guideline 108. National Institute for Health and Care Excellence.

NICE (2010b). Unstable angina and NSTEMI - the early management of unstable angina and non-ST-segment-elevation myocardial infarction. NICE Clinical Guideline 94. National Institute for Health and Care Excellence.

NICE (2011). Ticagrelor for the treatment of acute coronary syndromes. NICE Technology Appraisal 236. National Institute for Health and Care Excellence.

NICE (2012). Acute upper gastrointestinal bleeding. NICE Clinical Guideline 141. National Institute for Health and Care Excellence.

NICE (2013). MI - secondary prevention. NICE Clinical Guideline 172. National Institute for Health and Care Excellence.

NICE (2014a). Cardiovascular disease: risk assessment and reduction, including lipid modification. NICE Clinical Guideline 181. National Institute for Health and Care Excellence.

NICE (2016). Alirocumab for treating primary hypercholesterolaemia and mixed dyslipidaemia. NICE Technology Appraisal Guidance 393. National Institute for Health and Care Excellence.

NICE (2016). Evolocumab for treating primary hypercholesterolaemia and mixed dyslipidaemia. NICE Technology Appraisal Guidance 394. National Institute for Health and Care Excellence.

NICE (2014b). Implantable cardioverter defibrillators and cardiac resynchronisation therapy for arrhythmias and heart failure. NICE Technology Appraisal 314. National Institute for Health and Care Excellence.

Nichols, M., Townsend, N., Scarborough, P., and Rayner, M. (2012). European Cardiovascular Disease Statistics 2012. European Society of Cardiology.

O'Brien, E., Asmar, R., Beilin, L. et al. (2003). European Society of Hypertension recommendations for conventional, ambulatory and home blood pressure measurement. *Journal of Hypertension* 21 (5): 821–848.

Pedersen, S.S., van Domburg, R.T., Theuns, D.A. et al. (2005). Concerns about the implantable cardioverter defibrillator: a determinant of anxiety and depressive symptoms independent of experienced shocks. *American Heart Journal* 149 (4): 664–669.

Pigozzi, F., Alabiso, A., Parisi, A. et al. (2004). Vigorous exercise training is not associated with prevalence of ventricular arrhythmias in elderly athletes. *The Journal of Sports Medicine and Physical Fitness* 44 (1): 92–97.

Pitt, B., Remme, W., Zannad, F. et al. (2003). Eplerenone, a selective aldosterone blocker, in patients with left ventricular dysfunction after myocardial infarction. *The New England Journal of Medicine* 348: 1309–1321. https://doi.org/10.1056/NEJMoa030207.

Pitt, B., Zannad, F., Remme, W.J. et al. (1999). The effect of spironolactone on morbidity and mortality in patients with severe heart failure. Randomized Aldactone evaluation study investigators. *The New England Journal of Medicine* 341 (10): 709–717.

Ray, K.K., Seshasai, S.R., Wijesuriya, S. et al. (2009). Effect of intensive control of glucose on cardiovascular outcomes and death in patients with diabetes mellitus: a meta-analysis of randomised controlled trials. *Lancet* 373 (9677): 1765–1772.

Sabatine, M.S., Giugliano, R.P., Keech, A.C. et al. (2017). For the FOURIER Steering Committee and Investigators. *New England Journal of Medicine* 376: 1713–1722. doi: 10.1056/NEJMoa1615664.

Saha, S.A., Kizhakepunnur, L.G., Bahekar, A., and Arora, R.R. (2007). The role of fibrates in the prevention of cardiovascular disease – a pooled meta-analysis of long-term randomized placebo-controlled clinical trials. *American Heart Journal* 154 (5): 943–953.

Sears, S.F. Jr., Rauch, S., Handberg, E., and Conti, J.B. (2001). Fear of exertion following ICD storm: considering ICD shock and learning history. *Journal of Cardiopulmonary Rehabilitation* 21 (1): 47–49.

Short, P.M., Lipworth, S.I., Elder, D.H. et al. (2011). Effect of beta blockers in treatment of chronic obstructive pulmonary disease: a retrospective cohort study. *British Medical Journal* 342: d2549. https://doi.org/10.1136/bmj.d2549.

SIGN (2007). Management of chronic heart failure. SIGN Clinical Guideline 95. Scottish Intercollegiate Guidelines Network.

Storey, R.F., Becker, R.C., Harrington, R.A. et al. (2011). Characterization of dyspnoea in PLATO study patients treated with ticagrelor or clopidogrel and its association with clinical outcomes. *European Heart Journal* 32 (23): 2945–2953.

The AIM-HIGH Investigators (2011). Niacin in patients with low HDL cholesterol levels receiving intensive statin therapy. *New England Journal of Medicine* 365: 2255–2267.

The Diabetes Control and Complications Trial Research Group (1993). The effect of intensive treatment of diabetes on the development and progression of long-term complications in insulin-dependent diabetes mellitus. *New England Journal of Medicine* 329 (14): 977–986.

Turnbull, F.M., Abraira, C., Anderson, R.J. et al. (2009). Intensive glucose control and macrovascular outcomes in type 2 diabetes. *Diabetologia* 52 (11): 2288–2298.

UK Prospective Diabetes Study (UKPDS) Group (1998). Intensive blood-glucose control with sulphonylureas or insulin compared with conventional treatment and risk of complications in patients with type 2 diabetes (UKPDS 33). *Lancet* 352 (9131): 837–853.

Unal, B., Critchley, J.A., and Capewell, S. (2004). Explaining the decline in coronary heart disease mortality in England and Wales between 1981 and 2000. *Circulation* 109 (9): 1101–1107.

Vlachopoulos, C., Jackson, G., Stefanadis, C., and Montorsi, P. (2013). Erectile dysfunction in the cardiovascular patient. *European Heart Journal* 34 (27): 2034–2046. https://doi.org/10.1093/eurheartj/eht112.

Wallentin, L., Becker, R.C., Budaj, A. et al. (2009). Ticagrelor versus clopidogrel in patients with acute coronary syndromes. *The New England Journal of Medicine* 361: 1045–1057.

Wiviott, S.D., Braunwald, E., McCabe, C.H. et al. (2007). Prasugrel versus clopidogrel in patients with acute coronary syndromes. *The New England Journal of Medicine* 357: 2001–2015. https://doi.org/10.1056/NEJMoa0706482.

World Health Organization (2011). Use of glycated haemoglobin (HbA1c) in the diagnosis of diabetes mellitus. World Health Organization.

Yafi, F.A., Jenkins, L., Albersen, M. et al. (2016). Erectile dysfunction. *Nature Reviews. Disease Primers* 2 (16003): 2016.

Yusuf, S., Sleight, P., Pogue, J. et al. (2000). Effects of an angiotensin-converting-enzyme inhibitor, ramipril, on cardiovascular events in high-risk patients. The Heart Outcomes Prevention Evaluation Study Investigators. *The New England Journal of Medicine* 342 (3): 145–153.

CHAPTER 8

Long-term Management

Sally Hinton[1], Ann Marie Johnson[2], and Gail Sheppard[3]

[1] BACPR, London, UK
[2] Leeds Partnerships Clinical Commissioning, Leeds, UK
[3] Canterbury Christ Church University, Canterbury, UK

Abstract

The purpose of this chapter is to consider long-term strategies for the management of the cardiovascular patient, which is a core component of the BACPR Standards and Core Components. On completion of a cardio-vascular prevention and rehabilitation programme (CPRP) there should be a formal final assessment of the core components (as detailed within earlier chapters) together with agreement of long-term management goals. Patients will have been empowered and prepared to take ownership of their own responsibility to pursue a healthy lifestyle. Carers, spouses, and family should also be equipped to contribute to long-term adherence by helping and encouraging the individual to achieve their goals. This information should be communicated to the referrer, the patient and family, and those directly involved in the continuation of healthcare provision, ensuring seamless transition of care of the individual.

Keywords: *long-term strategies and management, lifestyle behaviour change, primary care, care planning, self-monitoring, heart support group*

Cardiovascular Prevention and Rehabilitation in Practice, Second Edition.
Edited by Jennifer Jones, John Buckley, Gill Furze, and Gail Sheppard.
© 2020 John Wiley & Sons Ltd. Published 2020 by John Wiley & Sons Ltd.

Key Points

- Primary care systems play a key role in delivering long-term management support for people with cardiovascular disease (CVD). The differing systems across the nations of the United Kingdom are described.
- It is important to consider long-term behaviour change and long-term management of risk factors for people with CVD. Recommendations are made in relation to long-term management of physical activity, smoking cessation, and diet and weight management.
- Methods of self-monitoring are highlighted that can support long-term progress in health behaviour change.
- The contribution that heart support groups (HSGs) make to long-term management is discussed.

8.1   RATIONALE AND AIMS

Although mortality rates due to CVD have decreased in recent years, owing to improved interventions (both clinical and non-clinical), morbidity rates have increased. The fact remains that initial survival also implies future risk. The outcome of this is that more people are living with, and managing, CVD. Providing strategies for the long-term management and care of those diagnosed with CVD, as part of a continuum of care and support, is vital in secondary prevention. The desired goal of long-term management is long-term survival and optimal uptake of healthy lifestyle behaviours. The role of the healthcare professional in this process is to provide support and highlight opportunities for the patient to access evidence-based advice, supplementary services (physical activity and exercise sessions, smoking cessation, and diet and weight management options), and to refer on, when necessary, to appropriate primary and secondary care. The aim of this chapter is to emphasise current options available within long-term management and to increase awareness of the various elements of care along the CVD management continuum.

8.2   PRIMARY CARE SERVICES

The long-term care of an individual with CVD on completion of their cardiovascular prevention and rehabilitation programme (CPRP) will be continued in the community. The information from the final cardiovascular assessment will ideally be electronically transferred into the individual's clinical record, and made available for the primary care healthcare team who will continue to support the individual.

The primary healthcare team consists of general practitioners, nurses, practice managers, allied health professionals, healthcare assistants, and the reception team. Primary care has been managing long-term conditions for many years and, through the necessity of improving efficiencies and sometimes despite a lack of resources, many primary care teams have developed long-term condition clinics in practice that deliver holistic, patient-centred care.

Structured care for patients with long-term conditions (CVD, diabetes, and respiratory disease) in primary care began formally in the 1990s with the general practice contract, which promoted registers, protocols, and regular follow-up.

The delivery of cardiac rehabilitation services currently remains outside the scope of primary care teams in the majority of GP practices, and the services that are delivered now in primary care are varied across the UK and are outlined below.

8.2.1 England

In 2016 NHS England published the 'General Practice Forward View', which proposed that electronic transmission of clinic letters be available within 24 hours of discharge (NHS England 2016) and outlined the Multispecialty Community Provider (MCP) contract, which aims to create a new clinical business model for the integrated provision of primary and community services, based on the GP registered list. The MCP contract aims to fully integrate a wider range of services and include relevant specialists wherever required irrespective of current institutional arrangements, to improve patient outcomes and reduce hospital admissions.

This MCP contract is an example of a New Model of Care, and is an opportunity to develop an inclusive integrated cardiovascular prevention and rehabilitation model delivered using the principles of the Year of Care approach, which could result in a productive partnership between patients and clinicians. This approach can deliver more effective self-management, better coordinated care, and improved outcomes for people living with a long-term condition (Coulter et al. 2013). There are many people with diverse long-term conditions that would benefit from an 'integrated cardiovascular prevention and rehabilitation model', for example people with: peripheral arterial disease, stroke and transient ischaemic attack, coronary heart disease (including heart failure), diabetes, hypertension, and for primary prevention in those at high risk of developing one of these conditions (e.g. those with a cardiovascular risk >10% and non-diabetic hyperglycaemia).

8.2.2 Northern Ireland

Health and social care (HSC) in Northern Ireland are provided as an integrated service. There are a number of organisations who work together to plan, deliver, and monitor HSC across Northern Ireland.

The HSC Board is responsible for commissioning services, resource management, and performance management and service improvement. It works to identify and meet the needs of the Northern Ireland population through its five Local Commissioning Groups, which cover the same geographical areas as the HSC Trusts. These HSC Trusts manage and administer hospitals, health centres, residential homes, day centres and other HSC facilities and they provide a wide range of HSC services to the community.

8.2.3   Scotland

The Scottish Government's vision for the future of primary care services is for multidisciplinary teams, made up of a variety of health professionals, to work together to support people in the community and free up GPs to spend more time with patients in specific need of their expertise.

The Scottish Government is working to transform primary care in order to develop new ways of working that will help to put in place long-term, sustainable change within primary care services that can better meet changing needs and demands:

- Putting general practice and primary care at the heart of the healthcare system.
- Ensuring people who need care are more informed and empowered than ever, with access to the right person at the right time, and remaining at or near home wherever possible.
- Developing multidisciplinary teams in every locality, both in and out of hours, involved in the strategic planning and delivery of services.

8.2.4   Wales

Healthcare in Wales is delivered by seven Local Health Boards (LHBs) and each board has a primary care directorate. GP practices are grouped into clusters that have a small amount of funding to develop local services. These clusters in turn are grouped into localities that have a greater amount of administrative support and can develop some services on a bigger scale. For example, in Cardiff and Vale LHB there are three GP locality groups each of which consist of three GP clusters and each cluster consisting of between 50 000 and 100 000 patients.

8.2.5   Community Care for Integrated Services

The cardiovascular prevention and rehabilitation team working in partnership with the wider community, for example, self-help groups, walking groups, stop smoking, and weight management services, can, together with the individual at the centre, deliver an integrated service for patients with long-term conditions.

Care and support planning is an on-going, often annual process to take stock, look forward, identify personal needs and goals, discuss options, and agree and coordinate a plan for how these goals will be met (Eaton et al. 2015). The benefits of care and support planning can improve quality of life, give patients with long-term conditions better health and better well-being, and improve outcomes.

It is vital that services are integrated and seamless across the continuum of care, with the patient at the centre and taking an active part in their care.

8.3   LONG-TERM MANAGEMENT OF RISK FACTORS

The multidisciplinary team in the early rehabilitation programme aim to positively influence attitudes, beliefs, and social efficacy in order for individuals to be equipped with the necessary skills and support to sustain the desired behaviour change over the long term.

As discussed in Chapter 4, effective health behaviour change techniques include three major variables: intention to undertake behaviour, skills needed to perform the behaviour, and presence or absence of environmental variables, which are outlined in the Major Theorists' Model (from Conner and Norman 2007). It is important to help individuals to be able to identify and use strategies which are client-centred to prevent relapses and sustain the desired behaviour.

8.3.1   Physical Activity and Exercise

Following completion and the final reassessment at a comprehensive CPRP, an individual should be encouraged to continue to undertake regular physical activity and exercise as part of their secondary prevention plan. There will be individualised long-term goals set by the CPRP team and prior to discharge from a programme the patient should be:

- Clinically stable
- Able to safely monitor and regulate the intensity of their activity
- Able to recognise their optimum level of exercise intensity
- Demonstrate commitment to modifying risk-related behaviour.

A clear outline of the programme undertaken during the early CPRP needs to be given to the patient at the end of the programme in order for them to continue with this independently, and where appropriate attend community group exercise sessions. The details of the exercise programme including total cardio-vascular (CV) time achieved will be transferred from the early rehabilitation programme to instructors who are supervising the community sessions to allow smooth transition (see Chapter 5c).

Long-term supervised group exercise sessions are run in the community in a variety of venues, e.g. community centres, local authority leisure facilities, and private health clubs. It is vital that the instructor who supervises these sessions has the correct qualifications in line with the UK Register of Exercise Professionals (The Register of Exercise Professionals 2016) and Chartered Institute for the Management of Sport and Physical Activity (CIMSPA 2012) in order to prescribe and deliver effective exercise programmes. The latest Resuscitation Council (UK) guidelines regarding resuscitation training and facilities for supervised CPRPs should be adhered to for these supervised sessions (Resuscitation Council (UK) 2018). The British Association for Cardiovascular Prevention and Rehabilitation (BACPR) deliver the Level 4 Cardiac Exercise Instructor Training qualification, which is considered the UK's leading training programme for exercise professionals who wish to lead these community sessions (BACPR 2016).

For these group sessions there will be many factors to consider for service delivery. These include risk stratification, inclusion/exclusion criteria, record-keeping, temperature of room, procedure for management of medical emergencies and exit strategies.

Good practice would include having a checklist at the start of the session – see Table 8.1 for an example.

TABLE 8.1   Pre-exercise checklist.

Pre-exercise checklist
Before starting your exercise session please ensure that you have advised the person in charge if you have: • Any change in symptoms, e.g. new or worsening chest pain • Any change in medication • Any test results, e.g. blood pressure or cholesterol level • Any new or worsening joint problems, e.g. back or knee pain • Any general feelings of being unwell, e.g. fever, sore throat
During your exercise session please tell the person in charge if you experience: • Any angina, chest discomfort, or dizziness • Any joint problems • Any general feelings of being unwell
If you have been prescribed GTN, please bring it to the class even if you do not use it on a regular basis
Always exercise at a level that represents exertion without discomfort

The aims of long-term physical activity programmes include:

- Providing regular supervised exercise sessions
- Establishing individualised exercise prescription for additional independent physical activity
- Offer general advice and support in maintaining lifestyle changes associated with risk factor reduction
- Encourage independence, self-help, and self-motivation
- Review on a regular basis participants' progress (or regression) and to alter the prescription accordingly
- In the case of new symptoms or deterioration in functional capacity of unknown cause, refer back to the primary care team.

As primary care has overall responsibility for an individual's long-term health, the instructor should be in close liaison with the primary care team and have a good communication pathway.

A detailed home programme is important for all patients to achieve the frequency, intensity, time, and type (FITT) principle and improve long-term compliance to regular physical activity. It is important to advise and encourage a home exercise programme, as regular exercise/physical activity is a difficult behaviour to move into the maintenance phase and is affected by many varying factors, e.g. exercise beliefs, barriers, insufficient time, and lack of support network.

Regular exercise can be seen as time consuming and possibly costly and being active is rarely a permanent characteristic. Individuals should be taught that lapses are normal and encourage them to be positive about their ability to resume regular activity. The Stages of Change in Exercise Behaviour model (Marcus and Simkin 1993) takes into consideration the decisional balance where an individual looks at the benefits and costs if new behaviour is continued. On leaving a programme individuals are more likely to drop out when supervision is discontinued so an established home programme becomes vital.

When developing a home exercise programme, consider:

- Individual values and beliefs
- Barriers to becoming more physically active
- Providing information on the benefits of physical activity
- Rating of perceived exertion (RPE) and monitoring exercise intensity (see Chapter 5c)
- Setting realistic goals
- Past and present activity levels
- The use of home activity diaries
- Regular reviews and record-keeping.

The home exercise programme should be:

- Safe and effective
- Evidence-based
- Individualised
- Progressive.

Prescription for unsupervised/independent activities should consider what:

- Is affordable, enjoyable, accessible
- Is realistically achievable
- Complements the exercise prescription undertaken at long-term management exercise sessions.

8.3.2   Diet and Weight Management

If identified in the final cardiac rehabilitation assessment patients should have access to community dietetic and weight management services. Health professionals should also be able to identify when the patient requires more in-depth support and hence a referral onto a dietetic department, weight management group, diabetes, or renal specialist team (see Chapter 5b).

8.3.3   Smoking Cessation and Relapse Prevention

Access to community smoking cessation clinics is important along with family and social support in order to prevent relapses, and again health professionals should also be able to identify when the patient requires referral on to specialist stop smoking services (see Chapter 5a).

8.4   SELF-MANAGEMENT

People with long-term conditions, with support from their families, undertake 80–90% of their own care. In an average year, an individual with a long-term condition will see a healthcare professional for three hours, and self-manage for the remaining 8757 hours each year. Ensuring the individual is at the centre of care improves health outcomes, but supporting self-management takes us one step further (Eaton et al. 2015). Self-management support recognises that people with long-term conditions are in charge of their own lives and are the primary decision-makers about the actions they take in relation to the management of their condition and improves health outcomes.

8.5   SELF-MONITORING AND TECHNOLOGY

The development of the ability to self-monitor during each stage of a CPRP can be an effective skill that potentially maintains and promotes health-related behaviour change (Chase 2011; Ferrier et al. 2011). The type and amount of self-monitoring experienced whilst attending a CPRP differs according to each specific programme, but typically includes a range of approaches, with the most frequently optimised options incorporating that of heart-rate monitoring and self-assessed level of exertion using Borg's RPE scale (Chapter 5c). The effectiveness of long-term adherence following the use of technological monitoring in a CPRP (for example ECG, heart-rate monitors) has been questioned (Carlson et al. 2001; Ilarraza et al. 2004); however, studies have also shown that those who self-monitor are able to maintain change for longer periods following the cessation of attendance at a CPRP (Arrigo et al. 2008; Izawa et al. 2005).

The use of devices to self-monitor health-related behaviour has become more popular over the past decade, due to the availability and affordability of a range of devices. The practice of tracking health-related behaviour, particularly that involving physical activity and nutritional intake (others include improvement of mood, stress management, and smoking cessation) is becoming increasingly popular, and can be used effectively as a further tool to maintain positive behaviour change, although current research has so far mainly looked at non-cardiac populations. Common ways of self-monitoring with technology are with the use of an application (app) on a mobile 'smartphone', or a 'body sensor' that is carried around by the user. The benefit of these 'on body' devices is that they are likely to be with the user for the majority of the day, may be free of charge from some programmes, and are easy to use. Further, they are increasingly used in conjunction with social networks and can typically include support, instruction, timely prompts/reminders, and advice. More significantly most of these devices require the individual to be interactive whilst monitoring and recording.

Smartphones have been recognised as an effective medium in which to promote health (Bert et al. 2014; Patrick et al. 2008). Smartphone features such as global positioning systems (GPS), Wifi connectivity, and built-in pedometers and accelerometers have the potential to create the technological environment for an integrated physical activity intervention system. Due to the modernity of the use of these apps, scientific research, particularly with regards to long-term maintenance, is limited.

It is important to remember that effective self-monitoring is more likely following a comprehensive delivery of education covering all the components of cardiovascular rehabilitation, during the earlier stages of contact. This foundation can then be maintained long term with or without the use of technology in order to support the individual with positive health behaviour practices. For example, when encouraging regular physical activity, the correct understanding of how to self-assess exercise frequency, intensity, and duration (see Chapter 5c) can be reinforced with a device that records that information, and adds further benefit such as a reminder when the activity has not been performed.

8.5.1 Self-monitoring Physical Activity

When deciding whether or not a self-monitoring device is appropriate for an individual, and consequently when deciding on the type of device most relevant, it is important to consider how the different kinds of devices differ, together with afford-ability. Also, there needs to be consideration of the level of familiarity of the individual with technology. The majority of physical activity monitoring devices have been developed to measure aerobic activity rather than strength and resistance activity.

8.5.1.1 Pedometers

The use of pedometers to monitor and record physical activity in cardiac patients has been found to both increase levels of physical activity (Furber et al. 2010) and enhance self-monitoring (Cupples et al. 2013). They are easy to use, small and inobtrusive, and can be low cost. At the most basic level the device will monitor and record the total number of steps taken. Pedometers are used most effectively when worn on the hip and can allow the individual to work regularly towards a pre-determined activity level (either the current public health recom-mendation or a tailored programme developed together with an exercise professional when attending the CPRP). Pedometers do not monitor intensity of physical activity, but can be used together with self-assessed perceived exertion with, for example, the Borg RPE scale. Many applications for smart phones have been developed to enable the mobile phone to be used as a pedometer, although the accuracy of this is dependent on how the device is positioned whilst walking.

8.5.1.2 Accelerometers

Previously, accelerometers have mainly been used for research purposes as they are more accurate than the mechanical pedometer, as they utilise microproces-sors to sense movement. Feedback is sometimes not readily accessible and data may need to be downloaded first. Although this type of device can be more expen-sive, there are now a wide range of previously unaffordable types available for the individual to purchase. In addition to the number of steps taken, this device can also measure intensity, heart rate (with or without a heart rate monitoring device), time spent in movement, distance travelled, calorific expenditure, and movement during sleep. Accelerometers can be worn as arm/wrist bands and often work together with software that allows the user to download data to an application on a smartphone or a computer. Some accelerometer devices are offered together with the capability to track dietary intake and assess sleep patterns.

Both pedometers and accelerometers can be effective in supporting continued adherence to regular physical activity in the long-term maintenance phase of the rehabilitative process.

8.5.1.3 Home Entertainment Physical Activity Systems

The popularity of physical activity video games (for example the Nintendo Wii Fit) has increased over recent years and many cardiac patients have questions about the suitability of these types of activities either during or following attendance at a CPRP. Rehabilitation professionals should aim to ensure that the individual fully understands the main concepts of the specific frequency, intensity, and duration principles of physical activity participation following diagnosis of a cardiac condition. If these principles are clear, then the suitability of the video game can be considered in a more informed way. What is absolutely essential is that it should be made clear that the game will probably not include an appropriate warm up or cool down for the cardiac individual, and these elements should be incorporated if the individual is utilising it as a means of exercise. Whilst not essential, the use of heart rate monitoring (either manual or device-based) could aid the monitoring of intensity during the activity, but this should be considered in relation to each individual with regards to suitability (refer to Chapter 5c for more information on the use of heart rate monitors).

8.6 HEART SUPPORT GROUPS

HSGs offer the opportunity, for those affected by cardiovascular disease and similar long-term conditions, to come together on a regular basis to provide mutual support and shared experiences for the benefit of all who attend. The groups are intended both for patients and their carers, families, and friends. Referral to the HSG can occur during any of the phases of the CPRP and health professionals should ensure that each patient is given details of their local group prior to discharge from the rehabilitation programme. One of the main aims of the HSG is to support health promotion interventional activities, in order to help the patient to maintain positive healthy lifestyle changes that they have achieved during rehabilitation, often in the 'outside' environments that present many competing needs, priorities, and influences. A structured HSG includes self-help activities that complement public health policy on cardiovascular health and rehabilitation.

Benefits of Heart Support Group membership:

- Supports empowerment of the individual and enables them to gain a sense of control over their condition
- Increased development of coping skills and sense of adjustment
- Allows the individual to share their experience with others in a similar position

- Can help to reduce stress and depression
- Option to add to a collection of health experiences
- Opportunity to develop the knowledge base required for further risk factor prevention (i.e. continued advice on healthy eating, physical activity, medication compliance, stress and relaxation techniques, smoking cessation).

HSGs facilitate the provision of continued lifestyle change and support on a long-term basis, and the opportunity to provide many health and social benefits, and the potential involvement of cardiovascular prevention and rehabilitation professionals.

The environment is essentially a social one, but with the added support of many other activities such as:

- Exercise classes supervised by qualified instructors
- Walking, swimming, cycling, yoga, or relaxation groups
- Potential direct link to cardiovascular prevention and rehabilitation professionals
- Social events
- Talks from guest speakers
- Organised outings to places of interest
- Coffee mornings.

In England and Wales, many HSGs are affiliated to the British Heart Foundation (British Heart Foundation 2017). In 2017 the number of affiliated groups was around 300, with a total membership of around 31 000 people.

The Cardiovascular Care Partnership (UK) (CCPUK) represents patients and carers within the process of cardiovascular service improvement and aims to encourage feedback from those who have experienced cardiovascular care in the UK (British Cardiovascular Society 2016).

8.7   CONCLUSION

Cardiovascular prevention and rehabilitation is a long-term continuum of care and aims to empower individuals to develop full biopsychosocial self-management skills, preparing them to develop ownership and understanding of their own responsibility to pursue a healthy lifestyle. Before progressing on from a supervised CPRP to long-term maintenance, all patients should be clinically stable and should have had a comprehensive risk factor assessment.

The uptake of healthy lifestyle practices such as regular physical activity, appropriate diet and weight management, and smoking cessation should be continually promoted and encouraged. All patients should be offered information on how to access their local Heart Support Group. An agreed system of communication, including shared databases, templates, and clinical coding, is vital to improve integrated service delivery across organisations.

REFERENCES

Arrigo, I., Brunner-LaRocca, H., Lefkovits, M. et al. (2008). Comparative outcome one year after formal cardiac rehabilitation: the effects of a randomized intervention to improve exercise adherence. *European Journal of Cardiovascular Prevention and Rehabilitation* 15 (3): 306–311.

Bert, F., Giacometti, M., Gualano, M.R., and Siliquini, R. (2014). Smartphones and health promotion: a review of the evidence. *Journal of Medical Systems* 38: 9995.

British Association for Cardiovascular Prevention and Rehabilitation (BACPR) (2016). *BACPR Specialist Exercise Instructor Level 4 Cardiac Qualification*. BACPR. http://www.bacpr.com/pages/page_box_contents.asp?pageid=851&navcatid=182 (accessed 28 August 2016).

British Cardiovascular Society (2016). *Cardiovascular Care Partnership (UK) (CCPUK)*. British Cardiovascular Society. https://www.bcs.com/pages/page_box_contents.asp?PageID=325 (accessed 28 August 2016).

British Heart Foundation (2017). Heart Support Groups. British Heart Foundation. https://www.bhf.org.uk/informationsupport/support/heart-support-groups (accessed 28 August 2017).

Carlson, J.J., Norman, G.J., Feltz, D.L. et al. (2001). Self-efficacy, psychosocial factors, and exercise behavior in traditional versus modified cardiac rehabilitation. *Journal of Cardiopulmonary Rehabilitation* 21 (6): 363–373.

Chartered Institute for the Management of Sport and Physical Activity (CIMSPA) (2012). Available at: www.cimspa.co.uk

Chase, J.A. (2011). Systematic review of physical activity intervention studies after cardiac rehabilitation. *Journal of Cardiovascular Nursing* 26 (5): 351–358.

Conner, M. and Norman, P. (2007). *Predicting Health Behaviour*, 2e. Maidenhead UK: Open University Press.

Coulter, A., Roberts, S., and Dixon, A. (2013). *Delivering Better Services for People with Long-Term Conditions: Building the House*. London: The Kings Fund.

Cupples, M., Dean, A., Tully, M. et al. (2013). Using pedometer step-count goals to promote physical activity in cardiac rehabilitation: a feasibility study of a controlled trial. *International Journal of Physical Medicine and Rehabilitation* 1: 157.

Eaton, S., Roberts, S., and Turner, B. (2015). Delivering person centred care in long-term conditions. *British Medical Journal* 350: h181.

Ferrier, S., Blanchard, C.M., Vallis, M., and Giacomantonio, N. (2011). Behavioural interventions to increase the physical activity of cardiac patients: a review. *European Journal of Cardiovascular Prevention and Rehabilitation* 18 (1): 15–32.

Furber, S., Butler, L., Phongsavan, P. et al. (2010). Randomised controlled trial of a pedometer-based telephone intervention to increase physical activity among cardiac patients not attending cardiac rehabilitation. *Patient Education and Counselling* 80 (2): 212–218.

Ilarraza, H., Myers, J., Kottman, W. et al. (2004). An evaluation of training responses using self-regulation in a residential rehabilitation program. *Journal of Cardiopulmonary Rehabilitation* 24 (1): 27–33.

Izawa, K.P., Watanabe, S., Omiya, K. et al. (2005). Effect of the self-monitoring approach on exercise maintenance during cardiac rehabilitation: a randomized, controlled trial. *American Journal of Physical Medicine & Rehabilitation* 84 (5): 313–321.

Marcus, B.H. and Simkin, L.R. (1993). The stages of exercise behaviour. *The Journal of Sports Medicine and Physical Fitness* 33 (1): 83–88.

NHS England (2016). *General Practice Forward View* (Gateway publication reference 05116). NHS England. https://www.england.nhs.uk/gp/gpfv.

Patrick, K., Griswold, W., Raab, F., and Intille, S. (2008). Health and the mobile phone. *American Journal of Preventive Medicine* 35 (2): 177–181.

Resuscitation Council (UK) (2018). *Resuscitation Guidelines*. Resuscitation Council (UK). https://www.resus.org.uk/cpr/requirements-for-resuscitation-training/.

The Register of Exercise Professionals (2016). *Register of Exercise Professionals*. http://www.exerciseregister.org (accessed 28 August 2016).

CHAPTER 9

Audit and Evaluation

Patrick Doherty, Alex Harrison, Corinna Petre, and Nerina Onion
Department of Health Sciences, University of York, York, UK

Abstract

Clinical audit can drive quality, evaluate practice, and improve service provision locally and nationally. In the UK, clinical audit of cardiovascular rehabilitation (CR) is achieved through the British Heart Foundation (BHF) National Audit of Cardiac Rehabilitation (NACR). The NACR published its first report on service provision in 2007 when uptake to CR was at 43% with limited data on service quality. Ten years on, the 2017 NACR report showed world-leading mean uptake at 51% alongside a robust methodology evaluating service level performance and patient outcomes at a programme level for England, Wales, and Northern Ireland.

The national clinical audit is dependent on strong working relationships between clinical teams, professional associations/societies, and informatics organisations including the NACR, BHF, BACPR, and NHS Digital. Collectively these organisations have supported clinicians and service providers to improve cardiovascular disease prevention and rehabilitation programmes in the UK.

Keywords: *clinical audit, quality service evaluation, research and improvement*

Key Points

- Clinical audit is a standard and core component of cardiovascular rehabilitation (CR).
- Quality assurance aids confidence in service delivery for patients and funders.
- Local and national level data helps providers improve and innovate.

9.1   CLINICAL AUDIT IN THE CONTEXT OF RESEARCH AND SERVICE EVALUATION

Modern-day clinical practice requires a mixture of an evidence-based approach alongside service innovation and service evaluation. A common feature of research, service evaluation, and clinical audit is that they are all based on a systematic methodology for collecting and utilising data. Where they differ is through the types of analyses performed and the interpretation of that data in respect of hypotheses testing, clinical outcomes, or benchmarking against agreed criteria or standards.

In this chapter the following operational definitions apply:

- Research – the generation of new knowledge or theories tested in controlled settings that take account of possible confounders with the results generalised to wider populations.
- Service evaluation – is used to define or measure current practice with an aim to monitor and improve a specific service and is, by definition, not expected to be generalised beyond the service in which the evaluation occurred.
- Clinical audit – is a systematic approach that collects data on existing practice and compares it against predefined standards or good practice criteria. In the case of CR in the UK, this is based on service standards formulated by the National Institute for Health and Care Excellence (NICE 2013) and the British Association for Cardiovascular Prevention and Rehabilitation (BACPR) Standards and Core Components (BACPR 2017). Clinical audit, at a national level, can be used to define good practice in a rapidly changing clinical landscape, which in turn can drive quality and improvement of services. Although audit, as a methodology, is often seen as distinct from research, audit data is often used to address research questions and test research hypotheses.

9.1.1   Quality Assurance and Equity of Access

Established good practice guidelines recommend that clinical services audit their practice through the collection of routine data recording the CR they provide (BACPR 2017; DH 2010; Department of Health (DH) Cardiovascular

Disease Team 2013; NICE 2013). Effective data collection and data quality is best achieved through an automated computer-based approach utilising direct data entry or data uploaded from third party software (imported data). This data is then electronically stored on safeguarded national servers underpinned by sound data governance. In the UK this is provided through National Audit for Cardiac Rehabilitation (NACR) working with NHS Digital, which is a designated 'Data Safe Haven' for NHS patient level data.

Cardiovascular prevention and rehabilitation services play a fundamental role in delivering clinical and cost effective management of patients with established cardiovascular disease (CVD) and in those following a cardiac event, a cardiac procedure, or cardiac surgery (Anderson et al. 2016; NICE 2013; Rauch et al. 2016). In the UK, cardiology and cardiac surgery centres tend to have independent audits funded by central government that is mandated as part of clinical practice. Although CR programmes are less well supported in terms of audit resources, they should nevertheless aim to embed audit as part of routine service delivery and support staff to input data in a timely fashion. The NHS has included NACR on the formal Quality Account list, which is a requirement for commissioners in England.

Irrespective of where CR is delivered, patients have a right to expect that the services they receive are of the highest quality in terms of delivery and outcome. Local cardiovascular prevention and rehabilitation programmes (CPRPs) are duty bound to ensure they evaluate their services and quality assure the care offered to patients. In the UK, cardiovascular services are funded through public investment, which places a further duty on providers to implement audit and service evaluation to ensure programmes are delivered to an agreed standard using an efficient and cost effective approach. Patients require assurances that service provision, in whichever part of a country they live, will not differ substantially in terms of quality of the service and the typical gains expected from attending. These assurances are best achieved through an independent national audit approach.

9.2   ROLE OF NATIONAL AUDITS

Collating data from local services, through an independent national audit, is vital to monitoring access, uptake, adherence, and outcomes of CR at a country level. Some countries have invested heavily in clinical audits to quality assure CR and quantify the benefits of routinely delivered services. The UK NACR monitors cardiovascular prevention and rehabilitation services using the following methods:

(a) Mapping the extent of CR provision within the geographical setting
(b) Monitoring quality indicators and clinical outcomes
(c) Highlighting inequalities in provision and outcome

(d) Establishing which factors best determine optimal access to CR and clinical outcome

(e) Aiding clinical decision-making locally and within health regions

(f) Disseminating audit findings to service providers, funders, commissioners, and the public

(g) Informing clinical guidance, policy-makers, and practice standards

(h) Supporting service evaluation and service improvement

(i) Using audit data to answer service-related research questions

(j) Mapping the extent of CR provision within the nations of the UK.

There are two aspects to mapping the extent of provision; the first relates to location and coverage of services, which should ideally be within relatively easy reach of patients, and the second is the expectation that patients accessing services in one part of the country should achieve similar benefits independent of the geographical location or postcode.

In the UK there are over 300 programmes covering most areas (Figure 9.1); however, there are certain regions that are not well represented compared to others. In some cases this might be explained by population density and in others the physical landscape (e.g. rural settings and remote regions) may have a bearing on the location of services. In some areas patients are required to travel long distances, which is known to create additional requirements in terms of time and cost and is associated with poor uptake and low compliance. As national audits start to report with greater detail (e.g. local service or commissioner level) there will be opportunities to investigate the impact of geographical location and travel in respect of attendance and patient outcomes.

9.2.1 Monitoring Quality Indicators and Clinical Outcomes

Mean uptake to CR is 51%, which puts the UK far ahead of European uptake values, which are around 30% (Bjarnason-Wehrens et al. 2010; BHF NACR 2017). Although uptake to services is important it should not, in isolation, be used to judge the quality of CR. Other quality indicators (e.g. wait time, proportion of patients with pre- and post-assessments, duration, staffing) and clinical outcomes are equally important. Uptake trends vary over time and between different treatment groups (e.g. coronary artery bypass graft [CABG], post-myocardial infarction [MI], and following percutaneous coronary intervention [PCI]) and these are important to capture so that inequalities in access can be monitored. These analyses should ideally be subdivided by gender, age, and mode of delivery, which are known to determine the likelihood of engaging and completing CR (Al Quait et al. 2017, Harrison and Doherty 2018, Sumner et al. 2017, Tang et al. 2017).

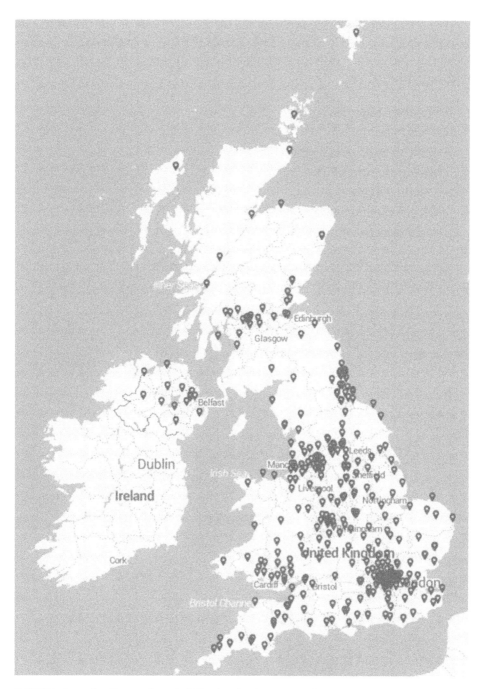

FIGURE 9.1   Cardiovascular rehabilitation (CR) provision for the UK.

The UK national audit recently started to report key service and performance indicators for Clinical Commissioning Groups (CCGs) in England, Health and Social Care Trusts in Northern Ireland, and Health Boards in Wales. The variables reported include:

- Numbers referred
- Time to referral
- Percentage of assessments completed
- Referral to start of CR
- Duration of CR
- CR completion figures
- Main reasons for not attending.

Large variation exists in how long patients wait to start CR. The median time for MI and/or PCI and post-CABG to starting the core delivery of rehabilitation

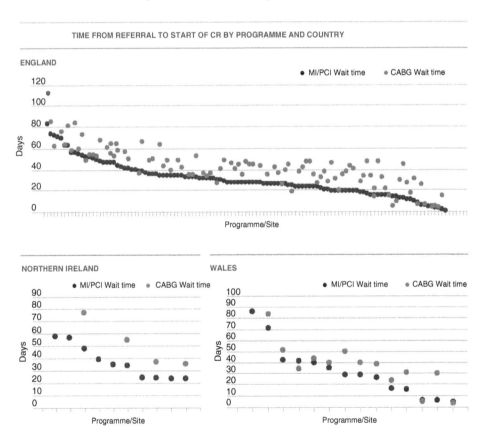

FIGURE 9.2   Time (median number of days) from initiating event to referral and commencing cardiovascular rehabilitation (CR) by country in 2017.

was 28 days and 41 days respectively (Figure 9.2). The Department of Health and the BACPR recommend 10 days as the period in which the formal core delivery of CR (i.e. outpatient) should commence (BACPR 2017; DH 2010). Such a huge difference between evidence-based recommendations (10 days) and median wait times in practice (28–41 days) should form the focus for future service improvement.

9.2.2   Highlight Inequalities in Provision and Outcome

As with many healthcare services the extent of access to, and outcomes from, these services varies across the social-economic spectrum. NACR collects data from NHS registries to determine the number of patients who suffered a cardiac event and were eligible for rehabilitation. This is particularly important as it enables the national audit to monitor equity of access and outcome in respect of patient demographics (e.g. age, gender, and ethnic origin). With so much pressure to reduce healthcare utilisation there is an increasing risk that scaled down services may not be taken up by patients, especially those with the most severe and complex presentations. From a national perspective, the demographic profile of UK-based CR is predominately British white (79%), retired (56%), and predominately male (70%) population (BHF NACR 2017). However, there are some programmes, in cities such as Birmingham, Manchester, and London, where the major ethnic group attending CR reflects the local demographic profile, for example South Asian older males. Younger patients (e.g. < 50 years) and females generally remain under-represented in UK CR.

It is incumbent on national audit to regularly monitor these trends and, where notable differences exist in access to CR and outcome, to liaise with programmes and relevant clinical networks to agree plans to remedy the situation. Where top performing services are identified for how they manage health inequalities it is equally important to liaise with them and national associations about sharing good practice with others.

9.3   ESTABLISH WHICH FACTORS BEST DETERMINE OPTIMAL ACCESS AND CLINICAL OUTCOME

Research evidence suggests that the mode and frequency of delivery impacts on outcome and patient satisfaction; however, little evidence exists to confirm this as part of routinely delivered practice. NACR, working with NHS Digital, BACPR, and other national associations, aims to use audit data to identify high and low performing services and to help disseminate positive CR delivery innovations into practice. An example from the UK is home-based, self-managed interventions where there is clear clinical and healthcare resource evidence recommending home-based CR as being equivalent to hospital-based programmes. However, there are presently fewer than 10% of patients receiving home-based and only 40%

of programmes support this mode of delivery (BHF NACR 2017; Harrison and Doherty 2018). Given the relatively low uptake figures for patients, it makes sense to offer greater evidence-based choices for intervention type and location of delivery. A future driver for promoting and supporting home-based approaches, as part of the CR menu, is the emerging evidence that patient preference is associated with improved clinical outcomes (Dalal et al. 2007; Harrison and Doherty 2018; Shanmugasegaram et al. 2013; Taylor et al. 2010).

There is always a risk that service innovations, working with finite resources, may fail to deliver an effective intervention, however, national audit is well positioned to verify the extent of service quality year-on-year. The NCP_CR now routinely monitors and reports on the quality of CR delivery against published standards and key performance indicators. This highlights that higher levels of service quality are achievable but more work is needed to reduce the variation that exists across the UK.

9.3.1 Aid Clinical Decision Making Locally and Within Regional Networks

The NACR has two modes of reporting used to aid clinical decision and support services:

(a) Clinician or service-focused reporting is where staff can request their patient level data through standardised reports that are used to show progress of patients and evaluate programme outcomes locally. This facility is offered to NACR users that input directly or upload to the audit through secure computer platforms. Local programme data can be tailored to clinician and provider specifications in respect to condition type, gender, race, etc.

(b) National audit reporting of key indicators at country level with subset analyses and reports in respect of Health Boards, Hospital Trusts, and CCGs benchmarked against established good practice. NACR produce annual statistical reports that are used by NICE (Quality Standard-QS99), the British Heart Foundation (BHF), BACPR, NHS England, Public Health England, and patient groups to inform guidance and create a case for change in service delivery.

9.3.2 Disseminate Audit Findings to Service Providers and the Public

NACR continues to expand its reporting mechanism, which starts at local programme level through to Health Regions, nationally for each country (England, Northern Ireland, and Wales) and finally for the UK. This is based primarily on electronic data entry supplemented by a short paper survey that informs the annual statistical report and is available online and as a hard copy. These reports have helped inform lobbying groups and have been used by government departments in identifying inequalities in CR services. As part of NACR's alignment with emerging NHS quality assurance and account-ability policy, CR audit reports have incrementally reported more detail, at local and regional levels, since 2012. This level of granularity, about CR ser-vices and outcomes, enables greater local and regional benchmarking and accountability.

The most recent NACR annual report is available electronically from the fol-lowing webpage: www.cardiacrehabilitation.org.uk/current-annual-report.htm.

9.3.3   Inform Clinical Guidance, Policy-makers, Commissioners, and Practice Standards

NICE and the Department of Health (DH) use anonymised NACR data for national benchmarking to help inform clinical guidance, service specifications, and policy. The NACR has worked with NHS Digital and NICE to agree key CR indicators (e.g. number of patients referred to CR and the number completing CR), which are collected through the national audit and reported to service pro-viders and healthcare commissioners. This is a real strength of the national audit that further enhances the emerging quality assurance and service improve-ment role of NACR.

9.3.4   Support Service Evaluation and Service Improvement

National audits tend to generate service level data and patient outcomes and carry out analyses to address specific service evaluation questions locally and within clinical networks.

Modern audits, like NACR, are proactive in driving change that improves the quality of services and generates better outcomes for patients. This role is increas-ingly aligned with service improvement opportunities whereby data and educational materials are produced, by NACR and other national associations, to support ser-vice change and staff continuing professional development opportunities. Service improvement is best done in collaboration with relevant stakeholders including staff, patients, funders, regional networks, and national associations.

9.3.5   Using Audit Data to Answer Research Questions

National audits and patient registries are used worldwide to implement obser-vational research to evaluate the effectiveness of routine CR. The most recent

UK-based RCT of CR (RAMIT) concluded that routine practice failed to yield the assumed benefits (West et al. 2011). RAMIT was a pragmatic trial of CR effectiveness in a real-life setting and not an efficacy trial testing whether CR works in an ideal setting. RAMIT aimed to randomise 8000 patients to rehab or usual care but only recruited a total of 1813 patients from, arguably, 14 atypical programmes. This meant that RAMIT was underpowered for mortality analysis and was non-representative of CR in the UK. RAMIT found no benefit in survival, physical activity, psychosocial status, or health-related quality of life, which conflicts with previous trials and systematic reviews and is contrary to established clinical guidance and cost effective evidence (Doherty and Lewin 2012; Doherty and Rauch 2013; Gore and Doherty 2017; Heran et al. 2011; NICE 2013; Perk et al. 2012; Wood 2012). What the RAMIT study does tell us is that we should not be complacent, as not all routine CPRPs automatically achieve the effectiveness seen in clinical trials. CPRPs need to ensure they deliver the core components using skilled professionals working to the evidence base.

Although clinical trials remain important in determining efficacy they fail to answer the question about the effectiveness of routinely delivered services. A valid next step in assessing effectiveness is to use an observational research approach whereby routinely collected audit data, from patients attending CR, is compared to a matched group of patients who were eligible for CR but did not take up the offer (non-attenders). NACR is in the process of securing data-sharing agreements, and governance approval, to investigate the effectiveness of routine CR for both attenders and non-attenders. This requires complex analysis, using propensity adjustment and controlling for confounders, and can yield results similar to those seen in RCTs (Dahabreh et al. 2012; Hannan 2008; Simms et al. 2013).

9.4   PROFILE AND OUTCOMES OF CR IN THE UK

This section uses national audit data to outline the typical profile and outcomes for CR programmes in the UK.

9.4.1   Multidisciplinary Approach to CR Programmes

Services continue to be delivered, for the most part, by a multidisciplinary (MDT) that aligns with the models underpinning research evidence. Although there are yearly variations in the proportional contribution for each professional group there remains a core group associated with the delivery of CR (Table 9.1). Given the emerging multi-morbid profile seen in the patients attending CR, the MDT mode of delivery continues to be important. The success of CR is underpinned

TABLE 9.1 CR staff profile.

Category	England		Northern Ireland		Wales		UK Total	
	N = 200		N = 11		N = 20		N = 234	
	N	%	N	%	N	%	N	%
Nurse	194	97	10	91	20	100	227	97
Physiotherapist	134	67	11	100	18	90	165	71
Dietician	94	47	7	64	11	55	114	49
Psychologist	29	15	6	55	2	10	37	16
Social worker	0	0	0	0	0	0	0	0
Counsellor	19	10	0	0	2	10	21	9
Doctor	16	8	4	36	0	0	21	9
Healthcare assistant	33	17	0	0	1	5	34	15
Secretary	153	77	8	73	19	95	181	77
Administrator	15	8	0	0	0	0	15	6
Exercise specialist	114	57	1	9	9	45	124	53
Occupational therapist	47	24	1	9	12	60	61	26
Pharmacist	72	36	10	91	11	55	95	41
Physiotherapy assistant	55	28	1	9	5	25	62	26

by sustained behaviour change making the low number of psychologists a serious issue for programmes. Innovative clinical and commissioning approaches are required to halt such a decline and proactively increase involvement from professionals with appropriate skills and competences to deliver the required psychological components.

The number of patients with co-morbidities has increased substantially over time with fewer than 18 000 in 2007 to over 43 000 patients with two or more co-morbidities managed by CPRPs in 2017. The range and percentage of co-morbidities (Table 9.2) remains high with over 50% of patients having two or more co-morbidities. Due to the increasing number of patients with more than three co-morbidities it is more appropriate, in these cases, to use the term multi-morbid population.

TABLE 9.2   Percentage of patients with co-morbidities.

Morbidity category	With two or more (%)
Angina	23
Arthritis	18
Cancer	9
Diabetes	32
Rheumatism	3
Stroke	7
Osteoporosis	2
Hypertension	63
Chronic bronchitis (COPD)	5
Emphysema	4
Asthma	10
Claudication	3
Chronic back problems	10
Anxiety	7
Depression	8
Family history of CVD	31
Erectile dysfunction	3
Hypercholesterolaemia/dyslipidaemia	42
Other morbidity	35

9.4.2   Clinical Outcomes from CR

The national audit reports expected 'typical gains' nationally and enabled local services to report clinical outcomes for their own services. The extent of change in key variables, for UK patients completing routine CR, is evident for most risk factors (Figure 9.3). This is especially so for psychosocial wellbeing, exercise, cholesterol, and quality of life but less so for BMI and waist circumference. The average dose of UK-based CR has yet to be confirmed. The small changes seen in BMI and waist measurement are less effective, suggesting that CR needs to offer greater intensity and/or greater volume of interventions to tackle elevated BMI. The NACR aims to aid clinical decision-making by producing patient reference values for key outcome variables, the first of which involved the incremental shuttle walk test (ISWT) as a measure of physical fitness (Alotaibi and Doherty 2017).

The ability to evaluate the impact of CR is made more difficult with an increasingly multi-morbid population. Around 60% of patients have one or more

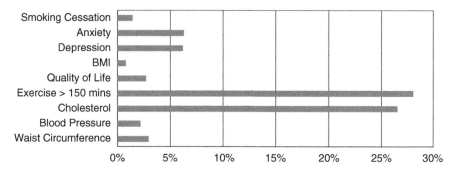

FIGURE 9.3   Percentage improvement for key variables following cardiovascular rehabilitation (CR).

co-morbidities and the extent of multi-morbid presentation is independent of age in both males and females (Table 9.3). The extent of benefit (percentage change) following CR is comparable across the six co-morbidity categories suggesting that a comprehensive MDT approach, as applied in the UK, is working. An example of this is shown in Table 9.4 in relation to the percentage of patients exercising for at least 150 minutes per week.

9.4.3   Uptake to Cardiac Rehabilitation Services in the UK and across Europe

The number of patients accessing services continues to grow and has achieved world-leading levels at 51% mean uptake (Table 9.5). UK CR is increasingly offering alternative modes of delivery including hospital, community, and home with combinations of supervised, facilitated, and self-management, all of which aligns with patient choice.

TABLE 9.3   Age and gender of patients by number of co-morbidities ($N = 101\,000$).

Number of co-morbidities	Males		Females		Total	
	Age (mean)	%	Age (mean)	%	Age	%
None	65	41.7%	69	39.4%	66	41.0%
One	65	16.9%	70	15.4%	66	16.4%
Two	66	16.8%	71	16.6%	68	16.7%
Three	67	12.5%	71	13.5%	68	12.8%
Four	67	6.9%	70	8.1%	68	7.2%
> Five	68	5.3%	70	7.0%	68	5.8%

TABLE 9.4 Percentage of patients exercising for at least 150 minutes per week.

Number of co-morbidities	Before CR	After CR	% Change
None	44%	72%	27%
One	45%	74%	29%
Two	42%	70%	28%
Three	40%	66%	27%
Four	36%	67%	30%
> Five	32%	57%	26%

TABLE 9.5 Percentage uptake for cardiovascular rehabilitation (CR)

	N	Receiving CR	Uptake %
Total UK			
MI	41 464	15 275	37
MI + PCI	43 979	26 045	59
PCI	29 434	14 927	51
CABG	19 021	12 307	65
Total	**133 898**	**68 554**	**51**
England			
MI	36 433	14 182	39
MI + PCI	40 872	23 554	58
PCI	26 495	13 893	52
CABG	17 699	11 193	63
Total	**121 499**	**62 822**	**52**
Northern Ireland			
MI	1779	363	20
MI + PCI	1533	985	64
PCI	1852	554	30
CABG	534	432	81
Total	**5698**	**2334**	**41**
Wales			
MI	3252	730	22
MI + PCI	1574	1506	96
PCI	1087	480	44
CABG	788	682	87
Total	**6701**	**3398**	**51**

Although uptake to CR in the UK is at a much higher level than most countries it is far from ideal, with almost half (49%) of eligible patients not taking up services. A European survey of 21 countries, in 2010, found uptake to CR ranged from as low as 3% to over 50% (Bjarnason-Wehrens et al. 2010). This represents an unacceptable level of variation and further reiterates the need for national audits to monitor access, quality assure programmes, and define typical outcomes.

9.5   MONITORING STANDARDS THROUGH NATIONAL AUDIT

9.5.1   Definition of Clinical Standards

National standards represent an agreed starting point for CPRPs to benchmark their care provision. Standards should be measurable and describe the absolute minimum level of provision and outcome expected of a service. Standards are best developed by national associations using experts in the area and should take account of the established evidence base, clinical expertise, quality service provision, and patient experience. In the UK the Department of Health and the BACPR have both contributed to the development of national standards (BACPR 2017; DH 2010). NACR is responsible for monitoring standards of care, which it achieves through programme specific and national level reporting of key indicators to each of the nations in the UK.

9.5.2   The BACPR Standards (See Chapter 2)

The six standards for cardiac rehabilitation emphasise:

1. Standard one. The delivery of six core components by a qualified and competent multidisciplinary team, led by a clinical coordinator.
2. Standard two. Prompt identification, referral, and recruitment of eligible patient populations.
3. Standard three. Early initial assessment of individual patient needs that informs the agreed personalised goals that are reviewed regularly.
4. Standard four. Early provision of a structured CPRP, with a defined pathway of care, which meets the individual's goals and is aligned with patient preference and choice.
5. Standard five. Upon programme completion, a final assessment of individual patient needs and demonstration of sustainable health outcomes.
6. Standard six. Registration and submission of data to the NACR and participation in the National Certification Programme (NCP_CR).

In terms of the national audit, standard six stipulates that:

- Every CR programme should register with NACR and submit data that will be analysed as part of annual reporting.
- Formal audit and evaluation of CR should include service level and patient level data as part of assessment at baseline and CR completion.

9.6   NCP_CR THROUGH THE BACPR AND NACR

The BACPR and NACR embarked on an ambitious project to use NACR data, collected as part of routine practice, to implement a certification process to quality assure CR in the UK (Doherty et al. 2017; Furze et al. 2016). The attractiveness of this approach is that it is based on routinely collected data administered through NACR, which reduces cost. Programmes registered with NACR are reviewed annually against key performance indicators using recent data and awarded an appropriate certification rating. The aim is to ensure that all programmes achieve a basic minimum standard and to assist programmes to achieve high quality delivery and outcomes through timely audit reporting against key indicators. These processes are less about creating performance league tables and much more about supporting programmes, through audit, education, and training to quality assure and improve services to patients. Using published data from the BHF NACR 2014 to 2019, NCP_CR shows that CR quality has improved by an average of 31.7% across the UK (NACR 2019).

9.7   ONGOING AND FUTURE RESEARCH

The EuroHeart II survey (Nichols et al. 2012) suggests that around half of all deaths in the European region are caused by CVD and that much of the morbidity, seen in those living with CVD, is preventable. Research shows that CVD prevention and rehabilitation programmes can yield significant mortality, and clinical and economic benefit (Anderson et al. 2016; Fidan et al. 2007; NICE 2013; Rauch et al. 2016; Taylor et al. 2014), yet the recent national surveys found large variation in CR uptake in the UK (BHF NACR 2017) and Europe (e.g. Spain 3%, Lithuania 90%) (Bjarnason-Wehrens et al. 2010). The mean age of patients in CR clinical trials, from the 1980s to 2017, is 56 years (mostly male), which is much younger than patients attending CR in routine clinical practice where services, being more analogous with elderly care provision, have a mean age of 67 years with greater multi-morbidity (BHF NACR 2017). Trial research evidence is therefore biased towards younger predominately male patients compared to clinical practice where CR delivery is applied to an older multi-morbid population with increasingly more females seen compared to clinical trials.

Informed by clinical trial evidence, BACPR, the European Society of Cardiology, and European Association of Preventive Cardiology guidelines have, over the last 10 years, stressed that following a cardiac event all patients should be offered equitable and effective prevention and rehabilitation programmes. The number of patients eligible for CR interventions (i.e. those suffering a cardiac event or undergoing a planned cardiac-related procedure) is around 2 million per year yet less than 40% access these services each year (BHF NACR 2017; Bjarnason-Wehrens et al. 2010; Nichols et al. 2012).

Although considerable trial evidence exists for the efficacy of CR, the ageing trial evidence base and an increasing gap between the research participants compared to routine CR practice demographics means there is concern surrounding its applicability to modern CR. After 25 years of clinical trials, numerous meta-analyses, and 10 years of clinical guidance, mostly recommending CR, it is now time to evaluate the implementation and effectiveness of trial evidence in routine practice. The first major systematic review of registry-based research involved 24 robust studies (none from the UK) comprising of over 17 000 acute coronary syndrome (ACS), CABG, or mixed populations with coronary artery disease (CAD) patients (Rauch et al. 2016). A further study conducted by our research group focused on 9836 acute MI patients in six countries across Europe and the USA (Sumner et al. 2017). The results collectively show positive gains in terms of mortality and health-related quality of life.

NACR is leading the largest observational study in UK CR investigating routinely collected audit and registry data. The project will overcome the limitations seen in other large registry projects and aim to define the most effective and innovative modes of delivery for CPRPs across the UK.

9.8 CONCLUSION

This chapter will hopefully have clarified the rationale for service evaluation and highlighted how local audit plays a role in enabling programmes to quality assure their own service and effectively monitor patient progress. The role of national audit in helping participating nations meet clinical standards and drive up the quality of service delivery should be evident. The partnership between BACPR and NACR, in jointly running a national certification programme, is world leading and will enable patients, carers, healthcare providers, commissioners, and funders to make better choices. Finally, the ability of national audit data to answer important research questions about best practice and identify key determinants of successful CR is hugely promising.

The authors wish to acknowledge the contribution of the BHF in funding the audit and supporting service improvement; the University of York for providing a high-quality data and research infrastructure; the BACPR for promoting the quality of CR programmes and training of professional staff; NHS Digital for ensuring that our data is robust and safeguarded; and CR programmes for their professional approach to audit and evaluation.

REFERENCES

Al Quait, A.I.M., Doherty, P.J., Gutacker, N., and Mills, J. (2017). In the modern era of percutaneous coronary intervention: is cardiac rehabilitation engagement purely a patient or a service level decision? *European Journal of Preventive Cardiology* 24 (13): 1351–1357. https://doi.org/10.1177/2047487317717064.

Alotaibi, J.F.M. and Doherty, P.J. (2017). Evaluation of determinants of walking fitness in patients attending cardiac rehabilitation. *BMJ Open Sport & Exercise Medicine* 2: e000203, 1–6. DOI: http://dx.doi.org/10.1136/bmjsem-2016-000203.

Anderson, L., Oldridge, N., Thompson, D.R. et al. (2016). Exercise-based cardiac rehabilitation for coronary heart disease: Cochrane systematic review and meta-analysis. *Journal of the American College of Cardiology* 67 (1): 1–12.

Bjarnason-Wehrens, B., McGee, H., Zwisler, A.-D. et al. (2010). Cardiac rehabilitation in Europe: results from the European cardiac rehabilitation inventory survey. *European Journal of Cardiovascular Prevention and Rehabilitation* 17 (4): 410–418.

British Association for Cardiovascular Prevention and Rehabilitation (BACPR) (2017). *BACPR Standards and Core Components for Cardiovascular Disease Prevention and Rehabilitation.* London: BACPR. https://www.bacpr.com/pages/page_box_contents.asp?pageid=791.

British Heart Foundation National Audit of Cardiac Rehabilitation (BHF NACR) (2017). *NACR Quality and Outcomes Report 2017.* London: British Heart Foundation. http://www.cardiacrehabilitation.org.uk/reports.htm

British Heart Foundation National Audit of Cardiac Rehabilitation (BHF NACR) (2019). *NACR Quality and Outcomes Report 2019.* London: British Heart Foundation.

Dahabreh, I., Sheldrick, R., Paulus, J. et al. (2012). Do observational studies using propensity score methods agree with randomized trials? A systematic comparison of studies on acute coronary syndromes. *European Heart Journal* 33 (15): 1893–1901.

Dalal, H., Evans, P., Campbell, J. et al. (2007). Home-based versus hospital-based rehabilitation after myocardial infarction: a randomized trial with preference arms–Cornwall heart attack rehabilitation management study (CHARMS). *International Journal of Cardiology* 119 (2): 202–211.

Department of Health (DH) (2010). *Commissioning Pack for Cardiac Rehabilitation.* London: DH https://webarchive.nationalarchives.gov.uk/20110907132421/http://www.dh.gov.uk/en/Publicationsandstatistics/Publications/PublicationsPolicyAndGuidance/Browsable/DH_117504 (accessed January 2018).

Department of Health (DH) Cardiovascular Disease Team (2013). *Cardiovascular Disease Outcomes Strategy: Improving Outcomes for People with or at Risk of Cardiovascular Disease*. London: DH. https://assets.publishing.service.gov.uk/government/uploads/system/uploads/attachment_data/file/217118/9387-2900853-CVD-Outcomes_web1.pdf (accessed January 2018).

Doherty, P. and Lewin, R. (2012). The RAMIT trial, a pragmatic RCT of cardiac rehabilitation versus usual care: what does it tell us? *Heart* 98 (8): 605–606. http://dx.doi.org/10.1136/heartjnl-2012-301728.

Doherty, P. and Rauch, G. (2013). Cardiac rehabilitation mortality trends: how far from a true picture are we? *Heart* 99 (9): 593–595. http://dx.doi.org/10.1136/heartjnl-2012-303365.

Doherty, P.J., Salman, A., Furze, G. et al. (2017). Does cardiac rehabilitation meet minimum standards: an observational study using UK national audit? *Open Heart* 4: e000519, 1–5. DOI: https://dx.doi.org/10.1186/s12913-018-3831-1.

Fidan, D., Unal, B., Critchley, J., and Capewell, S. (2007). Economic analysis of treatments reducing coronary heart disease mortality in England and Wales, 2000-2010. *QJM: Monthly Journal of the Association of Physicians* 100 (5): 277–289.

Furze, G., Doherty, P.J., and Grant-Pearce, C. (2016). Development of a UK national certification programme for cardiac rehabilitation (NCP-CR). *British Journal of Cardiology* 23 (2): 102–105. https://doi.org/10.5837/bjc.2016.024.

Gore, L. and Doherty, P.J. (2017). Cardiac rehabilitation: making a business case based on the evidence. *British Journal of Cardiac Nursing* 12 (10) https://doi.org/10.12968/bjca.2017.12.10.499.

Hannan, E. (2008). Randomized clinical trials and observational studies: guidelines for assessing respective strengths and limitations. *JACC. Cardiovascular Interventions* 1 (3): 211–217.

Harrison, A.S. and Doherty, P. (2018). Does the mode of delivery in cardiac rehabilitation determine the extent of psychosocial health outcomes? *International Journal of Cardiology* 255: 136–139.

Heran, B., Chen, J., Ebrahim, S. et al. (2011). Exercise-based cardiac rehabilitation for coronary heart disease. *The Cochrane Database of Systematic Reviews* 6 (7): CD001800. https://doi.org/10.1002/14651858.CD001800.pub2.

National Institute for Health and Care Excellence (2013). *Secondary Prevention in Primary and Secondary Care for Patients Following a Myocardial Infarction. (CG 172.)*. London: NICE www.nice.org.uk/guidance/cg172.

Nichols, M., Townsend, N., Scarborough, P., and Rayner, M. (2012). European Cardiovascular Disease Statistics 2012 edition. European Society of Cardiology. https://www.escardio.org/static_file/Escardio/Press-media/press-releases/2013/EU-cardiovascular-disease-statistics-2012.pdf (accessed 29 August 2016).

Perk, J., de Backer, G., Gohlke, H. et al. (2012). European guidelines on cardiovascular disease prevention in clinical practice (version 2012): the fifth joint task force of the European Society of Cardiology and Other Societies on cardiovascular disease prevention in clinical practice (constituted by representatives of nine societies and by invited experts). *European Heart Journal* 33: 1635–1701.

Rauch, B., Davos, C.H., Doherty, P. et al. (2016). The prognostic effect of cardiac rehabilitation in the era of acute revascularisation and statin therapy: a systematic review and meta-analysis of randomized and non-randomized studies–the Cardiac Rehabilitation Outcome Study (CROS). *European Journal of Preventive Cardiology* 23 (18): 1914–1939.

Shanmugasegaram, S., Oh, P., Reid, R. et al. (2013). A comparison of barriers to use of home- versus site-based cardiac rehabilitation. *Journal of Cardiopulmonary Rehabilitation and Prevention* 33 (5): 297–302.

Simms, A., Reynolds, S., Pieper, K. et al. (2013). Evaluation of the NICE mini-GRACE risk scores for acute myocardial infarction using the myocardial ischaemia national audit project (MINAP) 2003–2009: national institute for cardiovascular outcomes research (NICOR). *Heart* 99 (1): 35–40.

Sumner, J., Böhnke, J.R., and Doherty, P. (2017). Does service timing matter for psychological outcomes in cardiac rehabilitation? Insights from the National Audit of cardiac rehabilitation. *European Journal of Preventive Cardiology* 25 (1): 19–28. https://doi.org/10.1177/2047487317740951.

Tang, L.H., Kikkenborg Berg, S., Christensen, J. et al. (2017). Patients' preference for exercise setting and its influence on the health benefits gained from exercise-based cardiac rehabilitation. *International Journal of Cardiology* 232: 33–39. https://doi.org/10.1016/j.ijcard.2017.01.126.

Taylor, R.S., Dalal, H., Jolly, K. et al. (2010). Home-based versus centre-based cardiac rehabilitation. *Cochrane Database of Systematic Reviews* 20 January (1): CD007130. https://doi.org/10.1002/14651858.CD007130.pub2.

Taylor, R.S., Sagar, V.A., Davies, E.J. et al. (2014). Exercise-based rehabilitation for heart failure. *Cochrane Database of Systematic Reviews* (4): CD003331. https://doi.org/10.1002/14651858.CD003331.pub4.

West, R., Jones, D., and Henderson, A. (2011). Rehabilitation after myocardial infarction trial (RAMIT): multi-centre randomised controlled trial of comprehensive cardiac rehabilitation in patients following acute myocardial infarction. *Heart* 98 (8): 637–644.

Wood, D. (2012). Is cardiac rehabilitation fit for purpose in the NHS: maybe not. *Heart* 98 (8): 607–608.

CHAPTER 10

Future Prospects and International Perspectives

Joe Mills[1], Sherry L. Grace[2,3], Marie-Kristelle Ross[4], Caroline Chessex[5,6], Robyn Gallagher[7], Cate Ferry[8], and Vicki Wade[9]

[1] Liverpool Heart & Chest Hospital NHS Foundation Trust, Liverpool, UK
[2] York University, Toronto, Ontario, Canada
[3] Cardiac Rehabilitation Research, University Health Network, University of Toronto, Toronto, Ontario, Canada
[4] Hotel-Dieu de Lévis, Universite Laval, Quebec City, Quebec, Canada
[5] Department of Medicine, University of Toronto, Toronto, Ontario, Canada
[6] Division of Cardiology, University Health Network/Sinai Health System, Toronto, Ontario, Canada
[7] The University of Sydney, Sydney, Australia
[8] National Heart Foundation of Australia, Sydney, Australia
[9] Rheumatic Heart Disease, Australia Menzies School of Health Research Casuarina, Australia

Abstract

This chapter presents a series of international viewpoints on perspectives of cardiovascular prevention and rehabilitation (CR) from professionals working in CR within International and Commonwealth health systems. The chapter commences with a look to the future with particular reference to CR in the UK. This is followed by commentary from leading professionals of three international organisations with a similar remit to that of the British Association for Cardiovascular Prevention and Rehabilitation (BACPR).

Cardiovascular Prevention and Rehabilitation in Practice, Second Edition.
Edited by Jennifer Jones, John Buckley, Gill Furze, and Gail Sheppard.
© 2020 John Wiley & Sons Ltd. Published 2020 by John Wiley & Sons Ltd.

They comment on the application of the BACPR standards and core components within their own health systems.

Keywords: *cardiovascular disease, cardiovascular prevention and rehabilitation, BACPR Standards and Core Components, global perspectives*

Key Points

- The number of elderly people is rising globally, with the effect that numbers with cardiovascular disease (CVD) will rise, requiring greater global attention on reducing mortality and morbidity from CVD.
- Cardiovascular prevention and rehabilitation programmes (CPRPs) deliver an evidence-based way to help reduce CVD mortality and morbidity but, internationally, require political support to overcome challenges.
- The international perspectives echo the striving for quality of CR delivery across the globe.

10.1   FUTURE PROSPECTS (JOE MILLS)

Cardiovascular disease prevention and rehabilitation has developed beyond recognition since the perceived wisdom of post-myocardial infarction bed-rest back in the 1940s. As evidence began to emerge, long spells of immobilisation were replaced with brief episodes of ambulation in the 1950s, until the advent of more exercise-based programmes of recovery in the 1960s. In the latter half of the twentieth century, consistent and persuasive scientific data emerged that reinforced the health benefits of physical activity and demonstrated the negative impact of sedentary behaviour, and as a consequence, exercise-based cardiac rehabilitation became an established therapy for patients with established CVD within most national and international guidelines. Interventional techniques and pharmacotherapies for patients with ischaemic heart disease and heart failure have become increasingly complex, clinically effective, and more rapidly delivered, thereby dramatically reducing the median length of hospital stay for patients experiencing myocardial infarction and/or requiring revascularisation/device implantation. Not surprisingly, the published standards support efforts to enrol patients within cardiovascular prevention and rehabilitation programmes (CPRPs) as soon as possible following a qualifying event or diagnosis and there does not appear to be any additional hazard associated with such a strategy.

During the 65th World Health Assembly (WHA) in May, 2012, all 194 World Health Organization (WHO) member states endorsed a historic target to reduce premature death from non-communicable diseases (NCDs) by 25% by the year 2025. NCDs – predominantly CVD, cancer, chronic respiratory disease, and diabetes – constitute the most common cause for mortality worldwide, accounting for 63% of global deaths, which includes 14 million people younger than 70 years of age. Most of these premature deaths are linked to common risk factors such as tobacco use, unhealthy diet, physical inactivity, and excessive alcohol intake, and it is believed that 80% of all premature CVD could be avoided by tackling/eliminating these and other known (and linked) CVD risk factors. The 66th WHA subsequently endorsed the WHO Global Action Plan (GAP) for the prevention and control of NCDs 2013–2020 (WHO 2013). This GAP offers a paradigm shift by providing a road map and menus of policy options for member states, WHO, United Nations, other inter-governmental organisations, non-governmental organisations, and the private sector. When implemented collectively between 2013 and 2020 the ultimate outcome should be the attainment of nine voluntary global targets, including that of a 25% relative reduction in premature mortality from NCDs by 2025. Given that CVD accounts for the largest portion of the overall burden of the NCDs then the focus of attention will inevitably be directed to those of us working in the field of cardiovascular medicine.

Such a bold strategic directive, which is fully adopted and supported by the World Heart Federation, provides the impetus for significant changes in health policy and this is timely given a number of other factors that are stimulating a reassessment of priorities within healthcare provision in the UK. The expanding elderly population (both in absolute numbers and as a percentage of the population as a whole), the impact of multi-morbidity, the costs of health and social care, the incurable nature of CVD, and the financial pressures of a struggling economy all demand a focus on prevention strategies – the prevention/avoidance of social, environmental, and metabolic risk factors and the prevention of acute/unstable events once CVD has developed. Whilst major contributions from public health agencies, local council authorities, and commissioning bodies will be required in order to affect any meaningful improvements in CVD prevention, existing CPRPs are well placed to act as both delivery vehicle and a means of integrating the prevention pathway. The risk, of course, is that our national government will not be able to resist ongoing and increasing financial support of front-line, acute care, such that funds will be diverted away from 'Cinderella' services such as prevention and rehabilitation. Yet, at least for the moment, the political rhetoric is quite the reverse and even suggests some degree of prioritisation of the prevention agenda and a genuine intent to commission for longer-term outcomes (NHS 2019).

The challenges for CPRPs will be to sustain quality outcomes whilst demonstrating resilience to financial pressures as well as becoming increasingly innovative regarding prevention/rehabilitation delivery methods to ever more complex individuals in greater numbers with a strict focus on measurable clinical end-points and costs. Across the UK, there already exist exemplars of novel practice, including more symptom-specific programmes ('breathlessness' programmes where pulmonary and cardiac services have been combined), the inclusion of individuals with other NCDs such as cancer, and the use of digital platforms to enhance communication and allow more flexibility. However, these innovations represent a mere early phase in the evolution of prevention/rehabilitation services and much more will be needed in order to accommodate the full spectrum of prevention interventions for all those who may, in reality, derive significant benefit.

Given the need for the UK to actively contribute to the global strategy for a reduction in premature CVD mortality, coupled with the delivery of prevention/rehabilitation to an ageing, multi-morbid population, and all at a time of relative economic hardship within the NHS, the future might appear somewhat daunting. However, as is often the case when apparently insurmountable challenges arise, there exists a real opportunity for CPRPs to take centre stage and demonstrate both efficacy and value. Despite a legacy of rather oblique funding and a decidedly lowly status when compared with other more physician-led and delivered services, cardiovascular rehabilitation (CR) in the UK is the envy of the developed world, in terms of both its structure and its function. Available to all individuals with a qualifying diagnosis, a truly multidisciplinary team of talented and motivated healthcare professionals deliver high quality care (based upon a robust set of performance standards and core components) to an ever increasing proportion of eligible patients within hospital, community, and domestic settings. This is underpinned by a comprehensive and detailed national audit of CR (NACR) that is funded by the British Heart Foundation and which allows a programme of quality assurance (via attainment of certification through the delivery of minimum standards) to be conducted. In addition, NACR provides programme specific datasets that include important measures of process as well as key clinical outcomes, which will become essential for demonstrating performance, efficacy, and value. Over time, the intention will surely be to fully integrate all the current national clinical audits of CVD (myocardial infarction, heart failure, coronary, and valve interventions), with both NACR and primary-care outputs detailing individuals with accrued CVD risk factors. This will then provide an overview of the entire CVD pathway and allow novel interventions (treatments, procedures, processes, technologies, etc.) to be scientifically 'tested' through registry-based trials with enormous statistical power. The operability of efficient, well resourced CPRPs will be fundamental to the effective development of evidence-based cardiovascular care whether or not the initiating hypothesis is directly related to prevention/rehabilitation.

'Medical science has made such tremendous progress that there is hardly a healthy human left' – the words of Aldous Huxley certainly resonate with all of us involved in the world of prevention/rehabilitation. Fortunately, our remit is to equip individuals with the skills to avoid the onset or progression of disease and, as such, we have a duty to ensure that the obsessive investment in sophisticated treatments of ill-health does not occur at the expense of those services which are dedicated to the maintenance of sustainable, good health.

10.2   COMMONWEALTH AND INTERNATIONAL PERSPECTIVES ON APPLICATIONS OF BACPR STANDARDS AND CORE COMPONENTS

10.2.1   The International Council of Cardiovascular Prevention and Rehabilitation (ICCPR) (Sherry L. Grace)

The British Association of Cardiovascular Prevention and Rehabilitation (BACPR) is a Foundational Member of the International Council of Cardiovascular Prevention and Rehabilitation (ICCPR). The ICCPR is comprised of approximately 36 additional named board members of national/regional cardiac rehabilitation (CR) associations globally. The ICCPR's work is based on its Charter, which, in accordance with BACPR 3rd Edition Standards and Core Components (BACPR 2017), aims to promote CR as an obligatory, not optional, service.

The ICCPR has developed a consensus statement on CR delivery in low-resource settings, which has been endorsed formally by 12 member associations (including BACPR) (Grace et al. 2016). It is comprised of the same core components as recommended by the BACPR, including audit and evaluation. The ICCPR commends the BACPR for its leadership in specifying evidence-based standards for service, and encourages programmes in low-resource settings to aspire to these standards where possible.

The BACPR has developed minimum standards to enable assessment of whether programmes meet them; more transparency in reporting is welcomed, as the global CR community could use this for benchmarking purposes. Indeed, the ICCPR recognises and appreciates the leadership internationally that the BACPR has shown through NACR. Some ICCPR member associations have developed CR quality indicators, namely Canada, the United States, Australia, and Japan, which are all quite consistent (http://globalcardiacrehab.com/public-resources/quality-indicators/).

The BACPR should be commended for its development of core competences for delivery of the core components, as well as a certification programme for quality assuring programmes. The American Association of Cardiovascular Prevention and Rehabilitation similarly has developed core competencies, and has more recently developed a registry, with the capability for certification. Most recently, the ICCPR has developed a certification programme for delivery of CR in low-resource settings (Moghei et al. 2019).

10.2.2 The Canadian Association of Cardiovascular Prevention and Rehabilitation (Marie Kristelle Ross and Caroline Chessex)

As a nation of 34 million, living across a vast land mass stretching 3000 miles from coast to coast, often inaccessible and covered in snow, the Canadian Association of Cardiovascular Prevention and Rehabilitation (CACPR) has advocated for innovative approaches to facilitate the delivery of standardised cardiovascular rehabilitation to Canadians. Moreover, our healthcare system is mainly administered on a provincial level, further leading to significant discrepancies in service provision across the country.

Like in many healthcare systems, we are faced with the need to actively advocate for a share of finite resources. There currently is no systematically dedicated national or provincial funding for cardiac rehabilitation. This has empowered us to be flexible and creative in the way we deliver services, be it in urban or rural/remote settings, through person-centred menu-based programming. The impressive commitment of the steadfast healthcare professionals involved allows us, despite the obstacles, to provide a very high level of care.

In an effort to standardise the delivery of cardiac rehabilitation across the country, the rehabilitation community developed 37 quality indicators focusing on the structure, process, and outcome dimensions of care, under the auspices of the Canadian Cardiovascular Society (https://www.ccs.ca/images/Health_Policy/Quality-Project/CCS_QualityIndicators.pdf#targetText=The%20Canadian%20Cardiovascular%20Society%20has,drive%20improvements%20in%20patient%20outcomes). These indicators overlap with the priorities outlined in the BACPR Standards and Core Components.

Looking ahead, we must continue to provide the evidence base for our practice to maintain its relevance and increase its importance within the broader medical community. CACPR is currently focusing its efforts on creating a national registry, which will prove of great value in terms of quality control, audit of our programmes, and research opportunities to further advance the field.

CACPR has been leading efforts to promote cardiovascular rehabilitation in Canada for over 25 years, and still faces many challenges ahead. Collaborating with, and being inspired by, organisations like the BACPR will certainly get us closer to our goals.

10.3   AUSTRALIAN CARDIOVASCULAR HEALTH AND REHABILITATION ASSOCIATION PERSPECTIVES ON THE BRITISH ASSOCIATION FOR CARDIOVASCULAR PREVENTION AND REHABILITATION STANDARDS AND CORE COMPONENTS 2018 (ROBYN GALLAGHER, CATE FERRY, AND VICKI WADE)

The Australian Cardiovascular Health and Rehabilitation Association (ACRA) (www.acra.net.au) congratulates the British Association for Cardiovascular Prevention and Rehabilitation (BACPR) on the publication of their 2017 edition of their Standards and Core Components (SCC) for cardiovascular disease prevention and rehabilitation. These standards are internationally relevant and provide an excellent and essential guide to support cardiac rehabilitation and prevention programmes to improve cardiac health outcomes in Australia. The SCC provide important guidance for a rapidly evolving field, which is consistent with the core components published by ACRA (Woodruffe et al. 2015) and the cardiac rehabilitation priorities identified by the National Heart Foundation of Australia (HFA) (Heart Foundation 2014).

Key elements within this text include a focus on behaviour at the heart of long-term outcomes and the inclusion of detailed support for patient self-management. Whilst exercise and rehabilitation remain central, there has been a shift to include links between primary and secondary care that appropriately reflects important changes in cardiac patient populations and treatments in recent years. Universal healthcare occurs in Australia and Britain, so many aspects related to referral and transitions across inpatient to outpatient and community-based care are similarly relevant. Further similarities are present in diverse populations that include both biological and social inequalities, in part derived from immigration and refugee groups, which are thoughtfully addressed in the SCC. Indigenous Australians experience these inequalities within a unique history of colonialism, slaughter, and removal of a generation of children for adoption that differs from voluntary migration and refugee experiences, and provide substantial sociocultural barriers to accessing healthcare. Despite high CVD morbidity and mortality, Indigenous Australians do not receive equitable healthcare and participation rates in cardiac rehabilitation and secondary prevention are extremely low (Australian Bureau of Statistics 2016). Similar challenges may also apply to our Commonwealth friends in Canada and their own 'first nations' people.

The BACPR SCC provide a solid framework to help address the healthcare gap (Australian Bureau of Statistics 2016). However, challenges and considerations need to be taken into account. Indigenous Australians comprise diverse and complex communities scattered around Australia, often living very remotely from health services, consequently meaning two to three days travel to reach cardiac rehabilitation services and thus depend on intermittent fly-in fly-out teams. This means alternative delivery models discussed in the SCC are crucial, as is the need to address cultural safety and include primary prevention for high-risk individuals (Taylor and Guerin 2014). Audit and evaluation of all cardiac rehabilitation and prevention programmes is needed to determine equity of access and delivery, but is currently lacking in Australia. The BACPR provides useful standards for this assessment and ACRA anticipates collaboration in this area. We recommend the SCC.

REFERENCES

Australian Bureau of Statistics (2016). Causes of death, Australia, 2015 (Cat. No. 3303.0). Australian Bureau of Statistics. www.abs.gov.au/ausstats/abs@.nsf/mf/3303.0 (accessed 15 March 2018).

BACPR (2017). *The BACPR Standards and Core Components for Cardiovascular Disease Prevention and Rehabilitation*, 3e. London: BACPR http://www.bacpr. com/pages/page_box_contents.asp?pageid=791

Grace, S.L., Turk-Adawi, K.I., Contractor, A. et al. (2016). Cardiac rehabilitation delivery model for low-resource settings: an International Council of Cardiovascular Prevention and Rehabilitation Consensus Statement. *Progress in Cardiovascular Disease* 59 (3): 303–322.

Heart Foundation (2014). Improving the delivery of cardiac rehabilitation in Australia. National Heart Foundation of Australia. http://www.heartfoundation. org.au/images/uploads/publications/Improving-the-delivery-of-cardiac-rehabilitation.pdf (accessed 15 March 2018).

Moghei, M., Oh, P., Chessex, C. et al. (2019). Cardiac rehabilitation quality improvement: a narrative review. *Journal of cardiopulmonary rehabilitation and prevention*, 39 (4): 226–234.

NHS (2019). The NHS long-term plan. January 2019. https://www.longtermplan. nhs.uk/wp-content/uploads/2019/01/nhs-long-term-plan.pdf.

Taylor, K. and Guerin, P. (2014). *Health Care and Indigenous Australians: Cultural Safety in Practice*, 2e. Melbourne: Palgrave Macmillan.

Woodruffe, S., Neubeck, L., Clark, R.A. et al. (2015). Australian Cardiovascular Health and Rehabilitation Association (ACRA) core components of cardiovascular disease secondary prevention and cardiac rehabilitation 2014. *Heart Lung Circulation* 24: 430Y441. https://www.ncbi.nlm.nih.gov/pubmed/25637253

World Health Organization (WHO) (2013). *Global action plan for the prevention and control of noncommunicable diseases 2013–2020*. Geneva: WHO.

Index

A

accelerometers 280, 281
acceptance and commitment
    therapy 209
ACE inhibitors 233, 235, 251–2, 261
action plans 13
adherence 13, 83
adult learning 86
aerobic activity 155, 156, 165, 172
alcohol intake 138–9, 215–16
alirocumab 243
alpha blockers 233, 263
alprostadil 264
amyl nitrate 264
angioplasty, exercise after 166–8
angiotensin-converting enzyme (ACE)
    inhibitors 233, 235, 251–2, 261
angiotensin receptor blockers 233, 235,
    251–2, 261
anti-coagulant therapy 254–5
antihypertensives 232–5
anti-platelet therapy 249
anxiety 195, 198–9
  questionnaires 202
artificial sweeteners 144
Asians, BMI 130
aspirin 248–9
assessment
  body composition 130–2
  dietary intake 129–30
  erectile dysfunction 260, 261, 263
  health behaviour change 93

psychosocial health 201–4
sexual concerns 211
tobacco use 106–10
atorvastatin 239
atrial fibrillation 165–6, 254
audit 40–1, 60–2, 173, 285–302
  benchmarking 293
  clinical decision making 292
  dissemination of findings 292–3
  monitoring standards 299–300
  National Audit of Cardiac
    Rehabilitation (NACR) xiii, 10, 11,
    29, 60–1,
    287–92, 300, 308
  profile and outcomes of cardiac
    rehabilitation 294–9
  research 286–7, 293–4
  service evaluation 286–7, 293
  service improvement 293
Australian Cardiovascular Health and
    Rehabilitation Association (ACRA)
    311–12
avanafil 263

B

behavioural support 111–12
benchmarking 293
beta-blockers 233, 235, 250–1, 261
blood pressure 5, 230–5
body composition 34–5, 130–2
body mass index (BMI) 130
Borg scales 157, 171

---

breath carbon monoxide 107
Brief Illness Perceptions Questionnaire 77, 203
British Association for Cardiac Prevention and Rehabilitation (BACPR)
  core components of services 3, 30–41
  formation xiii
  service standards 11, 23–9, 299–300
bumetanide 253–4
bupropion 110, 117, 118
business case 61–2

C
calcium channel blockers 233, 235, 261
Canadian Association of Cardiovascular Prevention and Rehabilitation (CACPR) 310
cancer 5
carbon monoxide monitoring 107
Cardiac Beliefs Questionnaire 77
cardiac misconceptions 77–8
cardiac rehabilitation, definition 6–7
cardiac resynchronisation therapy 38, 255–9
Cardiovascular Care Partnership (UK) 282
cardiovascular disease, burden 3–5
Cardiovascular Disease Outcomes Strategy (DoH) xiii–xiv, 15, 50, 53
cardiovascular prevention and rehabilitation programmes
  BACPR core components 3, 30–41
  BACPR standards 11, 23–9, 299–300
  definition 6–7
  evidence base 8–9
certification 29, 41, 62, 300
Champix *see* varenicline
chocolate 142
cholesterol 5, 143, 236–9
chronic disease management approach 176
chronic kidney disease 146–7
chronic liver disease 242
chronotropic incompetence 170
clinical audit *see* audit

clinical coordinator 24, 52–3
clinical decision making 292
clinical guidance 293
clinical outcomes 288–91, 296–7
clopidogrel 249, 255
cocaine 216
Cochrane Reviews
  adherence issues 83
  exercise-based cardiac rehabilitation 8, 156
  exercise-based rehabilitation for heart failure 169
  tobacco cessation drugs 118
cod liver oil 143
CoEnzyme Q10 143
coffee 143
cognitive behaviour therapy 211
colesevelam 244
commissioners 293
communication 75, 153
community settings 14, 175, 274–5
co-morbidities 110, 176, 295–7
competency-based approach 51–2
constructive worry 210
CO-OP Charts 202
coping
  plans 13
  self-statements 209
  skills 205
coronary artery bypass grafting
  depression 196
  exercise 164–5
coronary heart disease 4, 5, 229
COURAGE trial 8
creatine kinase 241
CYP3A4 inhibitors 240

D
delivery of programmes 14, 24–5, 49–53
denial 196–7
depression
  heart disease 195–6
  partners and spouses 198–9
  questionnaires 202
  tobacco cessation 110, 117
diabetes 5, 147, 245–7

diaries 130
diet 5, 127–47
  assessment of intake 129–30
  components of a cardioprotective
    diet 132–9
  Eatwell plate 141
  healthy eating 34–5
  long-term management 278
discharge letter 29, 39, 59
Distress Thermometer 202
diuretics
  loop 253–4
  thiazide-like 233, 235, 261
dreams 114
drug misuse 216
dual antiplatelet therapy 249
dysglycaemia 245–7

E
e-cigarettes 119–21
EAGLES trial 118
early initial assessment 26–7, 55–6
early provision of programmes 11–12,
    28, 56–8, 160, 162–71, 290–1
Eatwell plate 141
ECG 173
education 6, 32–3, 85–9
  physical activity and exercise 158–61
  psychosocial interventions 204–5
efficacy expectations 71
egg consumption 143
electronic cigarettes 119–21
'elicit–provide–elicit' principle 75
Emotion Thermometer 202
emotions 72, 205–6
employment 214
environment
health behaviour change 72
tobacco smoke 105
EPHESUS trial 252
eplerenone 252–3
equity of access 286–7
erectile dysfunction 38, 199, 260–4
ethnicity
  BMI 130
  smoking 103

EUROACTION plus varenicline
    study 121–2
EuroHeart II survey 300
evaluation 40–1, 93, 173, 285–302
evidence-based practice 48–9
evolocumab 243
exercise see physical activity
    and exercise
ezetimibe 243

F
Fagerstrom Test for Nicotine
    Dependence 108
familial heterozygous
    hyperlipidaemia 238
fats 133–5
fibrates 244
fibre 136
final assessment 28–9, 39, 58–9
fish oils 134, 135, 143, 244
food
  labelling 144
  media stories 144
  see also diet
Friedewald formula 237
fruit intake 135–6, 143
functional capacity 173
furosemide 253–4

G
garlic 142
General Practice Forward View 273
Global Action Plan (GAP) 307
glycaemic control 245–8
glycaemic index (GI) 136
glycated haemoglobin (HbA1c) 245–7
goal-setting 56, 78–83, 209
grapefruit juice 145
group settings
  closed versus open (rolling)
    groups 92–3
  guidelines for 90
  health behaviour change and
    education 80–1, 87–8, 90–2
  heart support groups 281–2
  progress feedback 91

group settings (*cont'd*)
  psychosocial
    interventions 211–12, 214
  visitors to 91
GTN patches/spray 264

H
habit formation 72
harm reduction 122
HbA1c 245–7
health behaviour change 31, 67–94
  adherence 83
  component lead 69
  goal-setting 78–83
  group settings 80–1, 90–2
  monitoring 93
  social support 83–5
  theoretical foundations 70–2
healthy eating 34–5 *see also* diet
heart failure
  diet 145
  exercise 169–71
  hospital admissions 9
heart rate 156–7, 170
heart rate reserve 156–7
heart support groups 281–2
Heavy Smoking Index 108
high-income countries 3–5
high intensity interval training
    (HIIT) 172
home-based programmes 11, 14,
    277–8, 291–2
home entertainment physical activity
    systems 281
hospital admissions 9
Hospital Anxiety and Depression Scale
    (HADS) 202
hypertension 5, 231–6
  resistant/pseudoresistant 235, 236

I
identification of patients 25–6, 53–5, 57
if–then plans 82
illness representations 74–5, 77–8, 203
implantable cardioverter
    defibrillators 38, 255–9

implementation intentions 73, 82
Increasing Access to Psychological
    Therapies (IAPT) 216
inequalities 291
initial assessment 26–7, 55–6
insomnia 114, 210–11
inspiratory muscle training 166
intentions 71–2
  implementation intentions 73, 82
INTERHEART study 195
International Council of Cardiovascular
    Prevention and
    Rehabilitation (ICCPR)
    7, 309–10
internet-based programmes 14
intracavernosal vasoactive
    injections 264
intraurethral suppositories of
    prostaglandin E1 264

K
kidney disease, chronic 146–7

L
LDL-cholesterol 143, 236–8
life events 205
lifestyle
  blood pressure 231–2
  erectile dysfunction 261
  lipid-lowering 238
  risk factor management 33–5
lipid-lowering therapy 238–44
lipids 236–8
liver disease 242
long-term management 39–40, 271–83
loop diuretics 253–4
low- and middle-income countries 3

M
MacNew Heart Disease
    Questionnaire 202
margarine, sterol-enriched 143
marketing 55
maximal exercise testing 173
maximal heart rate 157, 170
medical risk management 37–8, 227–64

Mediterranean diet 132–3
Mediterranean Diet Score 130
mental health service referral 215
menu-based approach 28, 58, 89
mineralocorticoid receptor
    antagonists 252–3
minimum standards 62–3
minority ethnic communities 89
mono-unsaturated fatty acids 133, 135
motivational interviewing 74–6
motivational invitation
    techniques 12, 55
multidisciplinary teams 24–5, 49–53,
    200–1, 294–5
multi-morbidities 295–7
Multispecialty Community Provider
    (MCP) contract 273
muscle aches, statin-related 240–2
myocardial infarction
    depression 196
    exercise 166–7

N
National Audit of Cardiac
    Rehabilitation (NACR) xiii, 10, 11,
    29, 60–1, 287–91, 292, 300, 308
National Certification Programme for
    Cardiac Rehabilitation 29,
    41, 62, 299
National Institute for Health and
    Clinical Excellence
    (NICE) guidance
    aspirin use 248–9
    blood pressure management 233
    blood pressure targets 230–1
    cardiac resynchronisation
        therapy 255–6
    discharge letters 59
    early commencement of
        rehabilitation 55, 56, 162
    fat intake 133
    health behaviour change 69
    lipid levels 236–7
    PCSK9 monoclonal
        antibody use 243–4
    recruitment of patients 54, 57

salt intake 137
tobacco harm reduction 122
nausea 114, 117
nebivolol 261
NHS Digital-NACR 40
niacin 244
nicotine 105
nicotine replacement therapy 115–19
nicotinic acid 244
nitrates 264
non-alcoholic fatty liver disease 242
non-HDL cholesterol 236–8
nuts 137

O
obesity 5, 126 *see also* weight
    management
observational research 294
obstructive sleep apnoea 210
occupational stress 195
oils 144
oily fish 134, 135
omega-3 134, 135
optimism 198, 209
oral glucose tolerance test 245–6
orientation appointment 12
Orlistat 141
outcome expectancies 71
overprotection 84, 213

P
partners 84–5, 198–9, 213–14
patient identification 25–6, 53–5, 57
patient journey 57
patient recruitment 26, 53–5, 57
patient referral
    cardiovascular
        rehabilitation 26, 53–5, 57
    psychosocial issues 214–17
patient responsibilities 39
PCSK9 monoclonal
    antibodies 243–4
PDE5 inhibitors 261–3
pedometers 280, 281
personality 200
phosphodiesterase-5 inhibitors 261–3

physical activity and exercise 6, 8,
    33–4, 151–81
  adherence 13
  aerobic activity 155, 156, 165, 172
  audit and evaluation 173
  cardiovascular disease
      prevention 154–5
  cardiovascular disease rehabilitation
      and secondary prevention 156–8
  case study 176–81
  communication 153
  co-morbidities 176
  early commencement 160, 162–71
  education 158–61
  functional capacity 173
  heart failure 169–71
  high intensity interval training 172
  home-based 277–8
  implantable devices 257–9
  location of programmes 175
  long-term management 275–8
  outcomes 173
  post-angioplasty 166–8
  post-MI 166–7
  post-surgery 164–6
  prehabilitation exercise 166
  recommended levels 155–7
  resistance strength training 155,
      157, 165, 172
  risk reduction 163–4
  risk stratification 173
  self-monitoring 280–1
  staffing 174–5
  Tai Chi 172
  traditional provision 161–2
  walking 172
  warm-up and cool-down 163–4
physical fitness 153, 173
plant stanols/sterols 143
PLATO trial 249
policy makers 293
poly-unsaturated fatty acids 133, 135
'poppers' 264
positive affect 198
post-angioplasty exercise 166–7
post-myocardial infarction

  depression 196
  exercise 166–7
post-surgery
  depression 196
  diet 145
  exercise 164–6
post-traumatic growth 197
post-traumatic stress disorder 197
practice standards 293
prasugrel 249
pravastatin 239
prehabilitation exercise 166
primary care services 272–5
problem solving 210
progress feedback 91
proprotein convertase subtilisin/kexin
      type 9 (PCSK9) monoclonal
      antibodies 243–4
prostaglandin E1, intraurethral
      suppositories 264
pseudoresistant hypertension 235–6
psychological distress 194, 202, 215
psychological factors
  heart disease 194–200
  implantable devices 256–7
  tobacco cessation 110, 117
psychological interventions 36–7
psychosocial health 36–7, 193–17
  assessment 201–4
  component lead 201
  education 204–5
  group participation 211–12, 214
  interventions 204–11
  referral to other services 214–17
  team-working 200–1

Q
quality assurance 286–7
quality indicators 288–91
quality of life 9
  questionnaires 202

R
RALES trial 252
RAMIT trial 294
rapport building 75

rating of perceived exertion 157, 170–1
readability statistics 89
recall methods 129–30
record method 130
recruitment of patients 26, 53–5, 57
referral
  cardiovascular
    rehabilitation 26, 53–5, 57
  psychosocial issues 214–17
rehabilitation 7
relaxation skills training 206–7
resilience 197–8, 205, 209
resistance strength training 155,
    157, 165, 172
resistant hypertension 235
respiratory conditions 5
return to work 214
Revised Illness Perceptions
  Questionnaire
  203
rosuvastatin 239

S
salt intake 137
saturated fats 133, 135
scaling question 204
Scientific Advisory Committee on
  Nutrition 138
sedentary behaviour 5, 153, 171–2
self-discrepancy 72
self-efficacy 71, 203–4
self-management 278
self-monitoring 279–81
service delivery 14, 24–5, 49–53
service evaluation 286–7, 293
service improvement 293
service provision 10–11
service responsibilities 39–40
service uptake 10–13, 297–9
sexual counselling 211
sexual health 37, 199–200, 211, 261
Sexual Health Inventory for Men/
  International Index of Erectile
  Function-5 260–1
Short-Form 36 (SF-36) 202
sildenafil 263

simvastatin 145, 239
sitting 154
skills 72
Skills for Health Workforce Report 50
sleep interventions 210–11
SMART goals 56, 132, 141
smartphones 14, 132, 279
smoke-free legislation 102
smoking 5
  ethnicity 103
  status 107
  see also tobacco cessation and relapse
    prevention
social control 84–5
social pressure 71
social support 36, 83–5, 212–14
solution-focused approach 74,
    79–80, 210
soya 143
spironolactone 253, 261
Stages of Change in Exercise
  Behaviour 277
standing 154, 171–2
Start Active Stay Active 155
statins 145, 239–42, 261
sterol-enriched margarine 143
strength training 155, 157, 165, 172
stress 195, 205
stress management 205–6
substance misuse 215–16
sugar intake 138
supplements 134, 135, 142
support groups 281–2
surgery
  depression 196
  diet 145
  exercise 164–6

T
tadalafil 263
Tai Chi 172
target heart rate 156–7
technology
  delivery models 14
  diet and weight management 132
  recruitment of patients 57

technology (*cont'd*)
  self-monitoring 279–81
telemedicine 14
thiazide-like diuretics 233, 261
thought patterns 207–9
ticagrelor 249
tobacco cessation and relapse
    prevention 35, 50, 101–22
  assessment 106–10
  behavioural support 111–12
  component leader 121
  cut down to stop 115–16
  dependence on tobacco 105, 107–8
  electronic cigarettes 119–21
  harm reduction 122
  long-term management 278
  motivation to quit 108–9
  nicotine replacement therapy 115–19
  past quit attempts 110
  pharmacological agents 110, 112–19
  psychological co-morbidities 110, 117
  weight gain 121–2
  withdrawal oriented
      approach 110–11
trans fatty acids 135
transaminase levels 242
Type A/D personality 200

U
uptake of services 10–13, 297–9

V
vardenafil 263
varenicline 110, 113–14, 117–19

vegetable intake 135–6, 143
video games 281
vitamin D 143
vocational interventions 214

W
waist circumference 131–2
waiting times 290–1
walking 172
warfarin 143, 255
weight management 34–5
  long-term management 278
  tobacco cessation 121–2
  weight cycling 139
  weight loss 34, 35, 139–41
whole grains 136
work
  return to 214
  stress 195
World Health Assembly (WHA)
    306–7
World Health Organisation (WHO)
  Global Action Plan 307
  non-communicable disease
      prevention 3, 306–7
  physical activity goal 155

Z
Zyban *see* bupropion